MW00449201

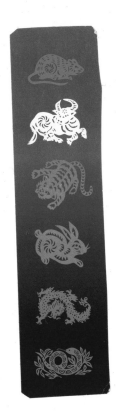

# Qigong Meditation

# Don't be afraid!
不用害怕！

# Dare to challenge.....
敢於挑戰.....

# Dare to accept.....
敢於接受.....

# Dare to dream.....
敢於夢想.....

## - Dare to emerge from the traditional matrix -
## - be free from spiritual bondage -

*"The philosopher should be a man willing to listen to every suggestion, but determined to judge for himself. He should not be biased by appearances, have no favorite hypothesis, be of no school, and in doctrine have no master. He should not be a respecter of persons, but of things. Truth should be his primary object. If to these qualities be added industry, he may indeed hope to walk within the veil of the temple of Nature."*

*- Michael Faraday (1791-1867)*

# Qigong
# Meditation

## Small Circulation

### Dr. Yang, Jwing-Ming

YMAA Publication Center
Boston, Mass. USA

**YMAA Publication Center, Inc.**
Main Office:
PO Box 480
Wolfeboro, New Hampshire 03894
1-800-669-8892 • www.ymaa.com • ymaa@aol.com

POD0410

Copyright ©2006 by Dr. Yang, Jwing-Ming
All rights reserved including the right of
reproduction in whole or in part in any form.

ISBN-13: 978- 1-59439-067-8
ISBN-10: 1-59439-067-3

Editor: David Silver
Cover Design: Tony Chee

**Publisher's Cataloging in Publication**

Yang, Jwing-Ming, 1946-

Qigong meditation : small circulation / Yang, Jwing-Ming. -- 1st ed. --
Boston, Mass. : YMAA Publication Center, 2006.

p. ; cm.

ISBN-13: 978-1-59439-67-8
ISBN-10: 1-59439-067-3
Text in English, with some Chinese characters included.
Includes bibliographical references, translation and glossary of
Chinese terms, and index.

1. Qi gong. 2. Qi (Chinese philosophy) 3. Meditation. I. Title.

RA781.8 .Y363 2006                    2006925695
613.7/148--dc22                       0605

Anatomy drawings copyright ©1994 by TechPool Studios Corp. USA, 1463 Warrensville
Center Road, Cleveland, OH 44121

Printed in USA.

Disclaimer:
The author and publisher of this material are NOT RESPONSIBLE in any manner whatsoever for
any injury which may occur through reading or following the instructions in this manual. The activities, physical or otherwise, described in this material may be too strenuous or dangerous for some
people, and the reader(s) should consult a physician before engaging in them.

# Contents

## PART I. FOUNDATIONS 根基
## Chapter 1. General Concepts 一般概念

## Chapter 2. Theoretical Foundations 理論基礎

## PART II. MEDITATION TRAINING PROCEDURES 靜坐訓練步驟
## Chapter 3. Four Refinements 四化

# Acknowledgments

Thanks to Tim Comrie for photography and typesetting, to Kyle McCauley for general help and to Erik Elsemans, David Silver, Roger Whidden, and Leslie Takao for proofing the manuscript and contributing valuable suggestions. Thanks to Tony Richard Chee for the drawings and cover design. Special thanks to Keith Brown for the first edit, and to David Silver for the final edit. Special thanks to Dr. Thomas G. Gutheil for the foreword.

## Romanization of Chinese Words

This book uses the Pinyin romanization system of Chinese to English. Pinyin is standard in the People's Republic of China, and in several world organizations, including the United Nations. Pinyin, which was introduced in China in the 1950's, replaces the Wade-Giles and Yale systems. In some cases, the more popular spelling of a word may be used for clarity.

Some common conversions:

| Pinyin | Also Spelled As | Pronunciation |
|---|---|---|
| Qi | Chi | chē |
| Qigong | Chi Kung | chē kǔng |
| Qin Na | Chin Na | chǐn nǎ |
| Jin | Jing | jǐn |
| Gongfu | Kung Fu | gōng foo |
| Taijiquan | Tai Chi Chuan | tī jē chüén |

For more information, please refer to *The People's Republic of China: Administrative Atlas, The Reform of the Chinese Written Language,* or a contemporary manual of style.

The author and publisher have taken the liberty of not italicizing words of foreign origin in this text. This decision was made to make the text easier to read. Please see the comprehensive glossary for definitions of Chinese words.

# Dedication

To my friend whom I can't forget
Mr. Wolfgang Pastore

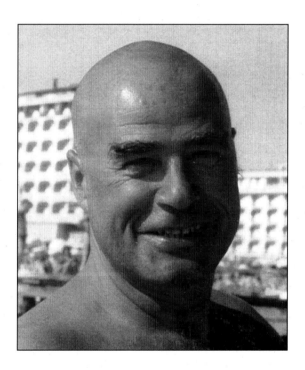

## About the Author

*Dr. Yang, Jwing-Ming, Ph.D.* 楊俊敏博士

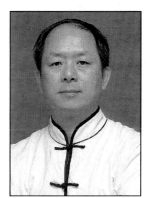

Dr. Yang, Jwing-Ming was born on August 11th, 1946, in Xinzhu Xian ( 新竹縣 ), Taiwan ( 台灣 ), Republic of China ( 中華民國 ). He started his Wushu ( 武術, Gongfu, 功夫 ) training at fifteen under Shaolin White Crane (Bai He, 少林白鶴 ) Master Cheng, Gin-Gsao ( 曾金灶, 1911-1976). As a child, Master Cheng learned Taizuquan ( 太祖拳 ) from his grandfather, and at fifteen started learning White Crane from Master Jin, Shao-Feng ( 金紹峰 ), following him for twenty-three years until Master Jin's death.

In thirteen years of study (1961-1974) under Master Cheng, Dr. Yang became an expert in the White Crane style of Chinese martial arts, including the use of barehands and various weapons such as saber, staff, spear, trident, two short rods and many other weapons. With the same master he studied White Crane Qigong ( 氣功 ), Qin Na ( 擒拿 ), Tui Na ( 推拿 ) and Dian Xue ( 點穴按摩 ) massage, and herbal treatment.

At sixteen he began the study of Yang Style Taijiquan ( 楊氏太極拳 ) under Master Gao, Tao ( 高濤 ). He later continued his study of Taijiquan with several masters and senior practitioners such as Master Li, Mao-Ching ( 李茂清 ) and Mr. Wilson Chen ( 陳威伸 ) in Taipei ( 台北 ). Master Li learned Taijiquan from the well known Master Han, Ching-Tang ( 韓慶堂 ), and Mr. Chen learned his from Master Zhang, Xiang-San ( 張祥三 ). Dr. Yang mastered the Taiji barehand sequence, pushing hands, the two-man fighting sequence, Taiji sword, Taiji saber and Taiji Qigong.

At the age of eighteen, he entered Tamkang College ( 淡江學院 ) in Taipei Xian ( 台北縣 ) to study Physics. In college he began studying traditional Shaolin Long Fist (Changquan, 少林長拳 ) with Master Li, Mao-Ching at the Tamkang College Guoshu Club ( 淡江國術社, 1964-1968), and became assistant instructor under Master Li. In 1971 he completed his M.S. degree in Physics at the National Taiwan University ( 台灣大學 ), then served in the Chinese Air Force from 1971 to 1972. There he taught Physics at the Junior Academy of the Chinese Air Force ( 空軍幼校 ) while also teaching Wushu. Honorably discharged in 1972, he returned to Tamkang College to teach Physics and resume study under Master Li, Mao-Ching. From Master Li, he learned Northern Style Wushu, including barehand and kicking techniques, and numerous weapons.

In 1974, he came to the United States to study mechanical engineering at Purdue University. At the request of a few students, he began to teach Gongfu, founding the Purdue University Chinese Gongfu Research Club in 1975. He also taught college-credited courses in Taijiquan. In May 1978, he was awarded a Ph.D. in Mechanical Engineering by Purdue.

In 1980, Dr. Yang moved to Houston to work for Texas Instruments, and founded Yang's Shaolin Kung Fu Academy, now under the direction of his disciple, Jeffery Bolt. In 1982 he moved to Boston, and founded Yang's Martial Arts Academy (YMAA). In 1984 he gave up his engineering career to devote himself to research, writing and teaching. In 1986 he purchased property in the Jamaica Plain area of Boston for the headquarters of YMAA. The organization has grown, and in 1989 YMAA became a division of Yang's Oriental Arts Association, Inc. (YOAA, Inc.).

In summary, Dr. Yang has been involved in Chinese Wushu since 1961. He spent thirteen years learning Shaolin White Crane (Bai He), Shaolin Long Fist (Changquan), and Taijiquan. He has taught for more than thirty-six years, seven in Taiwan, five at Purdue University, two in Houston, and twenty-two in Boston.

He has presented seminars around the world, to share his knowledge of Chinese martial arts and Qigong. He has visited Argentina, Austria, Barbados, Botswana, Belgium, Bermuda, Canada, China, Chile, England, Egypt, France, Germany, Holland, Qatar, South Africa, Switzerland, and Venezuela.

YMAA is an international organization, including 56 schools in Argentina, Belgium, Canada, Chile, France, Holland, Hungary, Iran, Ireland, Italy, Poland, Portugal, Spain, Sweden, South Africa, the United Kingdom, Switzerland, and the United States. Its books, videotapes, and DVDs have been translated into French, Italian, Spanish, Polish, Czech, Bulgarian, Russian, Hungarian, and Farsi.

Dr. Yang has published thirty-one other books on martial arts and Qigong:

1. Shaolin Chin Na; Unique Publications, Inc.,1980.

2. Shaolin Long Fist Kung Fu; Unique Publications, Inc., 1981.

3. Yang Style Tai Chi Chuan; Unique Publications, Inc., 1981.

4. Introduction to Ancient Chinese Weapons; Unique Publications, Inc., 1985.

5. Qigong for Health and Martial Arts; YMAA Publication Center, 1985.

6. Northern Shaolin Sword; YMAA Publication Center, 1985.

7. Tai Chi Theory and Martial Power; YMAA Publication Center, 1986.

8. Tai Chi Chuan Martial Applications; YMAA Publication Center, 1986.

9. Analysis of Shaolin Chin Na; YMAA Publication Center, 1987, second Edition—Analysis of Shaolin Chin Na, 2004.

10. Eight Simple Qigong Exercises for Health; YMAA Publication Center, 1988.

11. The Root of Chinese Qigong—The Secrets of Qigong Training; YMAA Publication Center, 1989.

12. Qigong—The Secret of Youth; YMAA Publication Center, 1989.

13. Xingyiquan—Theory and Applications; YMAA Publication Center, 1990.

14. The Essence of Taiji Qigong—Health and Martial Arts; YMAA Publication Center, 1990.

15. Qigong for Arthritis; YMAA Publication Center, 1991, third edition—Arthritis Relief, 2005.

16. Chinese Qigong Massage—General Massage; YMAA Publication Center, 1992, second edition—Qigong Massage, 2005.

17. How to Defend Yourself; YMAA Publication Center, 1992.

18. Baguazhang—Emei Baguazhang; YMAA Publication Center, 1994.

19. Comprehensive Applications of Shaolin Chin Na—The Practical Defense of Chinese Seizing Arts; YMAA Publication Center, 1995.

20. Taiji Chin Na—The Seizing Art of Taijiquan; YMAA Publication Center, 1995.

21. The Essence of Shaolin White Crane; YMAA Publication Center, 1996.

22. Back Pain—Chinese Qigong for Healing and Prevention; YMAA Publication Center, 1997. 2nd edition—Back Pain Relief, 2004.

23. Ancient Chinese Weapons; YMAA Publication Center, 1999.

24. Taijiquan—Classical Yang Style; YMAA Publication Center, 1999.

25. Tai Chi Secrets of Ancient Masters; YMAA Publication Center, 1999.

26. Taiji Sword—Classical Yang Style; YMAA Publication Center, 1999.

27. Tai Chi Secrets of Wǔ and Li Styles; YMAA Publication Center, 2001.

28. Tai Chi Secrets of Yang Style; YMAA Publication Center, 2001.

29. Tai Chi Secrets of Wu Style; YMAA Publication Center, 2002.

30. Taijiquan Theory of Dr. Yang, Jwing-Ming; YMAA Publication Center, 2003.

31. Qigong Meditation—Embryonic Breathing; YMAA Publication Center, 2004.


He has also published the following videotapes and DVDs:

Videotapes:

1. Yang Style Tai Chi Chuan and Its Applications; YMAA Publication Center, 1984.

2. Shaolin Long Fist Kung Fu—Lien Bu Chuan (Lian Bu Quan) and Its Applications; YMAA Publication Center,1985.

3. Shaolin Long Fist Kung Fu—Gung Li Chuan (Gong Li Quan) and Its Applications; YMAA Publication Center,1986.

4. Analysis of Shaolin Chin Na; YMAA Publication Center, 1987.

5. Eight Simple Qigong Exercises for Health (Wai Dan Chi Kung Vol. 1) The Eight Pieces of Brocade; YMAA Publication Center, 1987. 2nd Edition 2004.

6. The Essence of Tai Chi Chi Kung (Taiji Qigong); YMAA Publication Center, 1990.

7. Qigong for Arthritis; YMAA Publication Center, 1991. Arthritis Relief, 2005.

8. Qigong Massage—Self Massage; YMAA Publication Center, 1992.

9. Qigong Massage—With a Partner; YMAA Publication Center, 1992.

10. Defend Yourself 1—Unarmed Attack; YMAA Publication Center, 1992.

11. Defend Yourself 2—Knife Attack; YMAA Publication Center, 1992.

12. Comprehensive Applications of Shaolin Chin Na 1; YMAA Publication Center, 1995.

13. Comprehensive Applications of Shaolin Chin Na 2; YMAA Publication Center, 1995.

14. Shaolin Long Fist Kung Fu—Yi Lu Mai Fu & Er Lu Mai Fu; YMAA Publication Center, 1995.

15. Shaolin Long Fist Kung Fu—Shi Zi Tang; YMAA Publication Center, 1995.

16. Taiji Chin Na; YMAA Publication Center, 1995.

17. Emei Baguazhang—1; Basic Training, Qigong, Eight Palms, and Applications; YMAA Publication Center, 1995.

18. Emei Baguazhang—2; Swimming Body Baguazhang and Its Applications; YMAA Publication Center, 1995.

19. Emei Baguazhang—3; Bagua Deer Hook Sword and Its Applications YMAA Publication Center, 1995.

20. Xingyiquan—12 Animal Patterns and Their Applications; YMAA Publication Center, 1995.

21. 24 and 48 Simplified Taijiquan; YMAA Publication Center, 1995.

22. White Crane Hard Qigong; YMAA Publication Center, 1997.

23. White Crane Soft Qigong; YMAA Publication Center, 1997.

24. Xiao Hu Yan—Intermediate Level Long Fist Sequence; YMAA Publication Center, 1997.

25. Back Pain—Chinese Qigong for Healing and Prevention; YMAA Publication Center, 1997. Back Pain Relief, 2005.

26. Scientific Foundation of Chinese Qigong; YMAA Publication Center, 1997.

27. Taijiquan—Classical Yang Style; YMAA Publication Center, 1999.

28. Taiji Sword—Classical Yang Style; YMAA Publication Center, 1999.

29. Chin Na in Depth—1; YMAA Publication Center, 2000.

30. Chin Na in Depth—2; YMAA Publication Center, 2000.

31. San Cai Jian & Its Applications; YMAA Publication Center, 2000.

32. Kun Wu Jian & Its Applications; YMAA Publication Center, 2000.

33. Qi Men Jian & Its Applications; YMAA Publication Center, 2000.

34. Chin Na in Depth—3; YMAA Publication Center, 2001.

35. Chin Na in Depth—4; YMAA Publication Center, 2001.

36. Chin Na in Depth—5; YMAA Publication Center, 2001.

37. Chin Na in Depth—6; YMAA Publication Center, 2001.

38. 12 Routines of Tan Tui; YMAA Publication Center, 2001.

39. Chin Na in Depth—7; YMAA Publication Center, 2002.

40. Chin Na in Depth—8; YMAA Publication Center, 2002.

41. Chin Na in Depth—9; YMAA Publication Center, 2002.

42. Chin Na in Depth—10; YMAA Publication Center, 2002.

43. Chin Na in Depth—11; YMAA Publication Center, 2002.

44. Chin Na in Depth—12; YMAA Publication Center, 2002.

45. White Crane Gongfu—1; YMAA Publication Center, 2002.

46. White Crane Gongfu—2; YMAA Publication Center, 2002.

47. Taijiquan Pushing Hands—1; YMAA Publication Center, 2003.

48. Taijiquan Pushing Hands—2; YMAA Publication Center, 2003.

49. Taiji Saber and Its Applications; YMAA Publication Center, 2003.

50. Taiji Yin & Yang Symbol Sticking Hands—1; YMAA Publication Center, 2003.

51. Taiji Ball Qigong—1; YMAA Publication Center, 2003.

52. Taiji Ball Qigong—2; YMAA Publication Center, 2003.

53. Taijiquan Pushing Hands—3; YMAA Publication Center, 2004.

54. Taijiquan Pushing Hands—4; YMAA Publication Center, 2004.

55. Taiji & Shaolin Staff—Fundamental Training—1; YMAA Publication Center, 2004.

56. Shaolin Kung Fu—1, Fundamental Training; YMAA Publication Center, 2004.

57. Shaolin Kung Fu—2, Fundamental Training; YMAA Publication Center, 2004.

58. Taiji Ball Qigong—3; YMAA Publication Center, 2004.

59. Taiji Ball Qigong—4; YMAA Publication Center, 2004.

60. Advanced Practical Chin Na—1; YMAA Publication Center, 2004.

61. Advanced Practical Chin Na—2; YMAA Publication Center, 2004.

62. Taiji Yin & Yang Symbol Sticking Hands—2; YMAA Publication Center, 2004.

63. Taiji Chin Na In-Depth—1; YMAA Publication Center, 2004.

64. Taiji Chin Na In-Depth—2; YMAA Publication Center, 2004.

65. Taiji Chin Na In-Depth—3; YMAA Publication Center, 2004.

66. Taiji Chin Na In-Depth—4; YMAA Publication Center, 2004.

67. White Crane Gongfu—3; YMAA Publication Center, 2004.

68. Tai Chi Fighting Set; YMAA Publication Center, 2004.

69. Taiji & Shaolin Staff—Fundamental Training—2; YMAA Publication Center, 2005.

70. Taiji Wrestling—1; YMAA Publication Center, 2005.

71. Taiji Wrestling—2; YMAA Publication Center, 2005.

DVD:

1. Chin Na in Depth—1, 2, 3, 4; YMAA Publication Center, 2003.

2. White Crane Qigong—Hard & Soft; YMAA Publication Center, 2003.

3. Taijiquan, Classical Yang Style; YMAA Publication Center, 2003.

4. Chin Na in Depth—5, 6, 7, 8; YMAA Publication Center, 2003.

5. Chin Na in Depth—9, 10, 11, 12; YMAA Publication Center, 2003.

6. Eight Simple Qigong Exercises for Health; YMAA Publication Center, 2003.

7. Shaolin White Crane Gong Fu—1 & 2; YMAA Publication Center, 2004.

8. Analysis of Shaolin Chin Na; YMAA Publication Center, 2004.

9. Shaolin Long Fist Kung Fu—Basic Sequences; YMAA Publication Center, 2004.

10. Shaolin Kung Fu Fundamental Training 1 & 2; YMAA Publication Center, 2005.

11. Taiji Sword, Classical Yang Style; YMAA Publication Center, 2005.

12. The Essence of Taiji Qigong; YMAA Publication Center, 2005.

13. Qigong Massage—Fundamental Techniques for Health and Relaxation; YMAA Publication Center, 2005.

14. Taiji Pushing Hands 1&2—Yang Style Single and Double Pushing Hands; YMAA Publication Center, 2005.

15. Taiji Pushing Hands 3&4—Yang Style Single and Double Pushing Hands; YMAA Publication Center, 2006.

16. Tai Chi Fighting Set—Two Person Matching Set; YMAA Publication Center, 2006.

17. Taiji Ball Qigong Courses 1&2—16 Circling and 16 Rotating Patterns; YMAA Publication Center, 2006.

# Editor's Note

*David Silver*

Master Yang, Jwing-Ming has made it his life's purpose to research and translate all of the available ancient documents pertaining to the subjects of Qigong and Internal Cultivation. His extensive scientific background, paired with his training in Soft (Taiji), Hard (Long Fist), and Soft-Hard (White Crane) martial arts, empowers him with a comprehensive insight on the subjects of human physiology, universal electromagnetic energy, and the relationship between them.

Ancient Buddhist, Daoist, Qigong, and Martial Arts documents are often fragments; each discussing a certain aspect of its training, from the author's unique perspective based on his or her experience and contemplation. These documents are truly among the most precious artifacts of human history, sometimes passed down in the form of songs and poems, transmitted from teacher to student. Because many documents are only a piece of the puzzle, Qigong and Meditation are frequently misunderstood, or passed-down in an incomplete form. In an effort to preserve this accumulated knowledge, most of Master Yang's works are written as a stand-alone document, offering readers worldwide a complete overview to the subject matter, as he works toward a 'Unified Theory' of Qigong.

Several chapters in this book offer information discussed in Master Yang's previous works. If you have truly assimilated this information already, you are encouraged to move on to later chapters. However, as Master Yang's tireless research continues, his insight expands, and it may benefit the reader to humbly read each chapter and again immerse oneself entirely in the subject, starting with its general concepts and theories. Master Yang is fond of scolding his students for neglecting fundamental training, saying "Don't be a Jedi too soon".

Many cultural and spiritual centers have been destroyed in times of war. It is impossible to know how much knowledge, and how many written works, have been lost forever. It is impossible to know what the future holds for humanity, what humanity holds for itself, or how much of today's scientific and spiritual information will survive.

I share Master Yang's hope that the interrelated subjects of Qigong, meditation, and human bioelectricity will continue to be researched, and will become an important focus of scientific, medical and spiritual study. In 100 or 500 years, the situation on Earth (and other planets) will be so different that it is nearly impossible to conceive. We must hope that by then things have changed for the better; that humanity has rediscovered its common spirituality, reopened our third eye, and created a balanced and peaceful global society.

If not, I hope someone finds this book.

David Silver
Boston, April 2005

# Foreword

*Thomas G. Gutheil, MD*

*"Qigong is a science of inner feeling which relates to spiritual cultivation."*

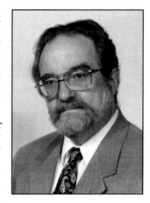

This definition may strike the Western reader as somewhat strange, since it fuses an Eastern concept of biologic energy and the idea of science, together with feeling and spirituality – concepts which are usually quite separate in Western thinking. But the very essence of Qigong is its union of physical, mental and spiritual issues into one discipline.

Western medicine is just beginning to explore the role of meditation in various forms as a legitimate adjunct to other approaches. The concept known as mindfulness, in which meditation consists of focus on breathing and the attempt to empty the mind of linear thought, is one such modern application. Though not as popular as it once was, transcendental mediation represents another form. Taiji, sometimes described as moving meditation, is, of course, one of the oldest forms but one which is enjoying a modern resurgence, even in alternative medicine where it is used to aid with a number of medical problems such as high blood pressure and ulcers. Yoga has also been practiced, sometimes in conjunction with mindfulness practice, to achieve some of the same states of tranquility. Finally, in the scientific community, studies of the so-called relaxation response represents another form that this method may take in current practice. Producing results ranging from feelings of inner harmony and tranquility to actual decreases in blood pressure, these techniques have gradually found a place in popular awareness and fields of healing.

In this work Dr. Yang, Jwing-Ming continues his astonishingly productive lifelong endeavor of unearthing hidden, secret, lost and otherwise unavailable ancient Chinese texts and translating them for the world of readers. The present book also takes its place in a series of works that explore almost every aspect of Qigong from its roots to its practical applications (see bibliography). Moreover, the present volume represents an updating of understanding of the fundamental principles of Qigong since publication of the predecessor volumes.

Based on the foundation of Internal Elixir Qigong practice, this book takes the reader to the next level of spiritual cultivation. Moving from an overview of the topic, Master Yang takes the reader through meditation training; then the specifics of Small Circulation, and then a look toward the future development of the subject.

While retaining the colorful and highly metaphoric language of the original texts, Dr. Yang makes the complex subject accessible and useful to the interested reader or practitioner. A helpful glossary furthers this accessibility. The thoughtful reader may thus gain a deep understanding of the basic sciences of this aspect of Qigong practice.

Thomas G. Gutheil, M.D.
Harvard Medical School

# Preface

Several friends have asked how I found time and energy to achieve proficiency in three Chinese martial arts styles, at the same time obtaining my Master's degree in Physics and Ph.D. in Mechanical Engineering. The main reason I could achieve each goal I set, was that I learned how to concentrate through meditation. I have practiced and studied meditation since I was seventeen. I could relax whenever I was tense, and ponder profoundly when I needed to. Meditation brought me another world—the world of spiritual awareness, which enabled me to build up self-confidence, wisdom and a better understanding of the world.

Small Circulation Meditation (Small Cyclic Heaven or Microcosmic Meditation, Xiao Zhou Tian Jing Zuo, 小周天静坐 ) has been well known for centuries throughout the East, including China, India, Indo-China, Korea, and Japan. According to ancient documents from Buddhist and Daoist monasteries, if one practices correctly under a master's guidance, it might take only 90 days to learn to circulate Qi in the Small Circulation path of the Conception and Governing Vessels. But I did not achieve this goal until I was 24 because I was young, and did not know the correct theory and technique. Documentary information was sparse, so I asked my White Crane and Taijiquan Masters. Due to lack of personal teaching experience, they refused to guide me. They simply advised me not to continue because of the danger involved. I could not calm down my mind to practice due to my school work and martial arts training. From the age of 15 to 19, in addition to school work, I trained Taijiquan in the early morning, and White Crane every evening. My meditation practice suffered as a result.

I finished my M.S. degree of science at Taiwan University. I was 23. Information was revealed to the public on meditation, and I could finally understand some theory. Then I was drafted into the Air Force as a military physics teacher. I had much time and little pressure, so I could calm my mind and put all my understanding into practicing every day for the whole year. I completed the Small Circulation path that summer, continuing until I married at age 27.

Being married, my life was very different and difficult, and my meditation was disrupted. I came to the United States in 1974 for Ph.D. study. I practiced a little, but could not advance further, due to the new environment and the pressure of studies. I only used meditation to calm my troubled mind. The following year, my wife arrived to join me from Taiwan, and in the year that followed, we lost our first child. Again I stopped meditating. I was sad and disappointed. Meditation had been part of my life and now I could not continue. After graduating with my Ph.D. from Purdue in 1978, my first son was born, then my daughter, followed by my second son. The financial pressure of supporting the family was so great, I almost forgot the pleasure and peace meditation could bring. But though I could not practice, I did not give up, and started collecting Qigong documents. Since 1980, many hidden

Qigong documents started to be revealed. I studied them and deepened my understanding of the subject.

To follow my dream, I resigned my engineering job in 1984 and dedicated my effort to writing and study. Life was great and the pressure of work was gone, but the financial reality of supporting my family worried me so much I could often not sleep at night. I developed pneumonia in the spring of 1984. Without health insurance, I did not see a doctor. One of my students studying as a medical doctor visited me and told me I had pneumonia for nearly two months, and was near death. My dentist brother in Taiwan sent me some antibiotics, and two weeks later my recurrent fever was disappearing. Three months later I published my first Qigong book, *Chi Kung— Health and Martial Arts*. The new edition is called *Qigong for Health and Martial Arts*. Surprisingly, this book started to bring some income, and I could smile again.

Since 1984, I continued to read, study and research. More books and ancient documents were revealed in Taiwan and mainland China. The second half of the 1980s became the most joyful of my life, as many more hidden documents were revealed. The most valuable to me were the secret classics, *Yi Jin Jing (Muscle/Tendon Changing*, 易筋經) and *Xi Sui Jing (Marrow/Brain Washing*, 洗髓經), said to have been written by Da Mo (達磨) around 500 A.D. in the Shaolin monastery. These classics are very profound. To many Qigong practitioners, their theory remains obscure, but to me they were the most precious knowledge I had ever received.

Studying them, I discovered the missing part of Qigong practice, its Yin side. Part of the Yi Jin Jing (Yang side) secret had previously been revealed through Shaolin martial arts, but not the Xi Sui Jing (Yin side). These two classics are two sides, Yin and Yang, of the same Qigong training. Both are required to reach the enlightenment or Buddhahood. Yi Jin Jing builds up and circulates Qi throughout the body to strengthen it (Yang side). Xi Sui Jing leads accumulated Qi from the Real Lower Dan Tian (Zhen Xia Dan Tian, 真下丹田) to the bone marrow, and also up to nourish the brain cells for spiritual enlightenment (Yin side).

To accumulate abundant Qi for Yi Jin Jing and Xi Sui Jing training, Small Circulation Meditation must first be practiced. This is the foundation of Internal Elixir Qigong (Nei Dan Qigong, 內丹氣功), without which Qi would be too weak to build up physical strength or to nurture spiritual enlightenment.

To fully comprehend the theory and training in these documents, I had to devote all my effort to it. This meant writing books about it. Through translating the documents, I was forced to ponder the meaning of every word. It also forced me to find related information with which to unravel the knots. My efforts came to fruition with publication of the books, *The Root of Chinese Qigong*, and *Qigong—The Secret of Youth* (previously *Muscle/Tendon Changing and Marrow/Brain Washing Chi Kung*.

Since 1984, countless Qigong documents, written by hundreds of ancient Qigong experts during the last four thousand years, have been compiled and published in mainland China. This has been a source of deep joy to me. I feel I am so lucky to have been born at this time, not only with access to these documents, but having a strong scientific background to understand and analyze them. Due to enhanced communication between East and West, great interest in this art of internal energy has also been aroused in Western society.

The more books I have written, the deeper I have understood this art. My mission in life is to present my Qigong knowledge in Western languages. All my children have grown up now, and my financial situation is stable. I resumed meditation practice in 1992, and can apply my understanding of Qigong theory in my practice. For the rest of my life I plan to enjoy reading and understanding these Qigong documents, the fruits of four thousand years of human feeling and spiritual cultivation. This will make my life meaningful and happy.

I have taught Small Circulation in the USA since 1981. After more than 20 years of teaching experience, I have modified some traditional practice methods, to make them safer and more suitable for practitioners in modern society. In this book, I share these methods with you. However, any book can only offer an opinion from the writer's point of view. You are the one who must collect more books, read and comprehend them, and finally arrive at a consistent scientific theory and method of practice, suitable to your lifestyle.

This book deals with vital new subject matter, including updated information and insights concerning subjects covered in earlier books. It focuses on profound discussion of the theory and practice of Small Circulation. Traditional training methods and modified ones are compared and analyzed. As long as you remain humble, and read and ponder carefully and sincerely, you should reach the goal of Small Circulation without risk. You should also discuss the subject with experienced practitioners.

The first part of the book reviews the general concepts and theory of Qigong. In the second part, traditional meditation training, procedures and theory are summarized, to show how traditional Qigong meditators reached the goal of enlightenment. The third part discusses the theory and practice of Small Circulation, especially Embryonic Breathing (Tai Xi, 胎息), the root of all Internal Elixir Qigong practice. More than 100 ancient documents discuss this important subject. For a deeper discussion of this subject, refer to my previous book, *Qigong Meditation—Embryonic Breathing*. In Part IV, we discuss the relevance of the subject matter to society.

Dr. Yang, Jwing-Ming

# Foundations 根基

## CHAPTER 1

# General Concepts
# 一般概念

## 1-1. INTRODUCTION 介紹

Qigong study and practice have become very popular since being introduced into Western society in the 1970s. However, many problems still remain:

1. Only a few books explain Qigong scientifically, bringing scientific theory and ancient experience together. So many people are still skeptical about Qigong science.

2. Few scholars and scientific researchers are willing to spend effort pursuing and verifying this Qigong science. Qigong is a newcomer to Western society, and few convincing scientific results are reported in scholarly studies and papers.

3. Many people are still in traditional and religious bondage, preventing them from opening their minds to another spiritual culture. Qigong is a science of inner feeling and spiritual cultivation. If one cannot or dares not jump out of the traditional matrix, one cannot accept this science which has been studied by Chinese and Indian society for more than four thousand years.

4. Few qualified Qigong practitioners can read, understand and accurately translate the abundant ancient Qigong documents into Western languages. I estimate that less than 1% of the ancient documents have been translated into Western languages. Most have been hidden in Buddhist and Daoist monasteries and only revealed in recent decades.

5. Many Qigong practitioners have used Qigong as a tool to abuse and mislead their followers. This has led people into superstitious belief and blind worship, making scientific scholars doubt the truth of Qigong practice.

Chinese Qigong derives from more than four thousand years of experience in healing and prevention of disease, and in spiritual cultivation. Four major schools have emerged: medical, scholar, religious, and martial. Qigong is one major essence of Chinese culture which cannot be separated from its people.

Western science has developed from its focus on the material world. That which can only be felt is considered unscientific, while inner feeling and development are ignored. But to Chinese, *feeling is a language which allows mind and body to communicate*, extending beyond the body to communicate with nature (heaven and earth) or Dao (道). This feeling has been studied and has become the core of Chinese culture, and is especially cultivated in Buddhist and Daoist society, where the final goal is to attain spiritual enlightenment, or Buddhahood. Through more than two thousand years of study and practice, this cultivation has reached such a high level that it cannot yet be interpreted by material science. I believe it will take some time to break through this barrier, and for Western scientists to accept this concept.

From my more than 42 years of Qigong practice, and from studying many ancient documents, I am confident at last that I have derived and understood the map of this Qigong science. As long as a "Dao searcher" (Xun Dao Zhe, 尋道者) is willing to study this map, even without guidance from a qualified master, one should still be able to stay on the correct path of study.

I have interpreted this map in several books:

1. *The Root of Chinese Qigong*. This book establishes a firm foundation for understanding Chinese Qigong.

2. *The Essence of Shaolin White Crane*. This is a martial Qigong book, and the theory is complete. However, the manifestation of this theory is in the White Crane style.

3. *Qigong—The Secret of Youth*. This book interpreted the crucial ancient classics, *Muscle/Tendon Changing* and *Marrow/Brain Washing Qigong* (*Yi Jin Jing, Xi Sui Jing*, 易筋經 · 洗髓經), passed down by the Indian monk Da Mo (達磨), around 500 A.D.

4. *Qigong Meditation—Embryonic Breathing* discusses Internal Elixir Qigong (Nei Dan, 內丹). Embryonic breathing (Tai Xi, 胎息) is a key practice in building and maintaining abundant inner energy. Without this practice as a foundation, the achievement of Internal Elixir would be shallow.

The practices described in these four books build a firm foundation for Internal Elixir Qigong (Nei Dan Qigong, 內丹氣功), making it possible for the next step in spiritual cultivation, Small Circulation, to be understood.

In this book, I introduce Small Circulation in four parts. Part I introduces and summarizes general Qigong knowledge of Small Circulation. Part II discusses traditional training procedures for Small Circulation and Enlightenment. Part III introduces Small Circulation training methods, while Part IV lists questions which remain to be answered someday. My next area of research will be on the topics of Grand Circulation and Spiritual Enlightenment Meditation, which will be published during the next few years in either one or two books.

## 1-2. What is Qi and What is Qigong? 何謂氣？何謂氣功？

We first discuss the general concept of Qi, both the traditional understanding and modern scientific paradigms and concepts explaining Qigong.

### A General Definition of Qi

Qi is the energy or natural force which fills the universe. The Chinese believe in Three Powers (San Cai, 三才) of the universe: Heaven (Tian, 天), Earth (Di, 地) and Man (Ren, 人). Heaven (the sky or universe) has Heaven Qi (Tian Qi, 天氣), the most important of the three, consisting of forces exerted by heavenly bodies, such as sunshine, moonlight, gravity and energy from the stars. Weather, climate and natural disasters are governed by Heaven Qi (Tian Qi, 天氣). Every energy field strives to stay in balance, so when the Heaven Qi loses its balance, it tries to rebalance itself, through wind, rain and even tornadoes and hurricanes which enable Heaven Qi to achieve a new energy balance.

Earth Qi (Di Qi, 地氣) is controlled by Heaven Qi. Too much rain forces a river to flood or change its path, but without rain, vegetation will die. The Chinese believe Earth Qi is made up of lines and patterns of energy, as well as the earth's magnetic field and the heat concealed underground. These energies must also be in balance, otherwise disasters such as earthquakes occur. When Earth Qi is balanced and harmonized, plants grow and animals thrive.

Finally, each individual person, animal, and plant has its own Qi field, which always seeks balance. Losing Qi balance, an individual sickens, dies and decomposes. All natural things, including mankind and our Human Qi (Ren Qi, 人氣), are determined by the natural cycles of Heaven Qi and Earth Qi. Throughout the history of Qigong, people have been most interested in Human Qi and its relationship with Heaven Qi and Earth Qi.

In China, Qi is also defined as any energy which demonstrates power and strength, be it electricity, magnetism, heat or light. Electric power is called electric Qi (Dian Qi, 電氣), and heat is called heat Qi (Re Qi, 熱氣). When a person is alive, his body's energy is called Human Qi (Ren Qi, 人氣).

Qi also expresses the energy state of something, especially of living things. The weather is called Heaven Qi (Tian Qi, 天氣) because it indicates the energy state of the heavens. When something is alive it has Vital Qi (Huo Qi, 活氣), and when dead it has Dead Qi (Si Qi, 死氣) or Ghost Qi (Gui Qi, 鬼氣). When a person is righteous and has the spiritual strength to do good, he is said to have Normal Qi or Righteous Qi (Zheng Qi, 正氣). The spiritual state or morale of an army is called its Energy State (Qi Shi, 氣勢).

Qi can represent energy itself, or else the state of the energy. It is important to understand this when you practice Qigong, so your mind is not channeled into a narrow understanding of Qi, limiting your future understanding and development.

## A Narrow Definition of Qi

Now let us look at how Qi is defined in Qigong society today. Among the Three Powers, the Chinese have been most concerned with Qi affecting health and longevity. After four thousand years emphasizing Human Qi, when people mention Qi they usually mean Qi circulating in our bodies.

In ancient Chinese medical and Qigong documents, the word Qi was written "炁". This character consists of two words, "旡" on top, which means "nothing", and "灬" at the bottom, which means "fire." So Qi was originally written as "no fire." In ancient times, *physicians and Qigong practitioners attempted to balance the Yin and Yang Qi circulating in the body, so there was "no fire" in the internal organs.* Each internal organ needs a specific amount of Qi to function properly. If it receives an improper amount, usually too much which makes it too Yang or on fire, it starts to malfunction, in time causing physical damage. The goal of Qigong was to attain a state of "no fire," which eventually became the word Qi.

But in more recent publications, the Qi of "no fire" has been replaced by the word "氣," again constructed of two words, "气" which means "air," and "米" which means "rice." Later practitioners realized that post-birth Qi is produced by breathing in air and consuming food. Air is called "Kong Qi" (空氣), literally "Space Energy."

For a long time, people debated what type of energy circulates in our bodies. Many believed it to be heat, others electricity, while others again assumed it was a mixture of heat, electricity and light. This debate continued into the 1980s, when the concept of Qi gradually became clear. Today, science postulates that, with the possible exception of gravity, there is actually only one type of energy in the universe, namely electromagnetic energy. Light and heat are also manifestations of electromagnetic energy. The Qi in our bodies is actually bioelectricity, and our bodies are a living electromagnetic field.[1] Thus, the Qi is affected by our thoughts, feelings, activities, the food we eat, the quality of the air we breathe, our lifestyles, the natural energy that surrounds us, and also the unnatural energy which modern science inflicts upon us.

The following scientific formula represents the major biochemical reaction in our body:

$$\text{glucose} + 6O_2 \longrightarrow 6CO_2 + 6H_2O$$

$$\Delta G^{o'} = -686 \text{ Kcal}$$

$$\longrightarrow \begin{array}{l} \text{Heat} \\ \text{Light} \\ \text{Bioelectricity (Qi)} \end{array}$$

As you can see, rice is glucose, oxygen is air, and bioelectricity is Qi.

**A General Definition of Qigong**

In China, the word "Gong" (功) is often used instead of "Gongfu" (Kung Fu, 功夫), meaning energy and time. *Any study or training which requires energy and time to achieve is called Gongfu.* It can be applied to any special skill or study requiring time, energy and patience. *Qigong is a science which studies the energy in nature.* The main difference between this energy science and Western energy science is that Qigong focuses on the inner energy of human beings, while Western energy science pays more attention to the energy outside the human body. When you study Qigong, it is worthwhile to consider the modern scientific point of view, and not restrict yourself to traditional beliefs.

The Chinese have studied Qi for thousands of years, recording information on the patterns and cycles of nature in books such as the *Yi Jing* (易經, *The Book of Changes*, 1122 B.C.), which describes the natural forces of Heaven (Tian, 天), Earth (Di, 地), and Man (Ren, 人). These Three Powers (San Cai, 三才) manifest as Heaven Qi, Earth Qi, and Human Qi, with their definite rules and cycles. The rules are unchanging, while the cycles return to repeat themselves. The *Yi Jing* applies these principles to calculate changes in natural Qi, through a process called The Eight Trigrams (Bagua, 八卦). From the Eight Trigrams are derived the 64 hexagrams. The *Yi Jing* was probably the first book describing Qi and its variations in nature and man. The relationship of the Three Natural Powers and their Qi variations were later discussed extensively in the book, *Theory of Qi's Variation* (*Qi Hua Lun*, 氣化論).

Understanding Heaven Qi is very difficult, and was especially so in ancient times. But since natural cycles recur, accumulated experience makes it possible to trace the natural patterns. Understanding the rules and cycles of Heavenly Timing (Tian Shi, 天時) helps describe changes in the seasons, climate, weather and other natural occurrences. Many of these routine patterns and cycles are caused by the rebalancing of Qi. Various natural cycles recur every day, month or year, while others return only every twelve or sixty years.

Earth Qi forms part of Heaven Qi. From understanding the rules and structure of the earth, you understand the process whereby mountains and rivers are formed, plants grow and rivers move, and also where it is best to build a house and which direction it should face to be a healthy place to live. In China, Geomancy Teachers (Di Li Shi, 地理師), or Wind Water Teachers (Feng Shui Shi, 風水師), make their living this way. The term Wind Water (Feng Shui, 風水) is used because the location and character of wind and water are the most important factors in evaluating a location. These experts use the accumulated body of geomantic knowledge and the *Yi Jing* to help make important decisions such as where and how to build a house, where to bury the dead, and how to rearrange homes and offices to be better and more prosperous places in which to live and work.

Human Qi has been studied most thoroughly, encompassing many different aspects. The Chinese believe Human Qi is affected and controlled by Heaven Qi and Earth Qi, and that they in fact determine your destiny. By understanding the relationship between nature and people, and also Human Relations (Ren Shi, 人事), you may predict wars, the destiny of a country, a person's desires and temperament, and even their future. The people who practice this profession are called Calculate Life Teachers (Suan Ming Shi, 算命師).

However, the greatest achievement in the study of Human Qi is in regard to health and longevity. Since Qi is the source of life, if you understand how Qi functions and know how to regulate it correctly, you may live a long and healthy life. As a part of nature, you are channeled into its cycles, and it is in your best interest to follow the way of nature. This is the meaning of *Dao* (道), which can be translated as *the Natural Way*.

Many different aspects of Human Qi have been researched, including acupuncture, massage, herbal treatment, meditation, and Qigong exercises. Their use in adjusting Human Qi flow has become the root of Chinese medical science. Meditation and moving Qigong exercises are used to improve health and cure certain illnesses. Daoists and Buddhists also use meditation and Qigong exercises in their pursuit of enlightenment.

In conclusion, *the study of any of the aspects of Qi including Heaven Qi, Earth Qi, and Human Qi should be called Qigong*. However, since the term is usually used today only in reference to the cultivation of Human Qi through meditation and exercises, we will conform to this narrower definition.

## A Narrow Definition of Qigong

The narrow definition of Qi is the energy circulating in the human body. Qigong studies and trains the Qi circulating in the body. Qigong includes how our bodies relate to Heaven Qi and Earth Qi, and the overlapping fields of acupuncture, herbal treatment, martial arts Qigong, Qigong massage and exercises, and religious enlightenment Qigong.

In ancient times, Qigong was called "Tu-Na" (吐納), meaning to "utter and admit," namely focused breathing. Qigong depends on correct breathing. Zhuang Zi (莊子) said, "Blowing to breathe, utter the old and admit the new. The bear's natural movement, and the bird's extending (of the neck), are all for longevity. This is favored by those living as long as Peng Zu (彭祖), who practice Dao-Yin (導引, guide and lead), and nourish the shape (cultivate the body)."[1] Peng Zu was a legendary Qigong practitioner during the reign of emperor Yao (堯, 2356 B.C.), said to have lived for 800 years. Qigong was also called Dao-Yin, *meaning to use the mind and physical movement to guide and lead Qi circulation*. The movements imitate natural movements of animals such as bears and birds. A famous medical Qigong set passed down from that time is called The Five Animal Sports (Wu Qin Xi, 五禽戲), which imitates the movements of the tiger, deer, bear, ape, and bird.

Qigong defines twelve major channels (Shi Er Jing, 十二經) in the body, branching into many secondary channels (Luo, 絡), similar to the blood circulatory system. The primary channels are like arteries and veins, while the secondary ones are like capillaries. The Twelve Primary Qi Channels are also like *rivers*, while the secondary channels are like *streams* flowing into and out of the rivers. Qi is distributed throughout the body through this network which connects the extremities to the internal organs, and the skin to the bone marrow. The internal organs of Chinese medicine do not necessarily correspond to the physical organs as understood in the West, but rather to a set of clinical functions related to the organ system.

The body also has Eight Vessels (Ba Mai, 八脈), called strange meridians (Qi Jing, 奇經), that function like *reservoirs* and regulate the Qi circulation. The famous Chinese Daoist medical doctor Li, Shi-Zhen (李時珍) described them in his book, *The Study of Strange Meridians and Eight Vessels* (奇經八脈考), "The regular meridians (12 Primary Qi Channels) are like rivers, while the strange meridians (Eight Vessels) are like lakes. When the Qi in the regular meridians is abundant and flourishing, they overflow into the strange meridians."[2]

When Qi in the eight reservoirs is full and strong, so is that in the rivers. Stagnation in any channel leads to irregularity in the Qi flow to the extremities and organs, and illness may develop. Every channel has its own particular Qi flow, its strength affected by your mind, the weather, time of day, food you have eaten, and even your mood. In dry weather, Qi in the lungs tends to be more positive and Yang than in wet weather. When you are angry, the Qi flow in your liver channel will be irregular. Qi strength in different channels varies throughout the day in a regular cycle, and at any particular time one channel is strongest. For example, between 11 A.M. and 1 P.M. the Qi flows most strongly in the heart channel. The Qi level of the same organ differs from one person to another. For more detail on the relationship of the Qi flow and time of day, refer to the YMAA book, *Qigong for Health and Martial Arts*.

When Qi flow in the twelve channels is irregular, the eight reservoirs regulate it back to normal. When one experiences a sudden shock, Qi in the bladder becomes deficient. The reservoir immediately regulates it to recover from the shock, unless the reservoir Qi is also deficient, or if the shock is too great. Then, the bladder contracts, causing urination.

A sick person's Qi tends to be either too positive (excess Yang, 陽) or too negative (deficient Yin, 陰). A Chinese physician would prescribe herbs to adjust the Qi, or else insert acupuncture needles at various points to adjust the flow and restore balance. The alternative is to practice Qigong, using physical and mental exercises to adjust the Qi.

In Scholar society, Qigong is defined differently, focusing on regulating disturbances of the emotional mind into a state of calm. This relaxes the body and enables

Qi to rebalance and circulate smoothly, so mental and physical health may be attained.

In Daoist and Buddhist society, Qigong is the method to lead Qi from the Lower Dan Tian (下丹田), or elixir field, to the brain for spiritual enlightenment or Buddhahood. This place in the abdomen stores Qi in a bioelectric battery. (We will discuss the Dan Tian in detail in section 2-3.) Religious Qigong is considered the highest and most rigorous level of Chinese Qigong training.

In martial arts society, Qigong is the theory and method of manifesting Qi to energize the physical body to its maximum efficiency and power. Martial arts Qigong originated from religious Qigong, especially Muscle/Tendon Changing and Marrow/Brain Washing Qigong (Yi Jin Jing and Xi Sui Jing, 易筋經、洗髓經), and the profoundest level of martial arts Qigong training is the same as that of religious Qigong, namely spiritual enlightenment.

## 1-3. CATEGORIES OF QIGONG 氣功之分類

I would like to discuss the scope of human Qigong, and the traditional concept of Nei Dan (內丹, Internal Elixir) and Wai Dan (外丹, External Elixir), to clarify the differences between the styles of Qigong practice around the world.

### A. Scope of Qigong Practice—Physical and Mental 氣功練習之規範

If we trace Qigong history back to before the Chinese Qin and Han Dynasties (255 B.C.-223 A.D., 秦、漢), we find the origin of many Qigong practices in dancing. Dancing exercises the body and maintains it in a healthy condition. Matching movement with music harmonizes the mind, either to energize it or calm it down. This Qigong dancing was later passed to Japan during the Han Dynasty, and became the very elegant, slow and refined dancing still practiced in the Japanese Royal Court today.

African and Native American dancing, in which the body is bounced up and down, also loosens the joints and improves Qi circulation. *Any activity which regulates Qi circulation in the body*, even jogging or weight-lifting, *may be regarded as Qigong*. Aspects of this include the food we eat, the air we breathe, and even our emotions and thoughts.

In Figure 1-1, the vertical axis to the left represents Qi use by the physical body (Yang), and the right vertex that of the mind (Yin). The more to the left an activity is represented, the more physical effort and the less mind is needed. This can be aerobics, dancing, walking or jogging in which the mind is used less than the body. This does not need special training, and is classified as secular Qigong. At the mid-point of the graph, mental and physical activity are combined in equal measure. This would be the slow-moving Qigong commonly practiced, in which the mind is used to lead Qi in coordination with movement. With slow, relaxed movements, the Qi led by the mind may reach deeper into the ligaments, marrow and internal organs.

Deep internal feeling can lead Qi there significantly. Taiji, White Crane, Snake, and Dragon are typical systems of Qigong, cultivated intensively in Chinese medical and martial arts societies.

At a deeper level of practice, the mind becomes critically important. It is actively involved while you are in deep relaxation. This is cultivated primarily by scholars and religious Qigong practitioners. There may be some physical movement in the lower abdomen, but *the main focus is cultivating a peaceful and neutral mind, and pursuing the final goal of spiritual enlightenment.* This practice includes Sitting Chan (Ren, 坐禪，忍), Embryonic Breathing (Tai Xi Jing Zuo, 胎息靜坐), Small Circulation (Xiao Zhou Tian, 小周天), Grand Circulation (Da Zhou Tian, 大周天), and Brain Washing Enlightenment Meditation (Xi Sui Gong, 洗髓功).

Different Qigong practices aim for different goals. For a long, happy life, you need health of mind and body. The best Qigong for health is at the middle of our model, to regulate both body and mind. You may practice the Yin side through still meditation, and the Yang side through physical activity. This balances Yin and Yang, and abundant Qi may be accumulated and circulated.

From this we may conclude:

1. Any activity able to improve Qi circulation is Qigong.

2. Qigong which emphasizes the physical more will improve physical strength and Qi circulation, conditioning the muscles, tendons, and ligaments.

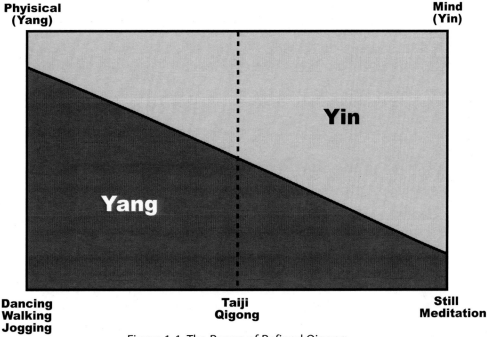

Figure 1-1. The Range of Refined Qigong

3. Qigong activating both physical and mental can reach deeper, enhancing physical strength and Qi circulation. By coordinating the relaxed physical body with the concentrated mind, Qi may circulate deep inside the joints, internal organs, and even the bone marrow.

4. Qigong which focuses on achieving a profound meditative state may however neglect physical movement, causing physical strength to degenerate.

### External and Internal Elixirs (Wai Dan and Nei Dan) 外丹與內丹

Qigong practices can be divided according to their training theory and methods into two general categories, Wai Dan (外丹, External Elixir) and Nei Dan (內丹, Internal Elixir). Understanding the differences between them gives you an overview of Qigong practice.

**Wai Dan (External Elixir)** 外丹. Wai means external, and Dan means elixir. External here means the skin and surface of the body, and also the limbs, as opposed to the torso at the center of the body, which includes the vital organs. Elixir is the life-prolonging substance for which Chinese Daoists searched for millennia. They first thought it was something physical which could be prepared from herbs or from chemicals purified in a furnace. After thousands of years of experimentation, they found the elixir within, namely Qi circulating in the body. To prolong your life, you must develop the elixir in your body, cultivating, protecting, and nourishing it.

In Wai Dan Qigong practice, you exercise to build Qi in your arms and legs. When enough Qi accumulates there, it flows through the Twelve Primary Qi Channels clearing obstructions, and into the center of the body to nourish the organs. A person who works out, or has a physical job, is generally healthier than one who sits around all day.

Massage, acupuncture, and herbal treatment are all Wai Dan practices. Massaging the body produces Qi, stimulating the cells to a more energized state. Qi is raised and circulation enhanced. After a massage you are relaxed, and the higher levels of Qi in the muscles and skin flow into the torso and internal organs. This is the theoretical foundation of Tui Na (推拿, push and grab) Qigong massage. Acupuncture may also enhance Qi, regulating the internal organs.

*Any stimulation or exercise that generates a high level of Qi in the limbs or at the surface of the body, which then flows into the center of the body, can be classified as Wai Dan* (Figure 1-2).

**Nei Dan (Internal Elixir)** 內丹. Nei means internal. Nei Dan means to build up the elixir internally, inside the body instead of in the limbs, in the vessels rather than the channels. Whereas in Wai Dan, Qi is built up in the limbs or skin, then moved into the body through primary Qi channels, *Nei Dan exercises build up Qi inside the body and lead it out to the limbs* (Figure 1-3). This is accomplished by special breath-

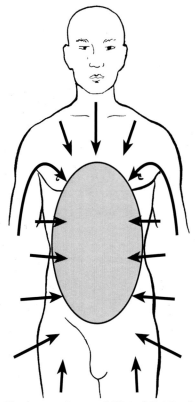

Figure 1-2. External Elixir (Wai Dan)

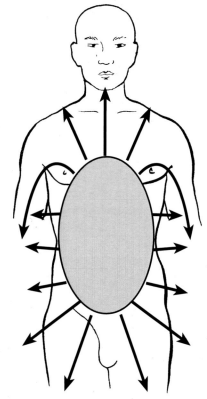

Figure 1-3. Internal Elixir (Nei Dan)

ing techniques during meditation. First one builds abundant Qi in the Lower Dan Tian, the bioelectric battery, then leads it to the Eight Vessels for storage. Then Qi in the Twelve Primary Channels can be regulated smoothly and efficiently.

Nei Dan is more profound than Wai Dan, and more difficult to understand and practice. Traditionally, Nei Dan Qigong practices were passed down more secretively than Wai Dan, especially at the highest levels such as Marrow/Brain Washing, which were passed down to only a few trusted disciples.

### Schools of Qigong Practice 氣功練習之門派

Qigong has four major categories according to the purpose of training—A. curing illness, B. maintaining health, C. enlightenment or Buddhahood, and D. martial arts. Most styles serve more than one of these purposes. For example, Daoist Qigong aims for longevity and enlightenment, but you need to maintain good health and cure sickness. Knowing the history and principles of each category helps understand their essence more clearly.

**Medical Qigong—for Healing.** In ancient China, most emperors respected scholars and their philosophy. Doctors were not highly regarded, because they made their diagnosis by touching the patient's body, considered characteristic of the lower social classes. Although doctors were commonly looked down on, they quietly passed down the results of their research to following generations. Of all the groups studying Qigong in China, doctors have been at it the longest. Since the discovery of Qi circulation in the human body about four thousand years ago, Chinese doctors have devoted major efforts to study it, developing acupuncture, acupressure, and herbal treatment.

Many Chinese doctors also created sets of Qigong for maintaining health or curing specific illnesses. Doing only sitting meditation with breathing, as in scholar Qigong or Buddhist Chan meditation, is not enough to cure illness, and they believed in movement to increase Qi circulation. Although a calm and peaceful mind is important for health, exercising the body is more important. They learned through practice that people who exercised properly got sick less often, and their bodies degenerated less quickly than people who just sat around. Specific movements increase Qi circulation in specific organs, and are used to treat specific illnesses and restore normal function.

Some movements are similar to the way certain animals move. For an animal to survive in the wild, it must instinctively protect its body, especially accumulating its Qi and preserving it. We humans have lost many of these instincts over time, in separating ourselves from nature.

A typical, well known set of such exercises is Wu Qin Xi (五禽戲, Five Animal Sports) created nearly two thousand years ago by Hua Tuo (華佗). (Others say it was by Jun Qing (君倩). Another famous set is Ba Duan Jin (八段錦), The Eight Pieces of Brocade. It was developed by Marshal Yue, Fei (岳飛) during the Southern Song Dynasty (1127-1280 A.D., 南宋), who was a soldier and scholar rather than a doctor.

Before physical damage manifests in an organ, there is first an abnormality in Qi circulation. Excess Yin or Yang is the root of illness and organ damage. In a specific channel, *abnormal Qi circulation leads to organ malfunction*. If the condition is not corrected, the organ degenerates. The best way to heal is to adjust and balance the Qi before there is any physical problem, the major goal of acupuncture and acupressure treatment. Herbs and special diets also help regulate the Qi.

As long as the illness is limited to Qi stagnation and there is no physical organ damage, Qigong exercises can be used to readjust Qi circulation and treat the problem. But if the sickness is already so serious that the organs have started to fail, the situation is critical and specific treatment is necessary. This can be acupuncture, herbs, or even an operation. Ulcers, asthma, and even certain kinds of cancer, are often treated effectively with simple exercises.

Over thousands of years of observing nature, Qigong practitioners went even deeper. Qi circulation changes with the seasons, so they helped the body during these periodic adjustments. In each season different organs have characteristic problems. For example, at the beginning of fall, the lungs adapt to breathing colder air, making them susceptible to colds. Other organs are also affected by seasonal changes, and by one another. Focusing on these seasonal Qi disorders, they developed movements to speed up the body's adjustment. These sets were originally created to maintain health, and later were also used for curing sickness.

**Scholar Qigong—for Maintaining Health.** Before the Han Dynasty (206 B.C.-221 A.D., 漢朝), two major scholar societies arose. One was founded by Confucius (551-479 B.C., Kong Zi, 孔子) during the Spring and Autumn Period (722-484 B.C., Chun Qiu, 春秋). His philosophy was popularized and expanded by Mencius (372-289 B.C., Meng Zi, 孟子) during the Warring States Period (403-222 B.C., Zhan Guo, 戰國). Scholars who practice his philosophy are called Confucians (Ru Jia, 儒家). Their basic philosophy consists of Loyalty (Zhong, 忠), Filial Piety (Xiao, 孝), Humanity (Ren, 仁), Kindness (Ai, 愛), Trust (Xin, 信), Justice (Yi, 義), Harmony (He, 和) and Peace (Ping, 平). Humanity and human feelings are the main subjects, and Confucian philosophy is the root of much of Chinese culture.

The second major scholar society was Daoism (Dao Jia, 道家), established by Lao Zi (老子) in the 6th century B.C. His classic, the *Dao De Jing* (道德經, *Classic on the Virtue of the Dao*), describes human morality. During the Warring States Period, his follower Zhuang Zhou (莊周) wrote a book called *Zhuang Zi* (莊子), which led to the forming of another strong branch of Daoism. Before the Han Dynasty, Daoism was considered a branch of scholarship. However, in the East Han Dynasty (25-168 A.D., 東漢), traditional Daoism was combined with Buddhism imported from India by Zhang, Dao-Ling (張道陵), and began to be treated as a religion. Daoism before the Han Dynasty should be considered scholarly Daoism rather than religious.

With regard to Qigong, both schools emphasized maintaining health and preventing disease. Many illnesses are caused by mental and emotional excesses. When one's mind is disturbed, the organs do not function normally. For example, depression may cause stomach ulcers and indigestion. Anger may cause the liver to malfunction. Sadness may lead to stagnation and tightness in the lungs, and fear can disturb the normal functioning of the kidneys and bladder. To avoid illness, you need to balance and relax your thoughts and emotions. This is called regulating the mind (Tiao Xin, 調心).

Both schools emphasize gaining a peaceful mind through meditation. In still meditation, the primary training is getting rid of thoughts, to clear the mind. As the flow of thoughts and emotions slows down, you feel mentally and emotionally neutral, leading to self-control. In this state of "no thought" you even relax deep down into your internal organs, and your Qi circulation is smooth and strong.

This still meditation is very common in Chinese scholar society, which focuses on regulating the mind, body, and breath, so Qi flows smoothly, and sickness may be averted. Their training is called Xiu Qi (修氣), which means cultivating Qi. This is very different from the religious Daoist Qigong since the East Han Dynasty, called Lian Qi (練氣), meaning to train Qi to make it stronger.

Qigong documents from Confucians and Daoists are mainly limited to maintaining health. Their aim is to follow natural destiny and maintain health. This is quite different from that of religious Daoists after the East Han Dynasty, who believed one's destiny could be changed. They believed it possible to train your Qi to make it stronger, and to extend your life. Scholar society maintained that "in human life, seventy is rare."[3] Few common people in ancient times reached seventy as a result of the harsh conditions. They also said, "peace with Heaven and delight in your destiny" (An Tian Le Ming, 安天樂命), and "cultivate the body and await destiny" (Xiu Shen Si Ming, 修身俟命). Compare this with the philosophy of the later Daoists, who said, "one hundred and twenty means dying young."[4] They proved by example that life can be extended, and destiny resisted and overcome.

**Religious Qigong for Enlightenment or Buddhahood.** Religious Qigong, though not as popular as other categories in China, has achieved the greatest accomplishments of all categories of Qigong. It was kept secret in the monasteries, and only revealed to seculars, or laypeople, in the last century.

It comprises mainly of Daoist and Buddhist Qigong. The main purpose of their training is striving for enlightenment or Buddhahood. They seek to rise above normal human suffering, and escape from the cycle of continual reincarnation. They believe all human suffering is caused by the seven passions and six desires (Qi Qing Liu Yu, 七情六慾). The seven passions are happiness (Xi, 喜), anger (Nu, 怒), sorrow (Ai, 哀), joy (Le, 樂), love (Ai, 愛), hate (Hen, 恨), and desire (Yu, 慾). The six desires are the six sensory pleasures of the eyes, ears, nose, tongue, body, and mind. If you are bound to them, you will reincarnate after death. To avoid this, they train to be spiritually independent of the body, and of physical attachments and circumstances. Thereby they enter the heavenly kingdom and gain eternal peace. This rigorous training is called Unification of Heaven and Man (Tian Ren He Yi, 天人合一). It is extremely difficult to achieve in the everyday world, so practitioners generally shun society and move into the solitude of the mountains, where they can concentrate all their energies on spiritual cultivation.

Religious Qigong practitioners train to strengthen internal Qi, to nourish their spirit (Shen) until it can survive the death of the body. Marrow/Brain Washing Qigong training enables them to lead Qi to the brain, where the spirit resides, and to raise the brain cells to a higher energy state. This training used to be restricted to only a few advanced priests in China and Tibet. Over the last two thousand years, Tibetan and Chinese Buddhists, and the religious Daoists, have followed the same principles to become the three major religious schools of Qigong training.

This religious striving toward enlightenment or Buddhahood is recognized as the highest and most difficult level of Qigong. Many practitioners reject the rigors of this religious striving, and practice Marrow/Brain Washing Qigong solely for longevity. It was these people who eventually revealed the secrets of Marrow/Brain Washing to the outside world, as described in *Qigong—The Secret of Youth*.

**Martial Qigong—for Fighting.** Chinese martial Qigong developed from Da Mo's *Muscle/Tendon Changing and Marrow/Brain Washing Qigong Classic* (*Yi Jin Jing, Xi Sui Jing*; 易筋經，洗髓經), written in the Shaolin Temple (Shaolin Si, 少林寺) during the Liang Dynasty (502-557 A.D., 梁朝). Shaolin monks training this Qigong improved their health and greatly increased their martial power and effectiveness. Since then, many martial styles have developed further Qigong sets, and many martial styles have been created based on Qigong theory. Martial artists have played a major role in Chinese Qigong society.

When Qigong theory was first applied to martial arts, it was used to increase the power and efficiency of the muscles. *The mind which is generated from clear thinking (Yi) leads Qi to the muscles to energize them to function more efficiently.* The average person generally uses his muscles at about 40% efficiency. Training a strong Yi to lead Qi to the muscles effectively, one may energize the muscles to a higher level, increasing fighting effectiveness.

Acupuncture theory enabled fighting techniques to reach even more advanced levels. Martial artists learned to attack vital cavities, disturbing the enemy's Qi flow to cause injury and death. Central to this is understanding the route and timing of Qi circulation in the body, to strike the cavities accurately and to the correct depth. These techniques are called Dian Xue (點穴, Pointing Cavities) or Dian Mai (點脈, Pointing Vessels).

While most martial Qigong practices also improve the practitioner's health, there are some which, although they build up some special skill useful for fighting, also damage the practitioner's health. An example of this is Iron Sand Palm (Tie Sha Zhang, 鐵砂掌). Although it builds amazing destructive power, it can also harm your hands and affect the Qi circulation in the hands and internal organs.

Many martial styles have developed from Da Mo's 6th century Qigong theory and methods. They can be roughly divided into external and internal styles. The external styles emphasize building Qi in the limbs for physical martial techniques, following the practices of Wai Dan Qigong. The concentrated mind is used during the exercises to energize the Qi. This significantly increases muscular strength and the effectiveness of the martial techniques. Qigong trains the body to resist punches and kicks, by leading Qi to energize the skin and the muscles, enabling them to resist a blow without injury. This training is called Iron Shirt (Tie Bu Shan, 鐵布衫) or Golden Bell Cover (Jin Zhong Zhao, 金鐘罩). Martial styles which use Wai Dan training are called external styles (Wai Jia, 外家). Hard Qigong training is called Hard Gong (Ying Gong, 硬功). Shaolin Gongfu is a typical example of a style using Wai Dan martial Qigong.

Although Wai Dan Qigong increases the martial artist's power, training the muscles can cause overdevelopment, leading to energy dispersion (San Gong, 散功). To prevent this, when an external martial artist reaches a high level of external training he will start training internal Qigong, which specializes in curing the energy dispersion problem. "The external styles are from external to internal and from hard to soft."[5]

By contrast, Internal Martial Qigong is based on the theory of Nei Dan. Qi is generated in the torso instead of the limbs, and later led to the limbs to increase power. To lead Qi to the limbs, the techniques must be soft and muscle use kept to a minimum. Nei Dan martial training is much more difficult than Wai Dan. For more detail refer to the book, *Tai Chi Theory and Martial Power*.

Several internal martial styles were created in the Wudang (武當山) and Emei (峨嵋山) Mountains. Popular ones are Taijiquan (太極拳), Baguazhang (八卦掌), Liu He Ba Fa (六合八法) and Xingyiquan (形意拳). Even internal martial styles, called Soft Styles, must sometimes use muscular strength while fighting. Utilizing strong power in a fight requires Qi to manifest externally, using harder, more external techniques. "Internal styles are from internal to external and from soft to hard."[6]

Although Qigong is widely studied in Chinese martial society, the main focus is on increasing fighting ability rather than on health. Good health is considered a byproduct of training. Only recently has health started receiving greater attention in martial Qigong, especially in the internal martial arts.

## 1-4. THEORY OF YIN AND YANG, KAN AND LI 陰陽坎離之理論

The most important concepts in Qigong practice are the theories of Yin and Yang, and of Kan and Li. These two different concepts have become confused in Qigong society, even in China. If you understand them clearly, you have grasped an important key to Qigong practice.

### What are Kan and Li?

The terms Kan (坎) and Li (離) occur frequently in Qigong documents. In the Eight Trigrams, Kan represents Water while Li represents Fire. Kan and Li training has long been of major importance to Qigong practitioners.

Although Kan-Li and Yin-Yang are related, Kan and Li are not Yin and Yang. Kan is Water, which cools your body down and makes it more Yin, while Li is Fire, which warms your body and makes it more Yang. *Kan and Li are the methods or causes, while Yin and Yang are the results.* When Kan and Li are adjusted correctly, Yin and Yang are balanced and interact harmoniously.

Qigong practitioners believe your body is always too Yang, unless you are sick or have not eaten for a long time. Excess Yang leads the body to degenerate and burn out, causing aging. Using Water to cool down your body, you can slow the aging process and lengthen your life. Qigong practitioners improve the quality of Water in their bodies, and reduce the quantity of Fire. You should always keep this subject at the top of your list for study and research. If you earnestly ponder and experiment, you will grasp the trick of adjusting them.

Water and Fire represent many things in the body. First, Qi is classified according to Fire or Water. When your Qi is not pure, causing your body to heat up and your mind to become unstable (Yang), it is classified as Fire Qi (Huo Qi, 火氣). The Qi which is pure and can cool your physical and spiritual bodies, making them more Yin, is Water Qi (Shui Qi, 水氣). Your Qi should never be purely Water. It may cool down the Fire, but should never quench it, which would signify death.

Fire Qi agitates and stimulates the emotions, generating from them the emotional mind called Xin (心), which is considered the Fire mind or Yang mind. On the other hand, the mind that Water Qi generates is calm, steady and wise. It is called Yi (意), and considered to be the Water mind or wisdom mind. If your spirit is nourished primarily by Fire Qi, although your spirit may be high, as a Yang spirit it will be scattered and confused. If the spirit is nourished and raised up mainly by Water Qi, it will be a firm, steady Yin mind. When your Yi governs your Xin effectively, your will, as strong emotional intention, can be firm.

Your Qi is the main cause of the Yin and Yang of your body, mind and spirit. To regulate Yin and Yang, you need to regulate Water and Fire Qi at their source.

To analyze Kan and Li and adjust them efficiently, apply modern science to marry the past and the present, and to give birth to the future. The reliance of modern medicine on drugs is the worst way to cure illness or gain health. The best way is to solve the problem at its root. Ancient China did not have our modern medical chemistry, and had to develop other ways to adjust the body's Water and Fire. We could learn much from them. For example, many arthritis patients today rely on medicine to reduce pain. While this may offer temporary relief from pain, it does not cure the problem. When the medicine is gone, the pain resumes. Chinese medical Qigong cures arthritis by rebuilding the strength of the joints. Patients increase Qi circulation with slow, easy exercises, and massage to strengthen the joints. These practices readjust the Yin and Yang balance, allowing the body to repair the damage and increase the strength of the joints. This approach addresses the root of the problem.

Nevertheless, many modern medical practices conform to Kan and Li theory. Fever is treated by applying medicine and ice cubes to reduce the temperature. Ice cubes are used to reduce swelling caused by injuries. Whether you follow ancient or modern medicine, the basic theory of healing remains the same, namely adjustment of Kan and Li. Medical chemistry has brought us much that is marvelous, but also many problems.

The key is understanding the circulation of Qi, or bioelectricity, in the body. Regulating it strengthens the body and maintains health, allowing doctors to correct irregular Qi even before the appearance of physical symptoms, and increasing the quality and duration of life.

## The Keys to Kan and Li Adjustment

Here we discuss how Kan and Li relate to your breathing, mind and spirit, and the keys to regulating them in Qigong practice. Combining them, we construct a secret key which leads to the Qigong treasure.

**Kan and Li of Breathing.** In Qigong, breathing is considered a strategy to lead the Qi. Directing your breath, you may lead Qi to the skin or marrow. Breathing slowly can calm the Qi flow, while rapid breathing can invigorate it. *When you are excited, your body is Yang, and you exhale longer than you inhale. This leads Qi to the skin, where excess Qi dissipates through sweat. When you are sad your body is Yin, and you inhale longer than you exhale. This preserves Qi by leading it inward, and you feel cold.* Through breathing you adjust the body's Yin and Yang, so breathing has Kan and Li.

Inhaling is a Water (Kan) activity, because you lead Qi inward to store it in the bone marrow. This reduces Guardian Qi (Wei Qi, 衛氣) and the Qi in the muscles and tendons, calming the body's Yang. Exhaling is a Fire (Li) activity because it brings Qi out to the muscles, tendons and skin to energize them, making the body more Yang, and enhancing Guardian Qi. When the body is more Yang than its surroundings, its Qi is dissipated.

Yin and Yang should be balanced so your body functions harmoniously. The trick is using breathing strategies. Usually inhalation and exhalation should be equal. When you are excited your body is too Yang, so you may inhale longer and deeper to calm your mind and lead Qi in, to make it more Yin.

Exhalation leads Qi to the skin and to the five extremities (the crown, the two Laogong (P-8, 勞宮) cavities at the center of the palms, and the two Yongquan (K-1, 湧泉) cavities near the centers of the soles), to exchange with your surroundings. Inhalation leads Qi deep inside your body to reach the internal organs and marrow. Table 1-1 summarizes how different breathing strategies affect Yin and Yang in their various manifestations.

**Kan and Li of the Mind.** According to Chinese tradition, one has two minds, Xin (心) and Yi (意). Xin means heart, the mind generated by emotional disturbance, or emotional mind. The Chinese word Yi comprises three characters. The top one means establish (Li, 立), the middle one means speaking (Yue, 曰), and the bottom one means heart (Xin, 心). That means the emotional mind is under control as you establish communication with your heart. Yi can be translated as wisdom mind. Xin makes you excited and disturbs your emotions, making your body Yang, so it is considered Li. Yi makes you calm, peaceful and able to think clearly (Yin), so it is considered Kan.

In Qigong training, the mind is the general who directs the battle, decides on fighting strategy (breathing), and directs the movement of the soldiers (Qi). As a general,

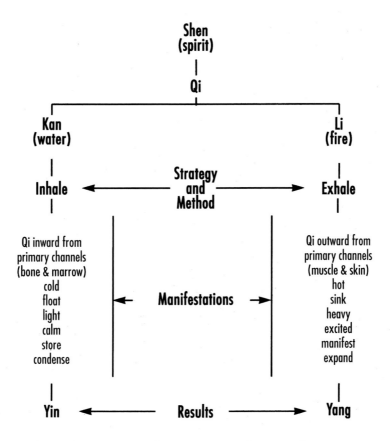

Table 1-1. The Effects of Breathing on the Body's Yin and Yang in their Various Manifestations

you control your Xin (emotional mind) and use your Yi (wisdom mind) to judge the situation and decide on the proper strategy.

In Qigong, your Yi dominates the situation and generates an idea. This idea generates and executes the strategy (breathing), and is the force moving the Qi. When your mind is excited and energized, the strategy (breathing) is more offensive (emphasizing exhalation) and Qi circulation is more vigorous and expansive. This aggressive mind is considered a Fire mind, making your body more Yang. When the strategy is more defensive (emphasizing inhalation), Qi circulation will be calmer and more condensed. A calm or depressed mind is a Water mind, since it makes your body more Yin.

The mind's Kan and Li are more important than breathing, since the mind determines the strategy. Regulating mind and breathing are the two basic techniques for controlling your body's Yin and Yang. Regulating mind and breathing cannot be separated. When the mind is regulated, the breathing can be too, and when breathing is regulated, the mind enters a deeper level of calm.

**Kan and Li of the Shen.** We now consider the most decisive element in winning a battle, the Shen (Spirit). Shen is the morale of the general's officers and soldiers. There are many cases throughout history of armies winning battles against great odds because the morale of their soldiers was high.

It is the same in Qigong training, where the Shen determines how successful your Qigong practice will be. Your Yi, the general who makes the strategy, must be concerned with raising up the fighting morale (Shen) of the soldiers (Qi). When morale is high the soldiers are led efficiently and strategy is executed effectively.

Using Yi to raise Shen is the primary key to successful Qigong training. Shen is the headquarters which governs Qi, together with the Yi. Yi and Shen are closely related and cannot be separated.

When Yi is energized, Shen is also raised. You want to raise up your Shen but not get it excited. When Shen is raised, strategy is carried out effectively, but if Shen is excited, the body becomes too Yang, which is not desirable in Qigong practice. When you practice Qigong, you want to keep your Shen high at all times, to govern the strategy and the Qi. This enables you to regulate Kan and Li.

Shen is the control tower which adjusts Kan and Li, but does not have Kan and Li itself. Some practitioners consider raised Shen to be Li (Fire) and calm Shen to be Kan (Water).

Now, let us draw a few important conclusions from this discussion:

- Kan (Water) and Li (Fire) are not Yin and Yang. Kan and Li are methods which regulate Yin or Yang.

- Qi itself is only a form of energy and does not have Kan and Li. When Qi is excessive or deficient, it can make the body too Yang or too Yin.

- When you adjust Kan and Li in the body, the mind is the first concern. The mind can be Kan or Li. It determines the strategy (breathing) for withdrawing Qi (Kan) or expanding it (Li).

- Breathing has Kan and Li. Inhaling is Kan as it makes the body more Yin, while exhaling, which makes the body more Yang, is Li.

- Shen does not have Kan and Li. Shen is the key to making the adjustment of Kan and Li effective.

### The Keys to Adjusting Kan and Li

The keys to Kan and Li adjustment are mentioned repeatedly in the ancient documents. The first key is that Shen and Breathing mutually rely on each other. The second key is that Shen and Qi mutually combine.

**Shen and Breathing Mutually Dependent (Shen Xi Xiang Yi,** 神息相依**).** Breathing is the strategy which directs Qi in various ways, controlling and adjusting Kan and Li, which in turn control the body's Yin and Yang. Shen is the controlling influence which makes strategy work most efficiently. Shen governs strategy directly, and controls Kan and Li and the body's Yin and Yang indirectly. The success of your Kan and Li adjustment depends upon your Shen.

When Shen matches respiration, it leads Qi directly to condense and expand in the most efficient way. Shen must match the breathing for it to be raised up or calmed down, and the breathing must rely on Shen to make the strategy work. It seems Shen and breathing are dependent on each other and cannot be separated. This training is called Shen Xi Xiang Yi, which means Shen and breathing depend on each other. When Shen and breathing match each other, it is called Shen Xi (神息) or spirit breathing, because it seems your Shen is actually doing the breathing.

Shen Xi Xiang Yi is a technique in which, when Shen and breathing are united, Shen controls the Qi directly.

**Shen and Qi Mutually Combine (Shen Qi Xiang He,** 神氣相合**).** When Shen and breathing match each other as one, the Qi is led directly, so Shen and Qi become one. This is called Shen Qi Xiang He, which means Shen and Qi mutually harmonized. Shen governs Qi directly and efficiently. Harmony of Shen and Qi is the result of Shen and breathing being mutually dependent.

Da Mo believed that to have a long and peaceful life, Shen and Qi must coordinate and harmonize with each other. He said, "If one does not keep mother (Qi) and son (Shen) together, though Qi breathes internally, Shen is labored and craves the external, so Shen is always debauched and dirty and thus not clear. If Shen is not clear, original harmonious Qi will disperse gradually, and they cannot be kept together."[7] The spirit is very important, and regulating Shen is one of the highest levels of Qigong practice. To reach a high level of harmony, first regulate your emotional mind, which is hard to achieve in secular society.

## 1-5. QIGONG AND HEALTH 氣功與健康

When we discuss the relationship between Qigong practice and health, we should first define health. There are two aspects of health, the Yang side of physical health which can be seen, and the Yin side of mental health which can only be felt. More than half of today's sickness is caused by mental problems such as depression, stress, and mental fatigue. There are several reasons:

1. Due to our changing social structure, the pressure of living in today's society is greater than ever. Our modern lifestyle only started in the 20th century. Before then, industry did not heavily dominate the social structure, and many people lived as farmers. The struggle of living in a society

demanding more money and material enjoyment dominates our thinking and generates great pressure. In a few short decades, we have become slaves to money. We have lost the original lifestyle which connected us with nature and spiritual feeling. We are facing a revolution which is changing the old life style to the new one, generating many mental problems.

2. Medical science has advanced to a high level and controls most common illnesses, but is still limited to the Yang side of understanding. It lacks interest in and knowledge of the bioenergetic aspect of body, mind, and spirit. Because of this, we miss half of human science, and are unable to solve several problems and illnesses. We cannot effectively cure problems such as cancer and aids. Also, lacking understanding of our mental and spiritual center, we cannot solve mental illness. Many scientists believe that we understand less than 12% of the function of the brain.

3. Due to the decline of religious belief, seculars have lost their guide in understanding the meaning of life. This is because knowledge of the general public has increased, and religious dogma is questioned more seriously than ever. Religious authorities cannot offer an educational program which is persuasive to the new open-minded generation. Most churches still preach with methods used for thousands of years. This is very unfortunate since many people have become lost in today's new society. Many Westerners cannot find new meaning in their lives from traditional religion, so turn to Eastern religions and philosophy, hoping to find answers and peace.

4. Internal cultivation, such as meditation, has been largely ignored. Many people build up a facade in order to hide their true selves from others around them. We lie, and hide our fears and guilty feelings deep in our subconscious mind. Going to confession (Western way), or removing our mask through meditation (Eastern way), were traditional ways of releasing pent-up emotions and balancing our feelings. Today, many people have lost these two most powerful methods of relieving mental imbalance induced by suppressed emotions and feelings of guilt.

Our mental condition is closely related to our health. Many diseases are caused by mental imbalance, which results in the disharmonious Qi circulation in the body. *To have good health, you need a strong body but also a healthy mind.* Qigong for healing and for maintaining health, is based on this concept.

To maintain physical strength, Qigong exercises which condition the muscles, tendons, ligaments and bones were developed. Before Da Mo (483 to 536 A.D., 達磨), many exercises were developed by doctors to regulate sickness and facilitate healing. Da Mo brought a different concept as recorded in the *Muscle/Tendon Changing Classic*

(*Yi Jin Jing*, 易筋經). Since then, based on this training, countless Wai Dan Qigong styles were created.

Meditation was developed by different schools to regulate the mind into peace and harmony. Meditation not only brings a peaceful mind, but also builds up abundant Qi to circulate in the body, through the Qi channels and vessels.

Modern medical science has improved health and extended lives significantly. But today's scientific achievement is still in its infancy. Many new problems have arisen due to the new social structure and environment. The pressure generated in today's society has caused many mental problems, and many new diseases have emerged. For example, the increase of breast cancer is caused by going against the course of nature. Even fifty years ago, many women could expect to bear at least ten children. There was a constant Qi exchange between mothers and babies. Today we control birth and most women will not bear more than three babies in their lifetime. Qi is trapped in the breast area and generates cancer cells. We should understand one important thing. The body we have now has developed through millions of years of evolution. It is impossible for us to fit into the new lifestyle created only in the last few decades.

Similarly, lower back pain is caused by lack of exercise. Physical labor was the traditional way of maintaining strength and health, but now machines have replaced most of it, and naturally, the torso degenerates rapidly. Again, common knee problems are generated by lack of walking, which was required in society until fifty years ago. Automobile transport has caused degeneration of our knees.

Other than that, human sperm production has decreased significantly over the last two decades, caused by our new lifestyle.[8] Traditionally, people went to bed shortly after sunset and woke up at dawn. Our bodies adapted to nature over millions of years. In our new lifestyle we often do not go to bed before midnight. According to Qigong theory, the Qi in our bodies manifests as physical action during daytime. Qi nourishes our brain and sexual organs through the spinal cord at night. If we go to sleep by 9 P.M., it takes two to three hours of natural breathing during sleep to lead Qi from the surface to nourish deep inside. By midnight it is ready to nourish the brain and sexual organs. Brain energy is recharged, and sperm and sexual hormones are produced. The modern lifestyle has introduced a new time schedule which precludes the natural production of hormones. Naturally, production of sperm has decreased over the last two decades. If it continues in this way, the problem will be even more significant and serious.

Countless other problems have been generated by new products which cause material and energetic pollution. Through lack of understanding of human energy and its vulnerability to this pollution, we live in a world at great risk of physical and mental imbalance. To solve these problems, we must first achieve awareness before we can awaken others. Profound and significant study and research needs to be conducted and acted upon.

## 1-6. QIGONG AND LONGEVITY 氣功與長壽

To many seculars, longevity means long life, without regard to health or the meaning of life. Most of the people today want to live long physically even though they are in pain mentally. Longevity is important to them, not happiness.

Others search for the meaning of life to make longevity more meaningful. They look for a way to extend physical life and at the same time keep mental peace in harmony with the physical body. For them, Qigong for longevity was developed.

To religious Daoists, longevity is considered very important and crucial to reaching enlightenment. They believe it takes many lifetimes to reach enlightenment to be reunited with the Dao. They believe, as do the Buddhists, that the physical body is only born for the spirit to reside in temporarily for further spiritual cultivation. The physical body has no further purpose or meaning. To Buddhists, the physical body is unimportant and they often ignore its condition, emphasizing only the cultivation of the mind and the spirit. But Daoists believe that if you live longer in each lifetime, you will have more time for spiritual cultivation, and need not reincarnate too many times before reaching enlightenment. So they take good care of the physical body. So to some religious people, the meaning of longevity is to provide a longer time for spiritual cultivation.

Then, what are the keys or requirements to reach longevity? How do we reach this goal? These questions have been searched in every human generations. Now let us summarize some key points of longevity from the past human experience.

**Key points:**

1. **The balance and harmony of the Qi body (Yin) with the physical body (Yang).** When there is balance and harmony of Yin and Yang, excess energy is minimized. Health is maintained and longevity reached through a healthy lifestyle, and by keeping Yin and Yang in balance through Qigong training.

2. **Follow the way of the Dao,** adjusting your body to fit in with natural cycles such as the time of day and the change of the seasons. Avoid artificial material or energetic pollution.

3. **Understand the physical body and Qi body scientifically.** Through this we can find a way to slow down the aging process, and the key to attaining spiritual enlightenment.

These concepts were also discussed in medical Qigong society. One of the oldest medical classics, *Yellow Emperor's Inner Classic: Simple Questions* (黃帝內經 · 素問) said, "The ancient people who knew the Dao, modeled themselves after Yin and Yang, matched the ways of nature, controlled their eating and drinking, lived with regularity, did not labor without knowing their limit, and so were able keep the shape (body) and the Shen (spirit) together. Therefore, they end their heaven years (the age granted by heaven) completely and pass hundred years, then gone."[9] For a healthy body, concern yourself with the harmony of Yin and Yang and follow the Natural Way. Only then can you reach longevity.

Let us summarize how we reach these goals with Qigong.

## Physical Body:

1. **Keep the bone marrow clean.** The majority of blood cells are produced by the bone marrow. Once we reach thirty, the bone marrow starts to degenerate rapidly and quality and quantity of blood production decreases. Blood cells carry nutrients, oxygen, and the Qi required to replace old cells with new ones. Without enough healthy blood cells, cell replacement stagnates and degeneration of the body sets in.

   Degeneration of bone marrow results from deficiency of Qi. Without abundant Qi, blood production from bone marrow is slow and deficient. Bone marrow washing Qigong teaches how to lead Qi to the bone marrow, as described in the book, *Qigong—The Secret of Youth.*

2. **Maintain health of the body, especially the torso.** For health and longevity, we need physical and mental health. Without a strong healthy body, even though you have abundant energy, you still cannot manifest this energy into physical form.

   A healthy physical body depends on the condition of your torso, especially the spine. Through the spinal cord our brain controls the whole body. Any spinal problem disturbs the smooth control by your brain. Along the spine there are two Qi vessels, one being the spinal cord (Thrusting Vessel, 衝脈) and the other outside spine, under the skin (Governing Vessel, 督脈). They distribute Qi to the central nervous system and out to the limbs. If your spine is healthy, Qi circulation will not be stagnant. Most blood cells are produced in the spinal marrow and the pelvis. When Qi circulates abundantly, degeneration of bone marrow is slowed, and production of healthy blood cells maintained.

3. **Provide the best quality food and air for cell replacement.** Approximately one trillion cells in our bodies die each day. To replace them, we must provide good quality food and air, else the new cells will be unhealthy and we will age faster. Deep breathing is one of the main keys to keeping cells healthy.

4. **Boost hormone production in the body.** Hormones (Original Essence) act as catalysts to expedite a smooth metabolism. When hormone production slows down, cell replacement does too, and our bodies degenerate faster.

## Qi and the Mind:

1. **Accumulate Qi at the Real Lower Dan Tian, which produces elixir Qi and also stores it.** From this energy center, Qi is distributed throughout the body. The Lower Dan Tian has a similar structure to the brain, with the capacity for memory.[10,11] They are connected through the spinal cord and the central nervous system, where electric conductivity is highest and resistance is lowest. Though there are two brains, their function can be considered as one. The lower brain can store bioelectricity. When the mind generates an idea (EMF, electromotive force), Qi is led to the body for action. When the Qi stored at the Real Lower Dan Tian is abundant, the life force is strong; otherwise we are weak and die young. We discuss this subject in more detail in Chapter 2.

2. **Accumulate Qi in the Eight Vessels.** With an abundant level of Qi in the Lower Dan Tian, distribute it to the Eight Vessels, or Qi reservoirs, and regulate it in the Twelve Primary Qi Channels, or Qi rivers. Small circulation meditation is one of the most important ways to increase Qi and circulate it. For more information on channels and vessels, refer to section 2-2.

3. **Circulate Qi smoothly in the Twelve Primary Qi Channels.** Only when Qi is distributed everywhere smoothly can the cells in the body obtain proper Qi nourishment and our life force be strong. To reach this goal, balance exercise (Yang) with relaxation (Yin).

4. **Maintain an emotionally neutral state.** To Chinese scholar Qigong, regulating the emotional mind is most important. Aging is caused by imbalance of Qi distributed in the body, caused in part by emotional disturbance. Set yourself free from emotional bondage to live peacefully and harmoniously.

5. **Raise up the spirit of vitality.** When your spirit is high, your life force is strong. To raise up the spirit of vitality, having stored abundant Qi at the Real Lower Dan Tian, lead it up to the brain to nourish the spirit. This raises the spirit up and leads to enlightenment.

6. **Understand the meaning of life.** Analyze your life and try to understand its meaning. Without understanding, you are rudderless and confused, leading to depression and low spirits. When you have a goal in life, your thinking and activities are meaningful.

## Possible Modern Methods for Longevity

This summarizes how Qigong relates to longevity. If we borrow the knowledge and experience of the past, we may find a modern, scientific path to longevity. Here are a few suggestions for today's medical scientists.

*Physically:*

1. **Investigate the human body electric.** Study the electric properties of the body to understand its electric circuitry. This will pinpoint Qi imbalances and stagnation, and enable external electromagnetic fields to correct them. Then we could prevent sickness before it manifests. In just fifty years, every household will have a scanner to scan the body's energetic condition and correct it. We will be able to preserve physical strength significantly.

2. **Maintain proper hormone level.** Artificial hormones can maintain our requirements. Many people already extend their lives with artificial human growth hormone.[12-15]

3. **Maintain blood production in the bone marrow.** Abundant Qi supply to the marrow is necessary. In the future we will clean the bone marrow using external electromagnetic intervention. We will have plenty of healthy blood cells to carry oxygen, Qi, and nutrients everywhere for cell replacement.

4. **Slow down the cell aging process.** Invent a machine or energy chamber to slow down the aging process of the cells, to extend life.

5. **Increase Qi storage in the Real Lower Dan Tian.** In the future, we may find a mechanical way to enhance Qi storage in the Real Lower Dan Tian; First to condition the battery itself, and then charge it externally.

*Mentally:*

1. **Humbly learn from ancient experiences which offer guidelines for the future.** They have shown what is possible and where the problem may be. If our scientific dignity ignores this accumulated experience, we may repeat their mistakes. One who is wise remembers both past successes and failures.

2. **Make life meaningful.** Many people have no meaning in their lives, making them depressed and unhealthy. To direct them we must establish non-religious spiritual centers, where they can meditate and recognize the spiritual role of their existence. Through meditation, the mind can be clear and peaceful, providing an environment for self-recognition. This is the first step to self-understanding and the path of spiritual enlightenment, and their minds will direct them to the right path in life.

3. **Raise up the spirit of vitality.** When one recognizes oneself, one will see how to fit into this society, and raise up the spirit of vitality. Using scientific methods to activate more brain cells and open the third eye, we may be able to shorten the path to enlightenment. Our spirit of vitality will be high, the most important invisible factor in longevity.

## Longevity and Spiritual Cultivation

According to Buddhism, one may need hundreds or even thousands of lifetimes to cultivate the spirit, and see the true nature of reality, to reach enlightenment. In each life, one might improve only a little. Before one is twenty years old, one starts to feel one's spiritual identity, the first step to spiritual recognition. Throughout life one collects information and experience, filters them, and finally understands their meaning. The spirit learns new ideas. If you die in your twenties you have only a few years for cultivation. The best time for spiritual cultivation is from the age of thirty, when one has a few advantages for spiritual cultivation:

1. **Understanding the world better.** By this age, one has been educated and has experienced the world. One may adjust their circumstances and become serious about spiritual life.

2. **Better financial situation.** With financial security, the mind is calmer, and not trapped in the circle of daily survival, so it can focus more on the spiritual than the material side.

3. **Better mental preparation.** By thirty, one is more mature both mentally and spiritually, and more ready for spiritual cultivation.

4. **A more logical mind.** By age thirty, one's knowledge and judgment have developed logical thinking, which is crucial for correct spiritual development. Spiritual cultivation guided by imagination can only lead you away from the true nature of reality, and into deeper bondage of emotional confusion.

The longer you live, the more time for cultivation and development of your spiritual understanding to a higher level. If you die young, you have only a short time for cultivation, and progress will be limited in this lifetime.

## 1-7. QIGONG AND SPIRITUAL ENLIGHTENMENT 氣功與神通

Even though both the Western and Eastern cultures have experienced and documented the existence of the spirit in the past, neither has been able to explain it clearly and satisfactorily. What, then, is the spirit? How do we define it? Since I am more familiar with Chinese concepts from the Buddhist and Daoist point of view, I will focus on their concept and understanding.

The ancient Chinese concept originated with *The Book of Change* (*Yi Jing*, 易經), believing there are two poles or dimensions coexisting in space. One is called Yin space (Yin Jian, 陰間) and the other Yang space (Yang Jian, 陽間). When these two poles or spaces coexist, Yin and Yang energy interact and exchange, from which process life is derived. The first derivation is spiritual life, and from this physical life is formed. Once physical lives are generated, spiritual lives can reside in them, uniting the Yin spiritual body and Yang physical body. The universe is alive, bearing both spiritual and physical existence at the same time. Every life formed or generated from this Yin-Yang space follows the patterns of nature and is a small universe within itself. It is said, "The universe is a large heaven and earth, man is a small heaven and earth."[16] Each life, even insects and animals, has its own heaven and earth.

In space, there are millions of universes, and within each there are millions of galaxies. Within each galaxy there are countless solar systems. Scientists postulate that our universe may be shaped like an egg with two poles (Figure 1-4).[17] It is believed that life derives from the energy interaction of these two poles.

We also have two poles in our bodies to sustain our lives. Since ancient times the Chinese have known the body has two poles, one called the Real Lower Dan Tian, at the the center of gravity, and the other called the Upper Dan Tian, in the brain where the spirit resides. These two poles are related to each other. When energy in the Lower Dan Tian is abundant, the spirit in the Upper Dan Tian will be high. Since ancient times Daoists have searched for ways of building up abundant Qi in the Real Lower Dan Tian. Today's science now recognizes that we have two brains, one in the head and the other in our gut.[10,11] This conforms to ancient experience.

What then is the spirit? The spirit is the true nature, or Dao (Taiji), of this universe. It is the essential energy from which lives are derived. It is the origin of all living beings. Dao may be what is called God in Western society. Like the universe, we also have this spirit within us.

Our Original Spirit, before birth, is pure and truthful. But after birth, our environment conditions us and we construct a conscious mind. We enter the bondage of emotional mud, and experience pain and happiness in life.

Daoists and Buddhists believe that to promote the spirit to a higher level, we must be born in physical form and borrow the body's sense organs to collect information about nature. This process generates confusion, but after filtering information through the wisdom mind, we gradually understand nature. To stimulate the spirit to learn and become aware, we lie, cheat, commit mistakes, experience pleasure and pain, and stay trapped in emotional bondage. Slowly and gradually, through emotional stimulation, we learn to be smart and truthful, and to keep a neutral mind. This is the path of returning our spirit to the neutral state, of unification with the natural spirit; since nature does not have this emotional bondage. You may reach the level of unification of heaven and man (Tian Ren He Yi, 天人合一), and will not reincarnate again, having gained eternal spiritual life.

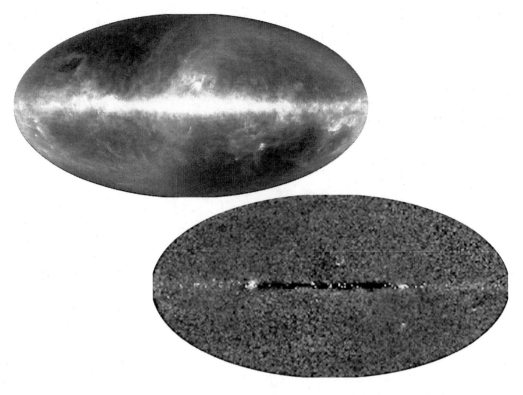

Figure 1-4. A Universe May be Shaped Like an Egg with Two Poles

By searching for the origin of the spirit, we may comprehend the meaning of spirit. In the same way, material scientists look for the most basic structure of matter, in order to unravel the mysteries of material science.

From more than two thousand years of experience in spiritual cultivation, Daoists and Buddhists discovered the way to achieve this unification of the human spirit with the universal spirit. The first step is to recognize our spiritual body and understand it, by first understanding the energetic body, which is associated with the spirit. In the past, Qi could only be felt, but now through bioelectric research it can be tested and measured, rather than regarded as a mysterious and obscure concept.

To unify our spirit with the natural spirit, we must also open the third eye (Upper Dan Tian or Tian Yan, 上丹田、天眼) at the lower center of the forehead. This opens the spiritual mind to be clear and see the true nature of reality, and to be able to access the natural spirit without obstacle. This step is called spiritual enlightenment.

To open this third eye, one first accumulates abundant Qi in the Real Lower Dan Tian. Only then does one have enough energy to be led up through the spinal cord to the brain, to activate and energize it to a high level of resonance. Since spirit resides in the brain, it can likewise be raised to a higher level. When more brain cells are activated, a halo will be seen. Years of Qi cultivation focus energy at the front of the brain, so the third eye can open. For more about this, refer to *Qigong—The Secret of Youth,* and also *Qigong Meditation—Embryonic Breathing.*

**Convert the essence and change it into Qi (Lian Jing Hua Qi, 練精化氣**. One absorbs healthy food and air (post-birth essence) and converts it into Qi, while generating hormone (pre-birth essence) production from your glands with Qigong. With higher hormone levels, you can convert food essence into Qi more efficiently. Once abundant Qi is converted, you store it in the Real Lower Dan Tian, which is considered the formation of the Holy Embryo (Sheng Tai, 聖胎). After this comes ten months carrying the baby (Shi Yue Hui Tai, 十月懷胎).

**Nourish the spirit with Qi (Lian Qi Hua Shen, 練氣化神).** Next you lead Qi up to the brain to nourish the brain cells, and raise up the spirit of vitality. You also lead Qi to the front of brain through the pituitary and pineal glands. This promotes smooth production of growth hormones and melatonin, the keys to longevity.

After many years, or many lifetimes, of meditation, you may finally open the third eye, allowing your spirit to leave your body while you are still alive. Your mind experiences gradual unification with the natural spirit, which it contacts directly. In Daoist cultivation, this is the birth of the holy baby embryo, as the spirit achieves enlightenment.

After the holy spirit baby is born, it must at first stay near your body to survive. Gradually it grows stronger. This step is called three years of nursing (San Nian Bu Ru, 三年哺乳).

**Refine the spirit and return it to nothingness (Lian Shen Fan Xu, 練神返虛).** To achieve unification with the natural spirit, you must completely free yourself from emotional bondage and remain neutral, which may take a long time. The spirit baby continues to grow stronger until it is mature and able to survive independently from you. It is said to take at least nine years of effort to do so. To keep your spiritual mind neutral, traditionally one must meditate facing the wall within a cave, which is called "nine years of facing the wall" (Jiu Nian Mian Bi, 九年面壁). Then, the spirit can have independent life without needing the physical body.

The independent spirit stays peacefully in the Yin space (Yin Jian, 陰間) for some time without emotional disturbance. This is spiritual sleep, the state of Wuji (無極, no extremity).

**Crush the nothingness (Fen Sui Xu Kong, 粉碎虛空).** The spirit can decide to remain in the neutral state of Wuji, but may want to reincarnate in physical form to accept the new challenge. The spirit faces a new environment to train it to a higher level. This is to "crush the emptiness" (Wuji state). After repeated cultivation, finally your spirit is united forever with the natural spirit.

This is only a brief summary of spiritual cultivation training. We will explain it in detail in later chapters, and in future publications on the topics of Grand Circulation and Spiritual Enlightenment Meditation.

## 1-8. BUDDHIST AND DAOIST QIGONG CONCEPTS 佛家與道家之氣功概念

Because it was kept so secret, religious Qigong did not become as popular as other categories in China before the Qing Dynasty (1644-1912 A.D., 清朝). Only in the 20th century were the secrets gradually revealed to the public, and religious Qigong became popular in China. Religious Qigong is mostly Daoist and Buddhist, and its main purpose is to assist the attainment of enlightenment, or what Buddhists refer to as Buddhahood.

### Buddhist Qigong

Three main schools of Buddhist Qigong developed in Asia during the last two thousand years: Indian, Chinese, and Tibetan. Buddhism was created in India by an Indian prince named Gautama between 558 B.C. and 478 B.C. Therefore, Indian Buddhist Qigong has the longest history. Buddhism was imported into China during the Eastern Han Dynasty (58 A.D., 東漢), and Chinese Buddhists gradually learned its methods of spiritual cultivation. Their practice was influenced by traditional Chinese scholar and medical Qigong, which had been developing for about two thousand years. What resulted was a unique system of training different from its antecedents.

According to the fragmentary records available, only the philosophy and doctrines of Buddhism were passed down to the Chinese during the first few centuries following its adoption. The actual methods of cultivation and Qigong training were not known. There are several reasons for this:

1. Because of the difficulty of transport and communication at that time, the transfer of Buddhist documents from India to China was limited. Although a few Indian priests were invited to China to preach, problems remained.

2. Even if the documents had been transferred, because of the profound theory and philosophy of Buddhism, very few people were qualified to really translate them accurately from Sanskrit to Chinese. This problem was exacerbated by the different cultural backgrounds. Even today, different cultural backgrounds are always the main problem in translating accurately from one language to another.

3. The main reason was probably that most of the actual training methods need to be taught and guided personally by an experienced master. Only a limited amount can be learned from documents. This problem was compounded by the tradition of passing information secretly from master to disciples.

The process was very slow and painful, especially with regard to the actual training methods. For several centuries it was believed that as long as you purified your mind and sincerely strove for Buddhahood, sooner or later you would succeed. This situation was not improved until Da Mo wrote the *Muscle/Tendon Changing and Marrow/Brain Washing Classics* (*Yi Jin Jing, Xi Sui Jing*, 易筋經、洗髓經). Then at last there was a firm direction in the training to reach Buddhahood.

Before Da Mo, Chinese Buddhist Qigong training was very similar to Chinese Scholar Qigong. The main difference was that while Scholar Qigong aimed at maintaining health, Buddhist Qigong aimed at becoming a Buddha. Meditation is a necessary process in training a priest to stay emotionally neutral. Buddhism believes all suffering is caused by the seven passions and six desires (Qi Qing Liu Yu, 七情六慾). The seven passions are happiness (Xi, 喜), anger (Nu, 怒), sorrow (Ai, 哀), joy (Le, 樂), love (Ai, 愛), hate (Hen, 恨), and desire (Yu, 慾). The six desires are the six sensory pleasures derived from the eyes, ears, nose, tongue, body, and mind. Buddhists also cultivate within themselves a neutral state separated from the four emptinesses of earth, water, fire, and wind (Si Da Jie Kong, 四大皆空). They believe that this training enables them to keep the spirit independent so it can escape from the recurring cycle of reincarnation, known as "the Wheel of Life and Death."

Tibetan Buddhism has always been kept secret and isolated from the outside world. Because of this, it is very difficult to determine precisely when Tibetan Buddhism was established. Because Tibet is near India, it is reasonable to assume that Tibetan Qigong training has had more influence from India than Chinese Qigong has. However, over thousands of years of study and research, the Tibetans established their own unique style of Qigong meditation. Tibetan priests are called Lamas (La Ma, 喇嘛), and many of them also learned martial arts. Because of the different cultural background, not only are the Lamas' meditation techniques different from those of the Chinese or Indian Buddhists, but so are their martial techniques. Tibetan Qigong meditation and martial arts were kept secret from the outside world, being called Mi Zong (秘宗) which means "secret style". Because of this, and because of the different language, there are only very limited documents available in Chinese. Tibetan Qigong and martial arts did not spread into Chinese society until almost the Qing Dynasty, but since then they have become popular.

## Daoist Qigong

Like Buddhists, Daoists believe in building up the spirit (Shen) so that it is independent and strong, to escape from the cycle of reincarnation. When a Daoist reaches this stage of enlightenment, it is said he has attained eternal life.

Daoist monks found that to enhance their spirit, they had to cultivate Qi which was converted from their Jing (Essence). Again, the Daoist Qigong training process is: 1. To convert the Jing (精, Essence) into Qi (Lian Jing Hua Qi, 練精化氣, 2. To nourish the Shen (Spirit, 神) with Qi (Lian Qi Hua Shen, 練氣化神), 3. To refine the Shen and return it to nothingness (Lian Shen Fan Xu, 練神返虛) and 4. To crush the nothingness (Fen Sui Xu Kong, 粉碎虛空).

The first step involves firming and strengthening the Jing (Gu Jing, 固精), converting it into Qi through meditation or other methods. This Qi is then led to the top of the head to nourish the brain and raise up the Shen. When a Daoist has reached this stage, it is called "the three flowers meet at the top" (San Hua Ju Ding, 三花聚頂). The three flowers are Jing (精), Qi (氣), and Shen (神). This stage achieves the necessary health and longevity for continued cultivation. Finally, the Daoist starts training to reach enlightenment. The biggest obstacle is emotional, affecting thought and upsetting spiritual balance. This is why Daoists retreat to the mountains, away from other people and distractions. Usually they also abstain from eating meat, feeling that is muddies thinking and intensifies the emotions, leading the spirit away from self-cultivation.

An important part of this training is Yi Jin Jing and Xi Sui Jing Qigong. Yi Jin Jing Qigong builds up abundant Qi in the Lower Dan Tian and strengthens the body. Xi Sui Jing Qigong leads Qi to the brain to raise up the spirit, and keeps Qi circulating in the marrow so it stays clean and healthy. Your marrow produces most of your blood cells, which bring nourishment to the whole body, and removes waste products. When your blood is healthy, your whole body is well-nourished and you can resist disease effectively. When the marrow is clean and fresh, it manufactures plenty of healthy blood cells which do their job efficiently. Your whole body stays healthy, and degeneration is slowed significantly.

Although the theory is simple, the training is very difficult. One accumulates Qi at the Real Lower Dan Tian and fills up your eight Qi vessels, then leads it into the bone to wash the marrow. Except for some Daoist monks, there are very few people who have lived more than 120 years, because the training is so arduous. You need a pure mind and a simple lifestyle to enable you to concentrate entirely on the training.

Many Daoist Qigong styles are based on the theory of cultivating both the spirit and the physical body. It is said, "Talking about human nature (spirit) and life, cultivate them both. Place the lead (Pb, Yin) and mercury (Hg, Yang) together. This secret is hard to comprehend. Cultivate human nature to refine self-being while cultivating life to return the essence (convert essence into Qi). Xin is the house of the spirit while the body is the residence of the Qi. Life is the Qi. Those who cultivate human nature blend the body and the Xin as a family. Jing, Qi, and spirit must combine into one unit. Then the cultivation of life can be approached."[18] This emphasizes that to reach enlightenment, you must cultivate both body and spirit. The key is to harmonize Yin and Yang. Yin is the spiritual body while Yang is the physical body. Only when they are harmonious and the three treasures (essence, Qi, and spirit) have reached the brain, can you reach enlightenment.

In Daoism, there are generally three ways of training: Golden Elixir Large Way (Jin Dan Da Dao, 金丹大道), Double Cultivation (Shuang Xiu, 雙修), and Herb Picking Outside the Dao (Dao Wai Cai Yao, 道外採藥).

Golden Elixir Large Way teaches training Qigong within yourself, to find the elixir of longevity and enlightenment within your own body.

In the second approach, Double Cultivation, a partner is used to balance one's Qi more quickly. Most people's Qi is not entirely balanced. Some are too positive, others too negative, and individual channels also are positive or negative. If you exchange Qi with a partner, you can speed your training. Double Cultivation has two meanings: one is to cultivate Qi with a partner, and the other means cultivation of both one's human nature and the physical body.

The third way, Herb Picking Outside of the Dao, uses herbs to accelerate and regulate cultivation. Herbs can be plants such as ginseng (Ren Sen, 人蔘), or animal products such as musk from the musk-deer. To many Daoists, the word "herbs" can also mean the Qi which can be obtained from sexual practices.

According to the training methods used, Daoist Qigong can again be divided into two major schools: Peaceful Cultivation Style (Qing Xiu Pai, 清修派), and Plant and Graft Style (Zai Jie Pai, 栽接派). This division was especially clear after the Song and Yuan Dynasties (960-1368 A.D., 宋、元朝). The meditation and methods of Peaceful Cultivation Style are similar to those of Buddhists. They believe the only way to reach enlightenment is Golden Elixir Large Way, according to which one builds up the elixir within the body. Using a partner for cultivation is considered immoral, and causes emotional problems which may significantly affect cultivation.

However, the Plant and Graft Style claims that their approach of using Double Cultivation and Herb Picking Outside of the Dao, in addition to Golden Elixir Large Way, makes the cultivation faster and more practical. For this reason, Daoist Qigong training is also commonly called Dan Ding Dao Gong (丹鼎道功) which means the Dao Training in the Elixir Crucible. Daoists originally believed they could find and purify the elixir from herbs, but later realized the only real elixir is in your body. Let us discuss these two styles in more detail.

**Peaceful Cultivation Style (Qing Xiu Pai, 清修派).** Qing means clear, pure, and peaceful. Xiu means cultivation, study, and training. Pai means style or division. The basic rules of Peaceful Cultivation Daoists are to follow tradition according to the Daoist bibles. All training and study are based on the fundamental principles which Lao Zi expounded, "Objects are many, each returns to its root. When it returns to its root, it means calmness. It also means repeating life."[19] All things have their origins, and ultimately return to them. Then they are calm and peaceful. From this state, life originates again. He also said, "Concentrate Qi to attain softness, can it be soft like a baby?"[20] These two sayings of Lao Zi demonstrate the emphasis on cultivating *calmness, peace, harmony, and softness*. These are the basic rules of traditional Daoism, which originated from observation of natural cycles. All life originates from the roots of calmness and peace.

Peaceful Cultivation Daoists emphasize, "the method of Yin and Yang, harmony of the numbers (according to the *Yi Jing*), and shape follows and combines with spirit."[21] Yin and Yang must be in harmony and balance each other, and the appearance of the body will follow the lead of the spirit. This style believes that spiritual cultivation alone can lead them to enlightenment, so a strong physical body is not important. The body is only a temporary ladder to reach the goal of spiritual enlightenment. They emphasize sitting meditation, through which they Regulate the Body (Tiao Shen, 調身), Regulate the Emotional Mind (Tiao Xin, 調心), Regulate the Breathing (Tiao Xi, 調息), Condense the Spirit (Ning Shen, 凝神), Tame the Qi (Fu Qi, 伏氣), Absorb the Essence (She Jing, 攝精), and Open the Crux (Kai Qiao, 開竅). These are their seven steps of Internal Gongfu (Nei Gong, 內功), by which they cultivate and trace back to their root, the point of calmness and peace within themselves, and finally cultivate for eternal spiritual life. Through this they endeavor to reach immortality and enlightenment.

The principles and training of Peaceful Cultivation Style are similar to those of Chan (禪, Zen, 忍) meditation in Buddhism. Once the mind is calm and peaceful, they look for the root and meaning of life, becoming emotionally neutral as they train to reach enlightenment.

**Plant and Graft Style (Zai Jie Pai, 栽接派)**. Zai means to plant, grow, or raise. Jie means to join, connect, or graft. Pai means style or division. Plant and Graft Style Daoists go in the opposite direction of Peaceful Cultivation Daoists. They maintain that the methods used by Peaceful Cultivation Style, such as still meditation alone, breathing, and swallowing saliva, using the Yi to lead Qi past the gates and open the vessels, are less effective and impractical. This view was expressed in the *Book on Awakening to the Truth* (悟真篇), "Within Yang, the quality of Yin essence is not tough. To cultivate one thing alone is wasteful. Working just on the shape (body) or leading (Qi) is not the Dao. To tame Qi and dine on rosy clouds is emptiness after all."[22] Meditation is the Yin side of cultivation, and the Yin essence in the Yang is not strong. You also need Yang training methods which are different from still meditation. This statement criticizes the Peaceful Cultivation Style Daoists for seeking longevity and enlightenment through meditation alone. Focusing exclusively on Yin training, such as the taming of Qi and enjoying beautiful scenery in meditation, is empty illusion after all.

The Daoist document *Maintaining Simplicity* (抱朴子) by Ge Hong (葛洪) said, "The Grand Ultimate (the emperor) knows Daoist secular techniques, which he carefully keeps and respects, of thoroughly studying the ultimate emptiness, enlivening all things, then viewing its repetition, finally obtaining the Dao and entering heaven."[23] Secular techniques are those used by Plant and Graft Daoists. When ultimate emptiness is reached, all things start again from the beginning and come to life. When you understand the cycles which occur continually throughout nature, you comprehend the real Dao. This sentence emphasizes that even the emperor practiced Daoist secular techniques to reach enlightenment.

What then are the secular techniques of the Plant and Graft Division? They said: "If the tree is not rooted, the flowers are few. If the tree is old and you join it to a fresh one, peach is grafted onto willow, mulberry is connected to plum. To pass down examples to those looking for the real (Dao), this is the ancient immortal's plant-grafting method. The man who is getting old has the medicine to cure after all. Visit the famous teacher, ask for prescriptions, immediately start to study and cultivate, do not delay."[24] This says that when you are getting old, you can gain new life from mutual Qi transportation through particular sexual practices and special types of meditation.

"When clothes are torn, use cloth to patch. When the tree is senile, cultivate the soil. When man is weakening, what should be used to patch? Use Heaven and Earth to create the opportunity of variations."[25] This asks how a weakened person is to regain his energy if not from another person? The purpose of Plant and Graft training is "similar types working together, spiritual communication between separate bodies."[26] People training together can help each other. Spiritual communication (Shen Jiao, 神交) uses shared feeling to guide your spirit and stimulate production of hormones. Qi is exchanged in communicating with your partner. Some sexual practices stimulate hormone production while protecting and storing the Qi, which is considered the "herb" to cure aging. When done correctly, neither partner loses Qi, and both obtain the benefits of longevity.

This style of Daoism encourages a proper sex life. With this approach it is more difficult to achieve emotional neutrality and enlightenment. As a result, it mainly emphasizes a long and happy life. *Han's Book of Art and Literature* (漢書藝文誌) says, "The activity in the bedroom is the ultimate of personality and emotions, the ultimate of reaching the Dao. To restrain external joy, is to forbid internal emotion. Harmony between husband and wife is the scholarship of longevity."[27] Correct sexuality promotes longevity, enabling you to balance your Qi and spirit.

In addition to sexual double cultivation, they also emphasize non-sexual double cultivation (Shuang Xiu, 雙修). Everyone has a different level of Qi, and no one's Qi is completely balanced. In your teens, your Qi is stronger and more abundant than afterwards. Once you pass forty, your Qi supply tends to weaken and become deficient. To be healthy, your Qi should be neither excessive nor deficient. Double Cultivation meditation helps balance each other's Qi. This can be done by two men, two women, or man and woman. It is said, "Yin and Yang are not necessarily male and female, the strength and weakness of Qi in the body are Yin and Yang."[28] "Two men can plant and graft and women can absorb and nourish."[29]

To Plant and Graft Daoists there are four requirements for reaching the Dao: money, partner, techniques, and place. Without money you spend too much time earning a living, and you will not have time to study and cultivate. Without the right partner, you cannot find the "herb" to balance your Qi. Without correct techniques you waste time. Without the right place to train, you cannot meditate to digest the "herb".

As a Plant and Graft Daoist, to balance Qi with your partner, you practice techniques of retaining semen, converting it into Qi, and using the Qi to nourish your Shen (spirit). Your energized Shen directs Qi into the five Yin organs, namely the heart, lungs, liver, kidneys, and spleen, to enhance their functions. This Qi is called Managing Qi (Ying Qi, 營氣). Your Shen also directs Qi to the skin, where it protects you against negative outside influences. This Qi is called Guardian Qi (Wei Qi, 衛氣), which may be what is known in the West as one's "aura". Your Shen also leads Qi into your bone marrow (Sui Qi, 髓氣).

Plant and Graft Daoists also use herbs to help Qi cultivation, believing they offer significant benefits. Peaceful Cultivation Daoists and Buddhists also use herbs, but usually only for healing.

Daoists at this level can have long and healthy lives. But to reach even higher and attain enlightenment, one must establish a baby Shen (Shen Tai, 神胎, Shen Ying, 神嬰) or spirit baby (Ling Tai, 靈胎), feed it, and teach it to be independent. To reach this higher level, one slowly regulates their emotions. One usually needs to leave normal society and become a hermit to be able to cultivate the mind.

Even though Plant and Graft techniques bring quick results, many Daoists and Buddhists oppose and even despise them. Since you are human, it is easy to fall back into emotional bondage during training, preventing you from clearing your mind. Also, many who practice these techniques do not balance Qi for the mutual benefit of both partners, but simply take what the partner offers, without giving anything in return. This is easy with a partner who does not know Qigong, and this kind of selfishness is considered immoral.

## GENERAL DIFFERENCES BETWEEN BUDDHIST AND DAOIST QIGONG

1. In view of training philosophy, Buddhism is conservative while Daoism is open-minded. Religious Daoism absorbed the imported Buddhist culture into traditional Scholar Daoism, their doctrine, which is generally open-minded. Whenever they found methods or theory which could enhance their cultivation, they adopted it. This was impossible for Buddhists, who believe that any philosophy other than Buddhism is not true. In Buddhist society, new ideas on cultivation would be considered a betrayal. The sixth Chan (禪) ancestor Hui Neng (慧能), who lived during the Tang Dynasty (713-907 A.D., 唐朝), changed some meditation methods and philosophy

and was considered a traitor for a long time. Because of this, Chan style divided into Northern and Southern styles. This is well known among Buddhists, and is called "Sixth ancestor disrupting the passed-down method" (Liu Zu Shuo Chuan Fa, 六祖說傳法). Daoists have had more opportunities to learn, compare and experience, and in many aspects have advanced faster than Buddhists. In health and longevity Qigong, Daoist methods are better organized and more effective than those of the Buddhists.

2. Though both Buddhists and Daoists kept their training secret for a long time, the Buddhists, especially Tibetans, were more strict than the Daoists. Before the Qing Dynasty, although both Buddhist and Daoist Qigong were kept secret from lay people, at least Daoist monks could learn from their masters more easily than Buddhists. In Buddhist society, only a few trusted disciples were selected to learn the deeper aspects of Qigong training.

3. Daoists and Buddhists have different training attitudes. Buddhist Qigong emphasizes cultivating the body (Xiu Shen, 修身) and cultivating the Qi (Xiu Qi, 修氣). Cultivation implies to maintain and to keep. However, Daoists focus on training the body (Lian Shen, 練身) and training the Qi (Lian Qi, 練氣). Training means to improve, build up, and strengthen. Daoists look for ways to resist destiny, to avoid illness, and to extend the usual limits of longevity.

4. Buddhist Qigong emphasizes striving for Buddhahood, while Daoist Qigong focuses on longevity and enlightenment. While striving for Buddhahood, most Buddhist monks concentrate all their attention only on cultivating their spirit, regarding the body as a "smelly skin bag" (Chou Pi Nang, 臭皮囊). The body is used for spiritual cultivation, and is not as important as the spirit, so physical health is widely ignored in Buddhist society. By contrast, Daoists insist on a healthy physical body to achieve the final goal, emphasizing both life and natural virtue. This is called Xing Ming Shuang Xiu (性命雙修), double cultivation of human nature and life. This is why more Daoists than Buddhists have had very long lives. "If only cultivates human nature and not (physical) life, this is the first illness of cultivation."[30] "Human nature is Yin while life is Yang. If only cultivating Yin Qi and not Yang Qi, it is like the rooster carry the egg by himself, the chicken will not be complete."[31] "Human nature is at the top (head)(Ni Wan, 泥丸) while the life is at the navel."[32]

Daoists found ways to strengthen the body and slow the degeneration of the organs, to achieve long life. They say, "One hundred and twenty means dying young."[4] Buddhists also do physical training, but generally only those doing martial arts, such as the Shaolin priests.

5. Buddhist spiritual cultivation has generally reached a higher level than that of the Daoists. For example, Chan meditation techniques have been highly developed, and Daoists can learn from them.

6. Almost all Buddhist monks are against such training methods as double cultivation (Shuang Xiu, 雙修) or picking the herb from outside the Dao (Dao Wai Cai Yao, 道外採藥) through sexual practices. Using someone else's Qi to nourish you leads to emotional involvement which may disturb your cultivation. The mind will not be pure and calm enough for spiritual cultivation. But, many Daoists train mainly for health and longevity instead of enlightenment, so they regard these methods as beneficial.

## 1-9. IMPORTANCE OF QIGONG STUDY TO THE HUMAN RACE
氣功研究對人類之重要

Qigong is an important science which has developed through thousands of years of observation, pondering, study, and experimentation. It is the product of the study of health, longevity, and spiritual growth, based on the generally applicable Daoist theory of Yin and Yang.

Before the 18th century, people generally followed the Natural Way (Dao) in their lifestyles. They went to bed soon after sunset and got up at dawn. They walked a lot and had sturdy limbs. Constant labor made their torsos strong. The human body developed over millions of years of harmony with nature into their present form.

Things changed quickly with the industrial revolution since the 18th century, when machines began to replace labor through mass production. Lifestyles are now very different from the Natural Way out of which we evolved, and since the 1950s they have been changing at a breathtaking pace. The great progress of material science has left our psyche and society in tatters, and has generated many problems. We need to re-evaluate the process objectively to find a wiser, more rational path for the future.

The discovery of electricity changed lifestyles significantly. It brought great convenience, but also many problems. With artificial light came changes in our sleeping patterns. How much has this new lifestyle influenced our physical and mental structure? What Qi imbalance is caused by working a night shift? Can this account for why human sperm count continues to decline?

With the invention of aircraft, we can relocate ourselves from one side of the earth to the other within hours. How does this affect Qi circulation? Will this cause us physical or mental problems?

Because we use automobiles, we walk much less than ever before in human history. Our knees have degenerated rapidly, with knee injuries becoming very common today. Foot injuries have also increased significantly. Now, with the creation of air-pump shoes, the feet are overprotected and the tendons weakened by lack of exercise. Use of the torso has seriously decreased, causing it also to weaken and degenerate. A very common problem is lower back pain and spinal injury.

Another serious problem caused by the new lifestyle is the increase of breast cancer. Only a few decades ago, a woman would usually bear about ten babies in her lifetime. Through a million years of evolution, women have developed breasts to produce milk for their babies. There is a great deal of Qi in a woman's breasts. Now, through the use of birth control, the average woman will have only one or two babies, and often will not breastfeed. The result is a great accumulation and stagnation of Qi in the breast area, which often triggers cancer. Many do not realize that human lifestyles have changed in a relatively short period, and do not know the consequences or how to solve the problems caused.

There are many other problems caused by the rapid development of material science. Microwave ovens, fluorescent light, and high tension powerlines are recent developments, which create artificial electromagnetic waves. Our body is a living electromagnetic field which can be influenced by external fields. A human brain contains 2.5 million tiny magnetic crystals. The brain is a magnetic unit like a computer floppy disk, with the capability of thought and memory. When the brain is exposed to a varying external magnetic field, it changes our moods, our thoughts, and we can even lose our memory.[33]

From more and more discovery, we realize how much risk we have exposed ourselves to in the new electromagnetic environment created by humans. How can we protect ourselves from the energy pollution of the new electromagnetic environment, which affects our thinking, judgment, and even our health?

We have also experienced a great loss of the human spirit, caused by wide-scale ignorance, a focus on material science and material possessions. Humans are ensnared in emotional bondage, having lost their spiritual center. To recover this lost spirituality, we must learn from the past, understand it, and bring it back into daily life.

We must educate the new generation about the importance of spirit. At the age of three years old, a child has become familiar with the body's balance, and learned to walk and run. This is the best age to teach them to feel the mental center of their being. For example, teaching them to walk with eyes closed, they establish a stronger inner feeling and body awareness. Next, teach them to locate the residence of the spirit and to communicate with it. This develops sensitivity to the subconscious mind. This kind of inner feeling is called Nei Shi Gongfu (內視功夫) which means Gongfu of internal vision. This kind of training is easier for children than adults since the child's mind has not yet been contaminated by the complex emotional world, and its thinking can be simple and pure. If we teach the new generation this meditation, we can bring them to a higher level of sensitivity and understanding of the spiritual world. From this recognition of spiritual identity, children will have less confusion and their lives will be more meaningful. Those methods which lead people to blind worship should be discouraged. Blind worship can only lead us back to the past of dictatorship and spiritual abuse.

However, we cannot deny that development of material science has also improved human life significantly. For example, the average age of men has increased from 47 in 1900 to 76 in 1998. We will soon be able to live to be 120 years old with the help of human growth hormone.[12-15] But we should also understand the side effects from injection of human growth hormone. If there are any cancer cells hidden in the body, growth hormone can help them spread. Hormones are catalysts in the body, which enhance its biochemical reaction, including the metabolism of bad cells. If blood circulation is not as abundant as it should be, growth hormone may keep the muscles and the surface of the body young, but the deep places such as the joints continue to age. Proper Qigong exercise and relaxation can minimize this problem.

From this we can summarize the importance of Qigong to society.

1. **Bring us better awareness.** When we understand the human electromagnetic field better, we can avoid exposing ourselves to harmful external electromagnetic fields.

2. **Alert us to harmful future developments.** Many chemicals and radioactive substances are harmful and should be forbidden, and we must prevent creation of such harmful products in the future. If we correct our wrong path now, we may lead ourselves to a safer and more peaceful environment.

3. **Educate the next generation about spirit.** Teach them how to meditate and develop the spiritual mind. Now we have reached a good level of material science and freed ourselves from material shortages. However, this also causes the danger of modern weapons. We face the complete destruction of the earth and human culture. If we cannot educate the next generation to be free from the emotional bondage, we will surely self-destruct. We have to wake up and enlighten our spirit, before we can expect harmony and peace on earth.

4. **Apply Qigong to solve today's problems.** Many sicknesses which cannot be cured by modern medicine respond to traditional Qigong methods. Cases of cancer or arthritis have been cured by Qigong. Spine and lower back pain is often cured by Qigong, which also rebuilds the strength of the torso. The greatest benefit in practicing Qigong is increasing the strength of your immune system and keeping you healthy.

5. **Help regain our spiritual center and understand the meaning of life.** Through Qigong practice, countless people have brought themselves back

from confusion and rootlessness, to a state of self-recognition. They regain their spiritual center and realize the role of their lives in society. This is the path of setting us free from emotional bondage and material slavery.

6. **From studying Qigong, we understand and develop the Yin side of science, that of energy and spirit.** We open the gate to understanding the spiritual side of the human being and comprehending the mission of our existence in this universe.

7. **By understanding past Qigong practice, we create a feasible way for future spiritual cultivation.** This will cultivate enlightenment for mankind, the unification of Heaven and Man (Tian Ren He Yi, 天人合一), of the natural spirit and the human spirit.

## 1-10. ABOUT THIS BOOK 關於這本書

Qigong is like an infinite garden which contains everything in nature, both material and spiritual, but we have never had a detailed map of it. Qigong masters each discovered some of the pathways to an understanding of this garden, and mysterious hidden places which manifest the beauty of nature were gradually discovered. They passed down their understanding through teaching students or through writing. Though each document may provide only a little information on how to reach a tiny area of the garden, it had taken a Qigong master's lifetime to obtain. Each document is a possible road sign to our goal. When they are combined, we can construct a map, a theory which might take us to places of our Qigong garden where nobody has ever gone before. It will probably take thousands of years of effort to obtain a detailed map of nature.

So far we have only limited information about material nature, and know very little about spiritual nature. We are still confused about the meaning of life, and far from understanding the truth of nature.

We need open minds to set us free from traditional brainwashing and bondage. We should humbly face the challenge and be willing to accept the truth and the mistakes we have already committed. Only then can we realize our dream of the future. Then we will be able to think with an open mind. If nobody can prove their ideas about the universe, we should dare to postulate a theory and explanation generated by the imagination. We try to prove our assumptions, and if proven wrong, we go back to modify the theory and try again. This is the scientific method: to *dare to dream, dare to accept the challenge, and dare to accept the facts and the truth.*

This book offers methods to establish a firm foundation of Small Circulation, a step on the path toward the ultimate goal of spiritual enlightenment.

Many explanations here originate from my personal understanding and scientific background. I cannot guarantee the correctness of my assumptions. It is quite possible that someone with deeper understanding of this subject may step in to modify or even completely change my theory. That is the natural course of scientific study. After the assumed theory has been tested repeatedly, we will be able to confirm what is correct and what is not, and the map will become clear.

The theory and practice methods introduced in this book only originate from Chinese study. You should keep an open mind and study the same subject in other cultures. A different view of the same topic could lead you to a clearer judgment. This is especially true for spiritual cultivation, as we are still at the beginning of understanding this subject. Any past experience could offer you more information and direct you to a better path of reaching the goal. This book is not an authority on this subject, and can only offer you one cultural viewpoint.

Even though we cannot yet prove the existence of the spirit in this universe by scientific method, it does not mean it does not exist. We should continue our research to untie this knot and open the gate of spiritual science experienced by people in all different cultures.

In the second chapter of part I, I offer a theoretic foundation of Qigong practice related to Small Circulation meditation. In Part II, training methods passed down from the past are introduced. From Part I and Part II, you will have a clear idea of how to approach the essence of this training. Meditation methods are introduced in Part III. Many remaining questions are listed in Part IV.

The theoretic foundation in this practice is like a map which could lead you to the final goal. You should first study it and understand it clearly. If you rush into practice without comprehending the theory, you may enter the wrong path and become confused, and endanger yourself through incorrect practice.

## References

1. 《莊子刻意》：〝吹呴呼吸，吐故納新，熊經鳥伸，為壽而已矣。此導引之士，養形之人，彭祖壽考者之所好也。〞

2. 李時珍《奇經八脈考》：〝蓋正經猶夫溝渠，奇經猶夫湖澤，正經之脈隆盛，則溢于奇經。〞

3. 人生七十古來稀。

4. 一百二十謂之天。

5. 外家由外而內，從硬到軟。

6. 內家由內而外，從軟到硬。

7. 《達摩大師住世留形內真妙用訣》：〝若不知子母相守，氣雖呼吸於于內，神常勞役于外，遂使神常穢濁而神不清，神既不清，即元和之氣漸散，而不能相守也。〞

8. "Silent Sperm," Lawrence Wright, p. 42, *The New Yorker,* January 15, 1996.

9. 《黃帝內經素問・上古天真論》：〝上古之人，知其道者，法于陰陽，和于術數，食飲有節，起居有常，不妄作勞，故能形與神俱，而盡終其天年度百歲乃去。〞

10. "Complex and Hidden Brain in the Gut Makes Cramps, Butterflies and Valium," Sandra Blakeslee, Science, *New York Times,* January 23.

11. *The Second Brain: The Scientific Basis of Gut Instinct and a Groundbreaking New Understanding of Nervous Disorders of the Stomach and Intestine,* Michael D. Gershon, New York: Harper Collins Publications, 1998.

12. "Effects of Human Growth Hormone in Men Over 60 Years Old," *New England Journal of Medicine,* Daniel Rudman, July, 1990.

13. "The Foundation of Youth", *Harvard Health Letter,* Vol. 17, Number 8, June, 1992.

14. "The Hormone That Makes Your Body 20 Years Younger," Bill Lawren, *Longevity,* Oct. 1990.

15. *Grow Young with HGH,* Dr. Ronald Klatz, Harper Collins Publishers, NY, 1997.

16. 宇宙是個大天地，人身是個小天地。

17. "Measuring Stardust's Glow," Earl Lane, *Newsday,* January 10, 1998.

18. 《性天風月通玄記・師徒傳道》：〝論性命，要雙修，將鉛汞，兩下投，這消息，難參透，修性即煉己，修命即還丹。心是神之舍，身是氣之宅。命即氣也，修性之人，把身心混作一家，精氣神打成一片。修命之能事備矣。〞

19. 老子云：夫物芸芸，各復歸其根，歸根曰靜，是謂復命。

20. 專氣致柔，能嬰兒乎。

21. 法於陰陽，和於術數，形與神俱。

22. 悟真篇云：陽裡陰精質不剛，獨修一物轉羸尪。勞形按引皆非道，服氣餐霞總是狂。

23. 抱朴子云：太上知玄素之術，守敬篤，致虛極，萬物並作，以觀其復而得道飛昇。

24. 無根樹，花正微，樹老將新接嫩枝，桃寄柳，桑接梅，傳於修真作樣兒，自古神仙栽接法，人老原來有藥醫。訪名師，問方兒，下手速修莫太遲。

25. 衣破用布補，樹衰以土培，人損將何補，乾坤造化機。

26. 同類施工，隔體神交。

27. 漢書藝文誌云：房中者，性情之極，至道之極，制外藥，禁內情，和夫婦，及壽考之學也。

28. 陰陽不必分男女，體氣強弱即陰陽。

29. 兩個男人可栽接，一對女人能採補。

30. 只知修性不修命，此是修行第一病。

31. 《道鄉集》：〝性為陰，命為陽，只修陰氣，不修陽氣，即〞牝雞自卵，其雛不全。〞

32. 性在泥丸，命在臍。〔性潛于頂，命歸于臍。〕

33. "Pulsing Magnets Offer New Method of Mapping Brain," Sandra Blakeslee, *New York Times,* May 21, 1996.

## CHAPTER 2

# Theoretical Foundations
# 理論基礎

## 2-1. INTRODUCTION 介紹

The Chinese concept of Dao (道) is commonly translated as the Natural Way. *Yi Jing* (易經, *The Book of Change*, 1122-1115 B.C.) said, "One Yin and One Yang is called Dao."[1] The fundamental concept of Dao is the coexistence of Yin and Yang aspects of nature. This concept was later refined by Lao Zi (老子, 604-531 B.C.). In his book *Dao De Jing* (道德經), Chapter 24, he said, "Dao begets one, one produces two, two generate three, and three derive into millions of objects."[2] Dao is the natural causative force which creates the first single object from emptiness, and later this (Wuji state of no extremity) divides into two aspects and continues to derive into millions of objects and lives.

Chapter 25 of *Dao De Jing* says, "There is an undiscriminated thing formed before the heaven and the earth (Yin and Yang). Extremely quiet, existing alone and without change, repeating cyclically without end, the mother of heaven and earth. I do not know its name and so call it Dao."[3] Dao exists since the very beginning, before heaven and earth, quietly, alone, and unchanging in its original virtue. When the Dao makes Wuji (no extremity) derive into Yin and Yang, it sets in motion the patterns of opposing forces and natural cycles. This derivation from Wuji to Yin and Yang is the origin of millions of things and therefore the mother of life.

Lao Zi believed Dao is responsible for all of creation and life. "Dao is the most mysterious of the mysterious, the door (origin) of all marvelousness."[4] "When Dao is born, the natural virtues are raised, objects are formed, and the natural state will be complete."[5] Millions of variations of nature derive from the Dao. Once this natural pattern is complete, the natural cycles are established and repeated. For us to fit into this nature, Lao Zi explained, "Man copies the earth, the earth follows heaven, heaven models itself after the Dao, the Dao follows nature."[6] It does not matter how big, such as heaven, or how small, such as a microbe, all follow the same energy patterns and the same Dao of nature.

Dao creates a single object from nothing, and from this single object, it divides into Yin and Yang. When Yin and Yang interact with each other harmoniously, millions of lives are created and derived. It is said in *Huai Nan Zi* (淮南子), "Dao begins from one, one does not beget, therefore dividing into Yin and Yang. When Yin and Yang harmonize with each other, millions of objects are born."[7]

Lao Zi pointed out the derivation from Wuji (無極) to Yin and Yang can proceed either way. Wuji can derive into Yin and Yang and Yin and Yang can be united to become Wuji. He said in Chapter 1, "Nothing, is the beginning of the pre-heaven (Wuji) state, the mother of millions of objects. Always nothing, wish to see its marvelousness, always existing, wish to see it expand."[8] Dao changes from nothing to something, and from something back to nothing, always changing from one to the other.

In order to understand the theoretical foundation of Chinese Qigong meditation, you must first study its history, tracing back the philosophic origins of Chinese culture. Qigong is an integral part of Chinese culture. If you separate them, you lose the root and essence of the art.

The oldest Chinese philosophy relates to the development of nature, especially human nature. The *Yi Jing* (*The Book of Changes*, 1122 B.C.) is the first book to offer a detailed clear discussion. Under its influence, the Dao (natural way) was followed by the Chinese people.

*Yi Jing, Great Biography* said,

> The ancestor named Bao Xi became king of heaven and earth. He looked up to see the phenomenal changes of the heavens, looked down to observe the natural rules of the earth, watched the instinctive behavior of birds and animals and how they interacted with the earth. He adapted to the changes of things he saw around him, he adopted the recurring cycles of objects, he then created the Eight Trigrams. This was used to understand the virtue of the divine and the behavior of millions of lives.

> 易大傳曰：「古者包羲氏之王天下也。仰則觀象於天，俯則觀法於地。觀鳥獸之文，與地之宜。近取諸身，遠取諸物。於是始作八卦，以通神明之德，以類萬物之情。」

Bao Xi (包羲, 2852-2737 B.C.) was the ruler of China. The heaven and the earth means the kingdom. After he carefully observed the patterns of natural cycles and the behavior of plants and animals, he created the Eight Trigrams (Bagua, 八卦), which are used to interpret and trace the patterns of nature. The theory of trigrams has significantly influenced Chinese culture.

*Yi Jing* also said,

> *Therefore, Yi (Change) has Taiji (Grand Ultimate), and begets two poles (Yin and Yang). Two poles produce four phases. Four phases give rise to Bagua (Eight Trigrams). Bagua determines good or bad fortune, from good or bad fortune, the great career is created.*

是故易有太極，是生兩儀，兩儀生四象，四象生八卦，
八卦定吉凶，吉凶生大業。

Only because there is Taiji, is there change. From Taiji, the Two Poles (Yin and Yang) are created from Wuji (no extremity or nothingness) and the two poles again derive into four phases. These four phases produce the Eight Trigrams. From the Eight Trigrams, the patterns of natural cycles can be understood, and good or bad fortune predicted. To be prosperous in business, follow the good luck patterns and avoid the bad luck patterns of nature. All derivations originate from Taiji. Taiji is the Dao or natural force which makes division and unification take place.

A Daoist classic, *Jin Si Lu* (近思錄) said,

> *Wuji begets Taiji. When Taiji moves, the Yang is born. When movement reaches its extremity, again calm, generating the Yin. When calmness reaches its extremity, again moving. One moves and one is calm, mutually as the root. Yin and Yang are discriminated and the two poles completed.*

無極生太極，太極動而生陽，動極復靜；靜而生陰，靜
極復動。一動一靜，互為其根，分陰分陽，兩儀至焉。

Through this recurring cycle of Yin and Yang, millions of lives are begotten. The causative force is called Taiji. The ancient Daoist classic, *Glossary Talking by Zhu Zi* (朱子語類) said, "What is called Taiji, is the root of millions of things in heaven and earth."[9]

Wang, Zong-Yue (王宗岳, 1750 A.D.) described Taiji,

> *What is Taiji? It is generated from Wuji and is a pivotal function of movement and stillness. It is the mother of Yin and Yang. When it moves, it divides. At rest it reunites.*

太極者，無極而生，動靜之機，陰陽之母也。動之則分，
靜之則合。

Taiji is neither Wuji nor Yin and Yang, but the natural force or Dao which makes the divisions and unifications happen. It is the cause and origin of life and death, the way of the natural cycle.

Chinese culture is based on the theory of Taiji, and of Yin and Yang. When the theory is applied to Qigong, the first important goal of practice is the harmony and balance of Yin and Yang (Yin Yang Xie Tiao, 陰陽諧調). To reach this harmonious state of balance, you adjust Yin and Yang, through the methods of Kan (坎, Water) and Li (離, Fire).

When this theory is applied to human health, the physical body is considered Yang, while the mental and the spiritual bodies are considered Yin. To have a long, healthy life, you must also consider your spiritual condition. Mind and spirit are the foundation of life, and although they cannot be seen, they are nevertheless the origins and the causes of physical manifestation. When this foundation is firm and strong, the manifestation of life can be strong. To achieve health and longevity, cultivate both mental and physical bodies. This is called double cultivation of human nature and life (Xing Ming Shuang Xiu, 性命雙修). Human nature means the inner nature, the original spirit carried with us since birth. Life here means the limited physical life.

When you adjust yourself into harmony internally and externally, it is called "balance the body and mind" (Shen Xin Ping Heng, 身心平衡). This allows you to live longer, enabling spiritual cultivation to reach enlightenment or Buddhahood, the final goal of cultivation.

Fortunately material science is highly developed, allowing us to verify things which were inexplicable in the past. Nevertheless, many mysteries remain that are waiting to be investigated from a scientific point of view. We live in a very exciting and challenging era, in which ancient mysteries and experiences can be comprehended using today's science. The documents passed down by thousands of Qigong experts provide us with clues, some more useful than others.

I am like a puzzle player. In front of me are thousands of pieces of the puzzle of Qigong practice. I try to choose those which are useful and valuable, discarding those which mislead. Through my efforts I have compiled a map of Qigong, not as detailed as I would like, but nevertheless a clear guide to prevent confusion and the fear of getting lost.

A clear and detailed map is necessary, but I cannot accomplish this mammoth task by myself in a single lifetime.

1. Thousands of ancient documents remain to be translated, interpreted and explained. This requires qualified scholars familiar with Qigong practice who are also masters of ancient Chinese writing, to understand the special terminology used.

2. We need experienced Qigong practitioners to translate these ancient documents into other languages correctly. This is no easy task since a Chinese word can have many different meanings, depending on where, how and when it is used.

3. We need open-minded scientists and medical experts to offer opinions on the merits of these ancient practices. They need to challenge and attempt to verify the ancient experience in a scientific context.

4. We need a foundation with strong financial support to bring the various experts together to discuss every aspect of Qigong practice. From these conferences, information would be compiled, studied, researched, experimented with, and finally published. Without government support, or the interest of various scientific groups, it will be hard to accomplish this task.

In this chapter, I try to explain many mysteries in Qigong practice based on my personal limited scientific background. These possible explanations remain to be verified, but until then they remain the most probable hypothesis.

We first review the Chinese medical concept of the Qi channels and vessels. With this foundation, we use the scientific view to discuss the concept of Chinese Qigong in section 3. In section 4, the meaning and the purpose of Qigong meditation is discussed.

The training theory of Muscle/Tendon Changing and Marrow/Brain Washing Qigong is summarized in section 5, followed by Small Circulation, Grand Circulation, and Enlightenment Meditation in sections 6, 7 and 8 respectively.

## 2-2. Qi Vessels and Channels 氣脈與經絡

We have two bodies, the physical body and the Qi (bioenergetic) body. The physical body can be seen, but Qi must be felt. The Qi body is the foundation of the physical body, of living cells, and of our lives. The Qi body is not only related to our cells, but also to our thinking and spirit, since it is the main energy source which maintains the brain's functioning. Therefore, Qi imbalance or stagnation are the root of any physical sickness or mental disorder.

Western medical science has long studied the physical body, while for the most part ignoring the Qi body. This has begun to change in the last two decades, but scientific understanding of the Qi body, and how it affects health and longevity, is still in its infancy. Under these circumstances, we may still accept the ancient Chinese understanding of our body's Qi network.

### Twelve Primary Qi Channels and the Eight Vessels

From the viewpoint of Chinese medicine, the Qi circulatory system in the body has Eight Vessels (Ba Mai, 八脈), Twelve Primary Qi Channels (Shi Er Jing, 十二經), and thousands of secondary channels branching out from the primary channels (Luo, 絡).

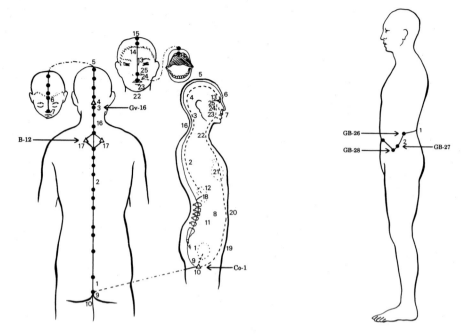

Figure 2-1. The Governing Vessel (Du Mai)　　Figure 2-2. The Girdle (Belt) Vessel (Dai Mai)

On two of the vessels (Governing and Conception Vessels) and the twelve primary Qi channels, there are more than seven hundred acupuncture cavities through which Qi can be adjusted. In this way, Qi circulation in the body, especially in the internal organs, can be regulated into a harmonious state, sickness cured ,and health maintained. Here, we briefly review these three circulatory networks. For more about this Qi network, refer to Chinese acupuncture books or my books, *The Root of Chinese Qigong* and *Qigong Massage*.

### Eight Vessels (Ba Mai, 八脈 )

a. The eight vessels include four Yang vessels and four Yin vessels, which balance each other.

b. The Four Yang Vessels are:

　　　Governing Vessel (Du Mai, 督脈 )(Figure 2-1)

　　　Girdle (or Belt) Vessel (Dai Mai, 帶脈 )(Figure 2-2)

　　　Yang Heel Vessel (Yangqiao Mai, 陽蹻脈 )(Figure 2-3)

　　　Yang Linking Vessel (Yangwei Mai, 陽維脈 )(Figure 2-4)

　The Four Yin Vessels are:

　　　Conception Vessel (Ren Mai, 任脈 )(Figure 2-5)

　　　Thrusting Vessel (Chong Mai, 衝脈 )(Figure 2-6)

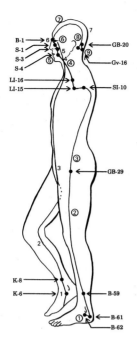

Figure 2-3. The Yang Heel Vessel (Yangqiao Mai) and The Yin Heel Vessel (Yinqiao Mai)

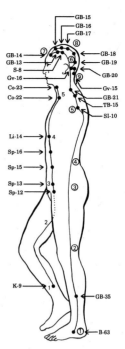

Figure 2-4. The Yang Linking Vessel (Yangwei Mai) and the Yin Linking Vessel (Yinwei Mai)

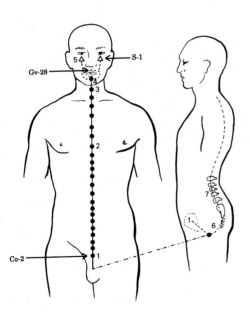

Figure 2-5. The Conception Vessel (Ren Mai)

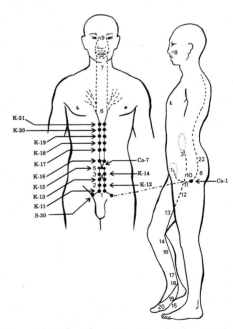

Figure 2-6. The Thrusting Vessel (Chong Mai)

Yin Heel Vessel (Yinqiao Mai, 陰蹻脈 )(Figure 2-3)

Yin Linking Vessel (Yinwei Mai, 陰維脈 )(Figure 2-4).

c. According to Chinese medicine, vessels function as reservoirs, connected to the twelve primary Qi channels and regulating Qi circulating in these channels. When the Qi level in some specific channel is too high, one or more of the reservoirs absorbs the excess, and if the Qi is too low, the shortfall will be supplied from these vessels. In this way, harmony is maintained.

d. Two Yang vessels, Governing and Girdle Vessels, and two Yin vessels, Conception and Thrusting Vessels, are in the torso. The other four vessels are in pairs, located in the legs. There are no vessels in the arms.

e. Among the eight vessels, the Governing and Conception Vessels are the most important, since they regulate the twelve primary Qi channels. The Governing Vessel regulates Qi in the six primary Yang channels, while the Conception Vessel regulates that in the six primary Yin channels. There are acupuncture cavities on these two vessels, but none on the other six. However, there are many cavities on the six vessels which belong to the twelve primary Qi channels, considered to be gates where Qi passes between the vessels and channels.

f. The methods for filling the vessels with Qi are very important. When their Qi is abundant, the regulating potential of the primary Qi channels is high. The Governing and Conception Vessels are the most important, since they regulate the twelve primary Qi channels. Qi circulates in them, and is distributed to the twelve primary Qi channels throughout the day.

g. In Religious Qigong meditation for enlightenment, the Thrusting Vessel (Spinal Cord) is very important. It connects the brain and the perineum, and Qi is abundant in this vessel around midnight. During these hours we sleep, and the body is very relaxed. The body does not need much Qi to support its activities, and Qi circulates abundantly in the spinal cord to nourish the brain and sexual organs. Hormone production increases at night. When the brain is nourished, the spirit is raised and enlightenment can be achieved. Again, for more detail, refer to my book, *Qigong—The Secret of Youth.*

h. The Governing Vessel, up the middle of the back, is the main vessel supplying Qi to the nervous system branching out from the spinal cord. The nervous system consists of physical cells which need to be nourished with Qi to function and stay alive. To maintain abundant Qi circulation in this vessel, your physical health is very important. Injury or damage along the course of this vessel, causes Qi supply to the nervous system to be stagnant and irregular. To have abundant Qi circulating in this vessel, increase the storage of Qi in the Lower Real Dan Tian (Zhen Xia Dan Tian, 真下丹田), which is the main Qi reservoir or bioelectric battery in our body. We discuss this subject in more detail in Chapter 6.

i. The Yang Girdle Vessel is very important, and is the only vessel in which Qi circulates horizontally. It is from this vessel that we feel our balance. Qi in this vessel is Yang and expands outwards. As with a tight-rope walker, the longer the balancing pole, the easier it is to keep balance. *Qigong practitioners and martial artists train this vessel to improve balance and stability of body and mind. Then you can find your center and be rooted, so your spirit can be raised.*

j. Li, Shi-Zhen (李時珍, 1518-1593 A.D.) said in his book, *The Study of Strange Meridians and Eight Vessels* (奇經八脈考), "The Yang Linking Vessel dominates the Qi of the surface (Guardian Qi) while the Yin Linking Vessel dominates the Qi of the inner body. The Yang Heel Vessel dominates the Yang of the body's left and right sides, while the Yin Heel Vessel dominates the Yin of the body's left and right sides. The Governing Vessel dominates the Yang at the back of the body, while the Conception and Thrusting Vessels dominate the Yin in front. The Girdle Vessel regulates all vessels horizontally."[10]

### The Twelve Primary Qi Channels and Their Branches (Shi Er Jing Luo, 十二經絡)

a. The six Yang channels and six Yin channels balance each other.

b. The six Yang channels are:

Arm Yang Brightness Large Intestine Channel (Shou Yang Ming Da Chang Jing, 手陽明大腸經)(Figure 2-7)

Leg Yang Brightness Stomach Channel (Zu Yang Ming Wei Jing, 足陽明胃經)(Figure 2-8)

Arm Greater Yang Small Intestine Channel (Shou Tai Yang Xiao Chang Jing, 手太陽小腸經)(Figure 2-9)

Leg Greater Yang Bladder Channel (Zu Tai Yang Pang Guang Jing, 足太陽膀胱經)(Figure 2-10)

Arm Lesser Yang Triple Burner Channel (Shou Shao Yang San Jiao Jing, 手少陽三焦經)(Figure 2-11)

Leg Lesser Yang Gall Bladder Channel (Zu Shao Yang Dan Jing, 足少陽膽經) (Figure 2-12)

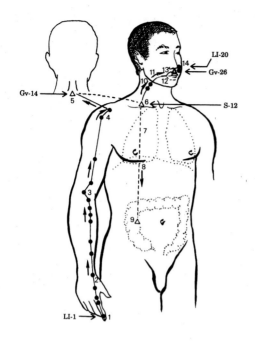

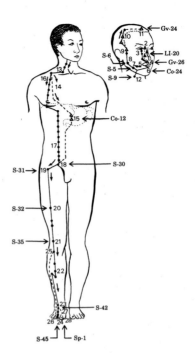

Figure 2-7. The Large Intestine Channel of the Hand-Yang Brightness

Figure 2-8. The Stomach Channel of the Foot-Yang Brightness

The Six Yin channels are:

Arm Greater Yin Lung Channel (Shou Tai Yin Fei Jing, 手太陰肺經) (Figure 2-13)

Leg Greater Yin Spleen Channel (Zu Tai Yin Pi Jing, 足太陰脾經) (Figure 2-14)

Arm Lesser Yin Heart Channel (Shou Shao Yin Xin Jing, 手少陰心經) (Figure 2-15)

Leg Lesser Yin Kidney Channel (Zu Shao Yin Shen Jing, 足少陰腎經) (Figure 2-16)

Arm Absolute Yin Pericardium Channel (Shou Jue Yin Xin Bao Luo Jing, 手厥陰心包絡經)( Figure 2-17)

Leg Absolute Yin Liver Channel (Zu Jue Yin Gan Jing, 足厥陰肝經) (Figure 2-18).

c. One end of each channel connects to an extremity, and the other end to an internal organ. Each channel has many acupuncture cavities through which its Qi can be regulated. This is the basic theory of acupuncture.

d. Thousands of secondary channels (Luo, 絡) branch out from each primary one. These lead Qi to the surface of the skin and to the bone

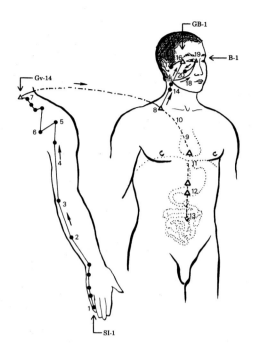

Figure 2-9. The Small Intestine Channel of the Hand-Greater Yang

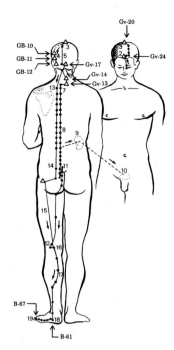

Figure 2-10. The Urinary Bladder Channel of the Foot-Greater Yang

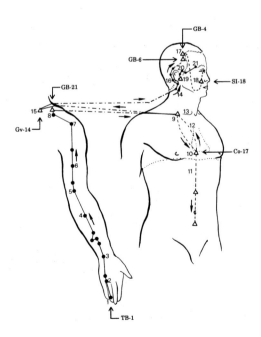

Figure 2-11. The Triple Burner Channel of the Hand-Lesser Yang

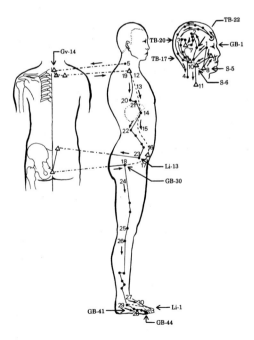

Figure 2-12. The Gall Bladder Channel of the Foot-Lesser Yang

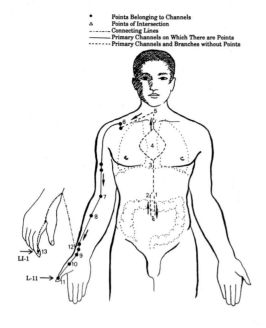

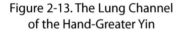

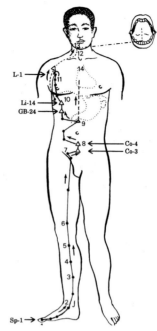

Figure 2-13. The Lung Channel of the Hand-Greater Yin

Figure 2-14. The Spleen Channel of the Foot-Greater Yin

marrow. This is very similar to the artery and capillary system. Instead of blood, Qi is distributed.

## 2-3. HUMAN QIGONG SCIENCE 人類之氣功科學

Modern science has started to accept Qigong concepts, but has far to go to reach profound understanding. The observations in this section are from my personal understanding, and from information already published. For a satisfactory explanation, many assumptions are needed, so use logic and a scientific mind to judge. Question all assumptions and explanations. Only once we have verified the theory can we trust it fully.

In this section, a human bioelectric network is postulated and compared to ancient Chinese medical concepts. We define the human biobattery, both in the traditional Chinese concept and also from the viewpoint of modern Western science.

### A Modern Definition of Qi

In ancient China, people had no knowledge of electricity. They only knew from acupuncture that when needles were inserted into acupuncture cavities, some kind of energy other than heat was produced, which often caused shock or a tickling sensation. When the Chinese became acquainted with electromagnetism, they realized

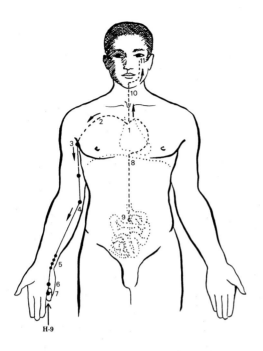

Figure 2-15. The Heart Channel
of the Hand-Lesser Yin

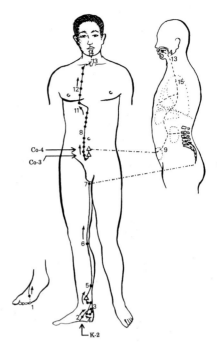

Figure 2-16. The Kidney Channel
of the Foot-Lesser Yin

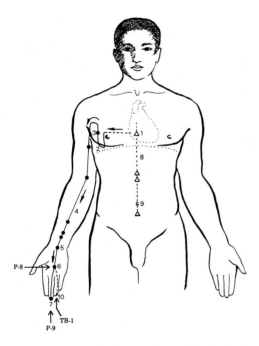

Figure 2-17. The Pericardium Channel
of the Hand-Absolute Yin

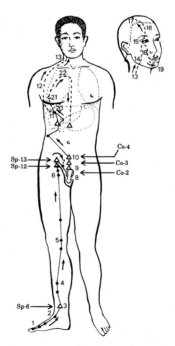

Figure 2-18. The Liver Channel
of the Foot-Absolute Yin

that this energy circulating in the body, which they called Qi, might be the same thing as what today's science calls bioelectricity.

The human body is constructed of many different electrically conductive materials, and forms a living electromagnetic circuit. Electromagnetic energy is continuously generated in the body through biochemical reaction, which assimilates food and air, and circulates electromotive force (EMF) within the body.

It is constantly affected by external electromagnetic fields such as that of the earth or electrical fields generated by clouds. When you practice Qigong, you need to be aware of these external factors and take them into account.

Countless experiments have been conducted in China and Japan to study how external electromagnetic fields affect the body's Qi field. Many acupuncturists use magnets and electricity in their treatment. They attach a magnet to the skin over a cavity and leave it there for a period of time, where its magnetic field gradually affects Qi circulation in that channel. Alternatively, they insert needles into cavities and then run an electric current through the needle to reach the Qi channels directly. Although researchers claim success in their experiments, they have not been able to explain the theory behind them. Conclusive proof remains elusive, and many unanswered questions remain. Of course, this theory is new, and will take more research before it is verified and understood. At present, many conservative acupuncturists are skeptical.

To unravel this knot, we look at what modern Western science has discovered about bioelectromagnetic energy. Many reports on bioelectricity research have been published, and frequently the results closely relate to what is experienced in Qigong training and Chinese medicine. During the electrophysiological research of the 1960s, investigators discovered that bones are piezoelectric. In other words, when they are stressed, mechanical energy is converted to electrical energy in the form of electric current.[11] This might explain one of the practices of Marrow Washing Qigong in which stress on the bones is increased to increase Qi circulation.

Dr. Robert O. Becker has done important work in this field. His book, *The Body Electric* reports on much of the research concerning the body's electric field.[12] It is presently believed that food and air are the fuels which generate electricity in the body through biochemical reaction. This electricity is circulated throughout the body by means of electrically conductive tissue, one of the main energy sources keeping cells alive.

When you are injured or sick, your body's electrical circulation is affected. If this circulation of electricity stops, you die. Bioelectric energy not only maintains life, it also repairs damage. Researchers seek ways of using external electromagnetic fields to speed up recovery from injury. Richard Leviton reports, "Researchers at Loma Linda University's School of Medicine in California have found, following studies in sixteen countries with over 1,000 patients, that low-frequency, low-intensity magnetic energy has been successful in treating chronic pain related to tissue ischemia, and has also worked well in clearing up slow-healing ulcers. In 90 percent of patients tested, it increased blood flow significantly."[13]

He reports that every cell functions like an electric battery, able to store electric charge. "Other biomagnetic investigators take an even closer look to find out what is happening, right down to the level of the blood, the organs, and the individual cell, which they regard as a small electric battery."[13] This convinces me that our entire body is essentially a big battery assembled from millions of small ones. All of them together activate the human electromagnetic field.

Much research relates to acupuncture. Dr. Becker reports that the conductivity of the skin is much higher at acupuncture cavities, and it is now possible to locate them precisely by measuring the skin's conductivity (Figure 2-19).[12] Many reports show a scientific basis for the acupuncture which has been done in China for thousands of years.

Some researchers use the theory of bioelectricity to explain ancient miracles attributed to the practice of Qigong. Albert Huebner reports, "These demonstrations of body electricity in human beings may also offer a new explanation of an ancient healing practice. If weak external fields can produce powerful physiological effects, it may be that fields from human tissues in one person are capable of producing clinical improvements in another. In short, the method of healing known as the laying on of hands could be an especially subtle form of electrical stimulation."[11]

Another phenomenon reported is the halo seen around the head of a Qigong practitioner who reaches a high level during meditation. This is commonly shown in paintings of Jesus Christ, Buddha, Orthodox and Catholic saints and various Oriental immortals. Frequently the light is pictured as surrounding the whole body. This phenomenon may be explained by the body electric theory. When one cultivates Qi to a high level, it may accumulate in the head. It may interact with the oxygen molecules in the air, ionize them and cause them to glow.

Although the link between the theory of The Body Electric and the Chinese theory of Qi is becoming more accepted, there are still many questions to be answered. For example, how does the mind actually generate EMF to circulate the electricity in the body? How is the human electromagnetic field affected by the multitude of other electric fields which surround us, such as radio or electrical appliances? How can we readjust our electromagnetic field and survive in outer space or on other planets where the magnetic fields are completely different from that on earth? The future of Qigong and bioelectric science is challenging and exciting. We need to use modern technology to understand the inner energy world which for the most part has been ignored by Western society.

## A Modern Definition of Qigong

If we accept the internal energy (Qi) circulating in our bodies is bioelectricity, we can formulate a definition of Qigong based on the principles of physics.

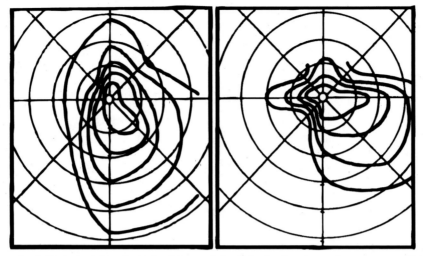

Figure 2-19. Electrical Conductivity Maps of the Skin Surface over Acupuncture Points

Let us assume that the circuit shown in Figure 2-20 is similar to that in our bodies. Although we now have some understanding of this circuit from acupuncture, we still do not know in detail exactly what the body's circuits looks like. We know there are Twelve Primary Qi Channels (Qi rivers) and Eight Vessels (Qi reservoirs). There are also thousands of small Qi channels (Luo, 络) which allow Qi to reach the skin and bone marrow. In this circuit, the twelve internal organs are connected and mutually related through these channels. There is also a Dan Tian (丹田, elixir field) bio-battery which stores the Qi.

In the illustration, you see that:

1. The Qi channels are like wires which carry electric current.

2. The internal organs are like electrical components such as resistors and solenoids.

3. The Qi vessels are like capacitors, which regulate the current in the circuit.

4. The Dan Tian is like a battery, which stores charge and provides EMF.

How do you keep this electrical circuit functioning efficiently? Your first concern is the resistance of the wires which carry current. In a machine, use a wire with high conductivity and low resistance, otherwise the current may melt it. It should be of a material like copper or even gold. In your body, you keep current flowing smoothly, removing anything which causes stagnation. Fat has low conductivity, so use diet and exercise to remove excess from your body. Relaxation to open the Qi channels is the first practice in Taijiquan and many Qigong exercises.

How do you maintain the electrical components, your internal organs? Your organs burn out from too much current (Yang) or too little (Yin). To avoid these

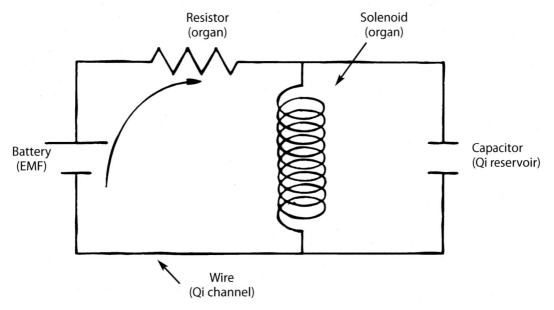

Figure 2-20. The Human Bioelectric Circuit is Similar to an Electric Circuit

problems in a machine, you use a capacitor to regulate the current. When there is too much current, the capacitor absorbs and stores the excess, and when it is weak, the capacitor supplies current to the circuit. The eight Qi vessels are your body's capacitors. Qigong increases their level of Qi to supply current when needed, and keep the internal organs functioning smoothly. This is especially important as you get older, when your Qi level is generally lower.

For a healthy circuit, you address the components themselves. If they are weak or of poor quality, the circuit suffers. Qigong maintains and rebuilds the internal organs. There is an important difference between the circuit in the diagram, and the Qi circuit in our bodies. The body is alive, and with proper Qi nourishment, all of the cells can be regrown and the state of health improved. For example, if you jog three miles today, and keep jogging regularly, you can gradually increase the distance to five miles, as your body rebuilds and adjusts to the circumstances.

If we increase Qi flow through our internal organs, they become stronger and healthier. The increase must be slow and gradual so they can adjust to it. To increase Qi flow you work with EMF. Imagine two containers filled with water and connected by a tube. If both have the same water level, water will not flow. However, if one side is higher than the other, the water will flow from that container to the other. In electricity, this potential difference is called electromotive force. The higher the EMF, the stronger the current will be.

The key to effective Qigong practice is reducing resistance in the Qi channels, and increasing the EMF in your body. There are six sources of EMF in the body which can increase the flow of bioelectricity.

1. **Natural energy.** Your body is made of conductive material, so its electro-magnetic field is affected by the sun, moon, clouds, gravity, and other energies around you. The sun, moon, and the earth's gravity affect Qi circulation significantly. We are now also affected by energy pollution by modern technology, such as radio, TV, microwave ovens, computers, and mobile telephone networks.

2. **Food and air.** To maintain life, we absorb food and air through our mouths and noses. These are converted into Qi through the biochemical reaction in the chest and digestive system (called the Triple Burner in Chinese medicine). EMF is generated which circulates Qi through the body. A major part of Qigong is devoted to getting proper food and fresh air.

3. **Thinking.** The mind is the most important source of bioelectric EMF. Any time you move to do something, you first generate an idea (Yi, 意). This idea generates EMF and leads Qi through the nervous system, to energize and move the appropriate muscles. The more you concentrate, the stronger the EMF, and the stronger the flow of Qi you lead to the muscles to energize them. The mind is the most important factor in Qigong training.

4. **Exercise.** Exercise converts stored food essence (fat) into Qi, building up EMF. Many Qigong styles utilize movement for this purpose.

5. **Converting Pre-Birth Essence into Qi.** The hormones produced by our endocrine glands are called Pre-Birth Essence in Chinese medicine. They are converted into Qi to stimulate the function of the body, increasing vitality. Balancing hormone production when you are young, and increasing its production when you are old, are important subjects in Chinese Qigong.

6. **Medical Methods.** In Chinese medicine, methods such as acupuncture, moxibustion and massage generate EMF to regulate irregular Qi in the body. These have become important methods of treatment in Chinese medicine.

The human body has an electrical circuit. To circulate bioelectricity requires a battery or power supply. There are three places which store Qi, called Dan Tians (elixir field). One is called the Lower Dan Tian, located one or two inches below the navel (Xia Dan Tian, 下丹田). The second is at the lower sternum, called the Middle Dan Tian (Zhong Dan Tian, 中丹田). The third is the lower central forehead, or third eye, called the Upper Dan Tian (Shang Dan Tian, 上丹田).

The Lower Dan Tian is the residence of Water Qi, called Original Qi (Yuan Qi, 元氣), generated from Original Essence (Yuan Jing, 元精). In this area is a cavity called Qihai (Co-6, 氣海, Qi ocean). This produces Qi elixir, abundant as the sea.

To accumulate Qi in the Lower Dan Tian, you move your abdomen (Lower Dan Tian) through abdominal breathing. This exercise is called Qi Huo ( 起火 ), which means starting the fire, also called "'back to childhood' breathing" (Fan Tong Hu Xi, 返童呼吸 ). After exercising the Lower Dan Tian for about ten minutes, you feel warmth in the lower abdomen, as Qi accumulates there. Daoists call the abdominal area Dan Lu ( 丹爐 ) which means elixir furnace.

What happens when the abdomen moves? It has about six layers of muscle and fat sandwiched between layers of fascia (Figure 2-21). When your mind moves the abdominal muscles, there is muscular contraction and relaxation, turning fat into bioelectricity. When bioelectricity encounters resistance from the fasciae, it turns into heat. Fat and fasciae are poor electrical conductors, while muscles are relatively good conductors.[11,12,13] When these materials are sandwiched together, they act like a battery. Through abdominal movement, energy is stored and manifests as warmth.

**Real Lower Dan Tian.** The front of the abdomen is not the real Dan Tian, but in fact a False Dan Tian (Jia Dan Tian, 假丹田 ). It generates Qi to a high level, but does not store it for long. It is located on the path of the Conception vessel, so whatever Qi builds up, circulates in the Conception and Governing Vessels. It cannot be a battery as we understand the term, as a real battery should store the Qi. Where then, is the Real Lower Dan Tian (Zhen Xia Dan Tian, 真下丹田 )?

Daoists teach that the Real Lower Dan Tian is at the center inside the abdomen, at the physical center of gravity in the large and small intestines (Figure 2-22).

Life begins with sperm from the father entering an egg from the mother, forming the original human cell (Figure 2-23).[14] This cell divides into two cells, then four, and so on. When this group of cells adheres to the internal wall of the uterus, the umbilical cord

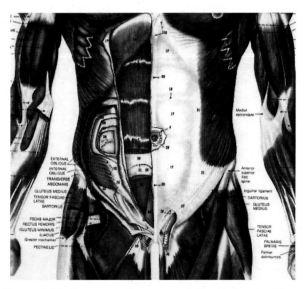

Figure 2-21. Anatomic Structure of the Abdominal Area

starts to develop. Nutrition and energy for further cell multiplication is absorbed from the mother through this cord. The baby's abdomen moves up and down, pumping nutrition and energy into its body. Immediately after birth, air and nutrition are taken in through the nose and mouth, through the mouth's sucking action and the lungs' breathing. The child slowly forgets the natural movement of the abdomen. This is why abdominal breathing is called 'back to childhood breathing.'

If your first human cell were still alive, where would it be? Most likely it died long ago. Approximately one trillion cells die in the body each day.[15] But if this first cell were still alive, it would be located at our center of gravity. From this center, the cells multiply evenly outwards until the body is fully constructed. To maintain this process, Qi must be centered here and radiate outward. In the embryonic state, this is the center of gravity and Qi. As we grow after birth, this center remains.

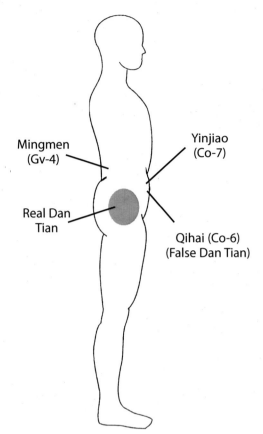

Figure 2-22. The Real Dan Tian and the False Dan Tian

The physical center of gravity is occupied by the Large and Small intestines (Figure 2-24). There are three kinds of muscle in our bodies, classified according to our ability to control them. The first is the heart muscle, in which the electrical conductivity is the highest. The heart beats all the time, regardless of our attention, and through practice and discipline, we can only regulate its beating, not start or stop it. The second category of muscles are those which contract automatically, but over which we can exert significant control if we make the effort. The diaphragm which controls breathing, our eyelids, and certain sexual responses are examples of this muscle type, and their electrical conductivity is lower than the first type. The third kind of muscle is directly controlled by our conscious mind. Their electric conductivity is the lowest of the three groups.

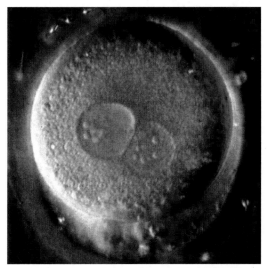

Figure 2-23. Original First Human Cell

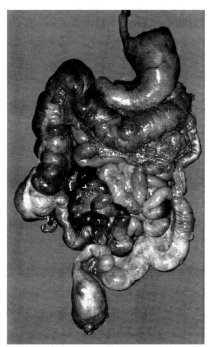

Figure 2-24. Anatomic Structure of the Real
Dan Tian—Large and Small Intestines

The total length of your Large and Small Intestines is approximately six times your body's height (Figure 2-25). With such long electrically conductive tissue sandwiched between the linings, which it is reasonable to believe are poor conductors, it acts like a huge battery in our body (Figure 2-26).[16] So the center of gravity, rather than the False Dan Tian, is the real battery in our body.

**Second Brain.** According to a 1996 report in *The New York Times*, the human body has two brains: one in the head, and the other in the digestive system, which is known as the *Enteric Nervous System*.[17,18] Though these two brains are separated physically, they function as one through the connection of the spinal cord, which is highly conductive tissue (Figure 2-27).

The article explained that the upper brain thinks and remembers, storing data, and uses electrochemical charges. The lower brain has memory but not the capacity for thought. This discovery confirms the Chinese belief that the Real Lower Dan Tian, in the large and small intestines, stores Qi, while the Upper Dan Tian governs thinking and directs the Qi. The upper brain thinks, so it should be able to generate EMF, while the lower brain should have a large capacity for storing this charge. In other words, the lower brain is the human battery in which the life force resides. Once the upper brain generates an idea (EMF), the charge is directed from the lower brain, through the spinal cord and nervous system, to activate the appropriate part of the body.[18]

According to Ohm's Law in physics,

$$\Delta V = i\,R$$

where $\Delta V$ is potential difference or EMF, $i$ is current, and $R$ is resistance.[19]

If $R$ is constant, then the higher the potential or EMF, the stronger the current generated. If we assume the resistance of our body remains constant, then the more we concentrate the EMF, the stronger the Qi flow will be. This parallels the Qigong concept that *the more you concentrate, the higher your energy level.* Qigong trains higher levels of concentration through still meditation. If EMF is constant, that means the mind's concentration remains the same. Then, the lower the $R$, the higher the current flow will be. According to Qigong, the more you relax, the more Qi can flow.

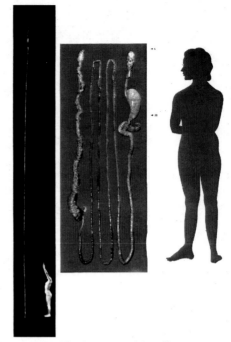

Figure 2-25. The Large and Small Intestines are About Six Times Your Height

We also examine the formula for manifestation of physical power:

$$\text{Power} = \Delta V \times i = i^2\,R$$

The power generated depends on the current and the resistance. When one manifests physical strength, one tenses the body. This increases the body's resistance, energy (current) is trapped in the muscles and power manifested. It is the same in external hard martial arts styles, such as Tiger and Eagle, which focus on building the muscles and tendons to manifest power to its highest level.

The approach of the soft internal martial styles and Internal Elixir Qigong is quite different. Current is the energy manifested, and its influence on power is much more significant, since current is squared in the formula, therefore practitioners pay more attention to cultivating a stronger flow of Qi. Meditation is vital for this, since it generates EMF to move the current. Smooth Qi circulation requires physical resistance or tension to be at a minimum, so relaxation is the key to the internal styles.

The most focused manifestation of power which can be generated should come from both energy and muscle, both the current and the resistance. Sacrifice either one, and power is reduced. Soft-hard martial styles of Qigong, such as White Crane,

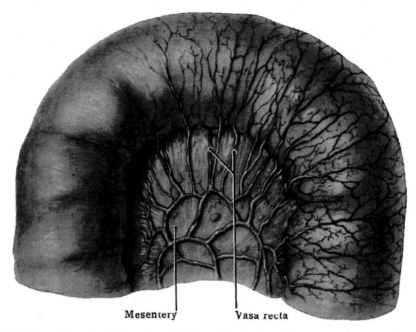

**Figure 2-26. Low Electrically Conductive Materials Such as Mesentery, Outer Casing, and Water in and Around the Intestines Makes the Entire Area Act Like a Battery**
(Used with permission: James E. Anderson, M.D., Grant's Atlas of Anatomy, 7th ed., ©Williams and Wilkins)

Xingyiquan, and Da Mo's Yi Jin Jing, emphasize both Qi (current) and tension (resistance). They do so by keeping the body as relaxed as possible, while using the concentrated mind to lead Qi to the body. Once Qi is led from the Lower Dan Tian to the limbs, right before impact, they suddenly tense the body. These are called soft-hard styles, emphasizing both internal and external manifestation of power.

**Middle Dan Tian.** The Middle Dan Tian is located at the diaphragm, which is a membranous muscular partition separating the abdominal and thoracic cavities (Figure 2-28). It functions in respiration and is a highly electrically conductive material. Above and below it are fasciae, which

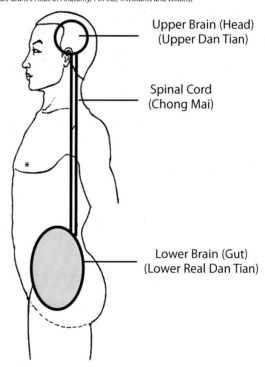

Figure 2-27. Two Polarities (Brains)
of a Human Body

71

isolate the internal organs from the diaphragm. Here again is a good electrical conductor isolated by poor electrical conductors, thus able to store electricity or Qi. Since it is between the lungs and the stomach, which assimilate Post-Birth Essence, namely air and food, into energy, the Qi accumulated in the Middle Dan Tian is classified as Fire Qi (Huo Qi, 火氣). Naturally, this Fire Qi can also agitate your emotional mind.

**Upper Dan Tian.** The brain is the Upper Dan Tian. The brain and the spinal cord constitute the central nervous system, having the highest electrical conductivity in the body. The brain is segregated into separate portions by the arachnoid mater, a delicate membrane of the spinal cord and brain, lying between the pia mater and dura mater (Figure 2-29). It is reasonable to assume that these tissues are poor elec-

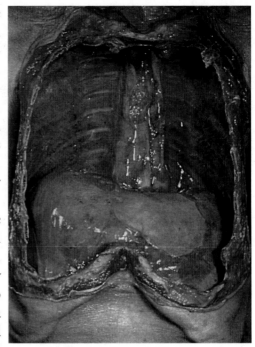

Figure 2-28. The Middle Dan Tian is Connected to the Diaphragm

trical conductors. This is another giant energy center which consumes a great amount of Qi, although it does not produce any itself.

In this way we can compare ancient experience with modern scientific understanding. Let us also look at Qigong from another scientific point of view, this time chemical.

**Cell Replacement.** When we breathe, we inhale oxygen and exhale a lot of carbon in the form of carbon dioxide (Figure 2-30). Where does this carbon come from, and how much is actually processed out through breathing? The first source of carbon is from the food (glucose) we eat. Food is converted into energy, yielding carbon dioxide.[20]

$$\text{glucose} + 6O_2 \longrightarrow 6CO_2 + 6H_2O$$

$$\Delta G^{o\prime} = -686 \text{ Kcal (energy content)}$$

The second source of carbon is from dead cells. The body is constructed mainly from carbon, hydrogen, oxygen and nitrogen, while other elements such as Calcium (Ca), Potassium (P), Chlorine (Cl), Sulfur (S), Potassium (K), Sodium (Na), Magnesium (Mg), Iodine (I), and Iron (Fe) comprise much less of our body weight.

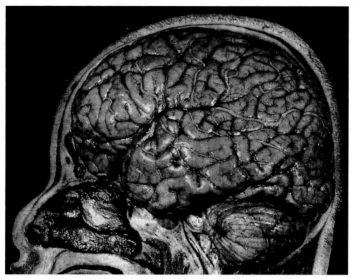

Figure 2-29. The Upper Dan Tian—The Human Brain

As many as a trillion cells die in the body every 24 hours.[15] The average lifespan of a skin cell is 28 days. Different cells such as those of the bone, marrow or liver each have their own individual lifespans. We rely on our respiration to expel the carbon from the dead cells and to supply living cells with fresh oxygen. Carbon and other minerals are replenished from the food we eat. This process is vital to the formation of new cells and the continuation of life.

The cell replacement process is ongoing and continuous. Health during our lifetime depends on how smoothly and quickly it is carried out. If there are more new healthy cells to replace the old cells, you live and grow. If the cells replaced are as healthy as the original cells, you remain young. If fewer cells are produced or if the new ones are not as healthy as the original ones, then you age.

To produce healthy cells requires hydrogen, oxygen, carbon, and other minerals which we absorb from air or food. Air quality, water purity, and the choice of food become critical factors when considering your health and longevity.

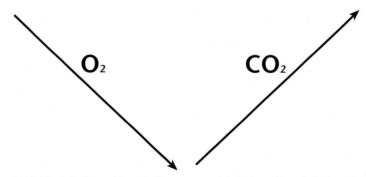

Figure 2-30. We Inhale to Absorb Oxygen and Exhale to Expel Carbon Dioxide

Air and water are being contaminated by pollution, especially in cities and industrial areas. The quality of food we eat depends on their source and processing methods. It is not easy to find the same pristine environment as in ancient times. However, we must adapt our new environment and choose our way of life wisely.

Since carbon comprises such a major part of our body, absorbing good quality carbon is an important issue in modern health. You may obtain it from animal products or from plants. Carbon from plants is generally more pure than that taken from animals.

Red meat is more contaminated then white meat, so is more likely to disturb and overstimulate your emotional mind and confuse your thinking. Fish is another good source of carbon, but of course some fish are better than others. Shrimp is high in cholesterol, which can increase the risk of high blood pressure.

Due to the high level of impurities in most animal products, Qigong practitioners have spent a lot of time and effort searching for ways to efficiently absorb the protein they needed from plants, such as peas and beans. Soy beans are one of the best of these sources. They are inexpensive and easy to grow, but for a non-vegetarian it can be difficult for the body to produce the enzymes required to digest an all-vegetable diet. Humans evolved as omnivores, and the craving for meat can be strong. Even today, we still have canine teeth, used to tear off raw meat in ancient times. The natural enzymes in the body are more tailored to digesting meat. If we placed meat and corn in human digestive enzymes, the meat would dissolve in a matter of minutes, while the corn could take hours. So it is generally easier for the body to absorb the carbon it needs from meat than from plants.

This does not mean that we are unable to absorb plant protein efficiently. The key is that if an enzyme is present to begin with, then its production can be increased within your body, but it will take time. If you wish to become a vegetarian, you must reduce the intake of meat products slowly and allow your body to adjust to it, otherwise you may experience protein deficiency.

We must consume a variety of foods instead of concentrating only on those that are high in protein, to ensure we absorb all the various vitamins and trace minerals the body requires. Although they comprise only a minor proportion of our bodies they are still essential in order for it to run smoothly. Calcium is important for bone development, and iron is crucial for healthy blood.

Nutrition is only one side of the coin. When a person ages quickly it may be due to poor Qi storage and circulation as opposed to malnourishment. Without an abundant supply, Qi circulation will not be regulated efficiently and your physical body will begin to degenerate. Qigong builds up the Qi in your Eight Vessels and helps you circulate it in your body. This Qigong training includes Wai Dan (External Elixir) and Nei Dan (Internal Elixir) practice, which we discuss in the next section.

While nutrition and Qi circulation are very important, the efficiency of the whole cell replacement process depends on the blood cells, which carry water, oxygen, and nutrients everywhere in the body through the blood circulatory network. From arteries and capillaries, the components for new cells are brought to even the most remote places in the body. The old cells absorb everything required from the blood stream and divide to produce new cells. The remaining material from the dead cells is brought back through the veins to the lungs. Through respiration, the dead cells are expelled as carbon dioxide. Qi is vital for the process of cell division. Every blood cell is actually a dipole or small battery, storing bioelectricity and releasing it.[11] In Chinese medicine, it is understood that blood and Qi are always together. Where there is blood, there is Qi, and vice versa. The term Qi-Xue (Qi-Blood, 氣血) is often used in Chinese medicine.

The arteries are located deep beneath the muscles, while the veins are near the skin surface. The color of the blood in the arteries is red, because of the presence of oxygen. In the veins it looks blue, due to the absence of this oxygen and the presence of carbon. Cell replacement starts inside the body, moving outward. If we tense more, blood circulation will be stagnant and the cell replacement process slower. Most cell replacement occurs at night, as we relax during sleep. So the importance of sleep in promoting health and longevity is obvious.

We must consider the means of ensuring steady production of healthy blood cells to maintain health and prevent premature aging. Without sufficient blood cells, the cell replacement process stagnates, and you degenerate swiftly.

Blood cells have a certain lifespan. When old ones die, new ones must be produced from the bone marrow to replace them. Bone marrow is the major blood factory of the body. When a person turns thirty, the marrow near the end of the bone cavities begins to turn yellow, as fat accumulates there. Red blood cells are no longer produced in the yellow area (Figure 2-31).[21] Qigong practitioners believe the degeneration of the bone marrow is due to insufficient Qi supply, and so Bone Marrow Washing Qigong was developed.

Hormone production also affects cell replacement. Hormones act as catalysts in the body. When hormone levels are high, we are more energized, and cell replacement proceeds faster and more smoothly. When hormone production is low, cell replacement will be slow and we age quickly. By increasing hormone levels, we extend life significantly.[22]

Maintaining healthy hormone production is a major concern in Qigong practice. Glands which produce hormones were recognized since ancient times, but hormones themselves were not well understood. They understood that the essence of life was stored in the kidneys. Today, we know this essence is actually the hormones produced by the adrenal glands on the top of the kidneys. They believed that through stimulation of the testicles and ovaries, the life force could be increased. From still meditation practice, they learned to lead Qi to the brain to raise up the spirit of vitality. It is led to the pituitary gland to stimulate growth hormone production. These practices are effective paths to longevity. Hormone levels decline significantly once our bones are complete, about the age of 30. Once the body has finished constructing itself, it triggers the reduction of hormone levels.

To prevent illness, we also consider our immune system. When Qi storage is abundant, you get sick less. Every white blood cell is like a fighting soldier who needs food to maintain his strength. When Qi is strong, the immune system is strong. Skin breathing was developed to lead Qi to the surface of the skin and strengthen the Guardian Qi (Wei Qi, 衛氣), the energetic component of the immune system near the skin surface.

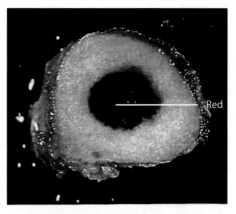

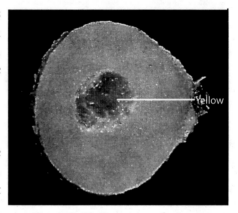

Figure 2-31. Structure of a Long Bone. Red Bone Marrow and Yellow Bone Marrow

## 2-4. Meaning and Purpose of Meditation
靜坐之意義與目的

Many different schools of meditation have developed to serve a wide range of purposes. Meditation has existed in some form in almost every culture around the world, especially in religious societies. In some of these societies religious meditation has reached a very high level.

In China, different schools of meditation exist in almost all levels of society. In medical and scholar society, meditation is called Jing Zuo (靜坐) which means to sit quietly. It is used to bring the mind to a neutral, harmonious, and calm state. Many illnesses and mental problems are caused by emotional disturbances, so if we neutralize these emotional imbalances, we remove the causes of illness and emotional pain. This meditation is considered suitable for lay society, and was designed for regulating the mind and not aggressively pursuing regulation of the spirit.

Chinese martial society also uses meditation to seek the meaning of life and raising up the spirit. When the meaning of life is comprehended during meditation, a peaceful mind is attained, namely Yin calmness. Then, Qi is led effectively to the body for Yang power manifestation. Balancing this Yin and Yang, a martial artist reaches a level of deep martial skill and profound understanding of harmony and peace. Most well known Chinese martial styles such as Shaolin 少林 ), Taiji (太極), Wudang (武當), Emei (峨嵋), Tianshan (天山), Qingcheng (青城), and Kunlun

(崑崙) were developed in the monasteries. Their meditation methods were influenced strongly by religious meditation and in many ways cannot be separated.

Religious meditation is called Zuo Chan (坐禪) in Buddhism, meaning sit for Chan, and Da Zuo (打坐) in Daoism, meaning to sit. Chan means to cultivate, refine or pursue the state of Buddhahood. In the Buddhist *A Han Classic* it says (阿含經), "Sit for Chan and ponder the origin, do not be neglectful and lazy."[23] Through Chan meditation, you search for the source of spiritual life.

The final goal of religious meditation is enlightenment (Daoist) or Buddhahood (Buddhism). Religious meditation is the highest level of meditation in Chinese society. Aspirants not only strive to achieve peace and harmony by neutralizing the emotional mind, but unification with the natural spirit (Tian Ren He Yi, 天人合一). To achieve this, abundant Qi storage in the Lower Real Dan Tian must strengthen the physical body and nourish the brain to an enlightened state. When the body is strong, life will be long, allowing you more time for spiritual cultivation. When the brain is nourished sufficiently, the third eye can be opened. Then the spirit is reunited with the natural spirit, and the purpose of life attained.

First establish the goal of your mediation training. Are you cultivating a peaceful mind, or martial arts, or enlightenment? Then determine the path to reach your goal. How do you find the correct way? How committed are you? Do you have enough patience, perseverance, and a strong enough will to actively pursue your goals? Without a clear idea of where you are going and how to get there you will soon lose your way and give up.

The Small Circulation Meditation introduced in this book originates from Chinese religious society. Its first goal is to store abundant Qi at the Lower Real Dan Tian. The second goal is leading Qi to circulate in the two major Qi vessels, the Conception and Governing Vessels (Ren Mai, Du Mai, 任脈・督脈). When the Qi is strong and circulating smoothly in these two vessels, the Qi circulating in the Twelve Primary Qi Channels is strong, and the body strong and healthy.

In the next section, we summarize the purposes of general meditation. Small Circulation, Grand Circulation, and Enlightenment meditation will be discussed later in this chapter.

## Purposes of General Meditation

**The search for a peaceful mind.** The most common purpose of meditation is to train the mind to be relaxed, calm and harmonious. Without meditation, the mind is generally emotionally agitated by surrounding circumstances, being scattered, confused, and excited. Through meditation with deep breathing, we can calm and clear the mind.

Using an EEG (Electroencephalogram), four separate groups of brainwaves (oscillating electrical currents) have been classified according to their frequency bands, with different activities related to each band.

These four categories are: (Figure 2-32)[24]

1. Beta activity (above 13 Hz): Occurs in bursts in the anterior part of the brain and is associated with mental activity.

2. Alpha activity (8-13 Hz): Relaxation, daydreaming.

3. Theta activity (4 to less than 8 Hz): Drowsy or asleep.

4. Delta activity (below 4 Hz): Deep sleep and coma.

When we are awake and thinking deeply (Beta), there is a lot of activity, but its amplitude is low. On average, 13 or more thoughts pass through our brain per second. By contrast, in the Alpha state of relaxation, although the signals are still almost as weak, the number of oscillations is significantly reduced. This implies that a calm mind has more clarity and focus. In the Theta state of drowsiness or sleep, the number of oscillations is also reduced, but the thoughts are more irregular. In deep, sound sleep (Delta), the number of oscillations is reduced substantially, while the amplitude is significantly increased. In scientific terms, the power of oscillation is as follows:[25]

$$P \propto Frequency^2 \times Amplitude^2$$

"Power is directly proportional to Frequency squared times Amplitude squared."

In deep sleep, although your conscious mind is not deeply involved in thought (frequency reduced), the brain cells obtain a large supply of nutrition, oxygen, and Qi nourishment. In this calm state, there is less disturbance in the brain. Under these

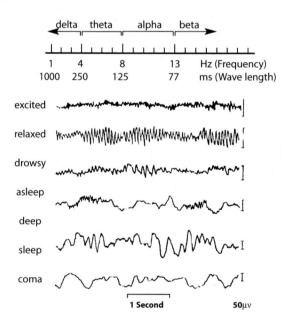

Figure 2-32. Typical Brain Wave Patterns from a
State of Excitement to One of Deep Coma

extremely calm and relaxed conditions, if you can control your consciousness without falling asleep, you can build up a better sensitivity for energy correspondence with the outside world. This is one of the desired states in meditation practice.

In meditation, you try to reach the stage at which the brainwaves are between Theta and Delta. It seems you are sleeping, yet your conscious mind is still governing the being. In this semi-sleeping or self-hypnotic state, the brain's sensitivity or energy correspondence with other brainwaves or natural vibrations reaches a peak. It is in this state that a meditator seeks the connection between his spiritual being and the spirit of nature.

**Improving health and healing.** When the mind is relaxed and calm, the body will be too. The more profound meditative state the mind reaches, the deeper the body can relax. When both mind and body relax, the Qi circulates smoothly and naturally. In this way, irregular Qi circulation due to illness or any other reason can be regulated to a healthy state of harmony. This is the main method used in Chinese medicine for healing and maintaining health. During deep meditation and relaxation, mind-body communication is efficient, Qi circulation is stronger, and the healing process faster.

During deep meditation, the breathing will be deep, soft and slender, which enables you to absorb oxygen and expel carbon dioxide more efficiently. Each brain cell consumes about twelve times as much oxygen as other cells, so a steady oxygen supply is crucial to keep the brain healthy. Deep exhalation of carbon dioxide disposes of waste from remote parts of the body. This is important for replacement of cells in the body.

**To find the center of self-being.** When you calm down, your mind becomes clearer and your thought processes more logical. You must prevent your mind from wandering to memories or into fantasy, called entering the devil (Ru Mo, 入魔). The best is to pay attention to the breathing, and keep the mind honest and truthful.

There are four steps to reach the final goal of spiritual freedom. The first is self-recognition (Zi Shi, 自識), where the mask you wear starts to drop off, allowing you to recognize your spiritual being more clearly. Mistakes you have made and lies you have told are buried in your subconscious and will gradually arise in your conscious awareness. Your subconscious mind is always truthful and associated with the spiritual being. Once you discard the mask you have been wearing, you must face the real you. You encounter the past and analyze it. Not only that, to attain deep emotional balance, you search for ways to release feelings of guilt hidden deep inside. This process makes you humble, helps you understand yourself better, and finally helps you find the center of your being.

The next step is self-awareness (Zi Jue, 自覺). By paying attention, you become aware of your spiritual being and the problems existing within yourself. You become more aware of your thinking and behavior, as well as that of others. You analyze your existence, your problems, and the role you should play in society. Through this self-awareness meditation process, you establish a calm and peaceful mind which harmonizes you with others and with nature.

**To search for and understand the meaning of our lives.** The third stage of cultivation is called self-awakening (Zi Xing, Zi Wu, 自醒・自悟). Through this stage you pay attention, collect information, and understand yourself and your environment. Many people, after this awakening process, see how ugly human nature is and decide to separate from lay society and become hermits or monks. Others build up their self-confidence and make their lives more meaningful.

**The search for spiritual freedom.** Realizing that we are being abused by political and spiritual leaders, the search begins for freedom from spiritual bondage (Jie Tuo, 解脫), known as spiritual independence. When you reach this stage, your spiritual being can be independent and does not need to rely on others.

**To comprehend the meaning of the universe.** Many non-religious people try through meditation to comprehend the meaning, root, or origin of nature, searching for the truth of the Dao. The first step is to search for the root of our lives (Sheng Ming Zhi Ben, 生命之本). Since our lives are a part of nature, from understanding the root of our lives, we comprehend the meaning of nature. To keep and cherish this root is called embracing the origin (Bao Yuan, Bao Yi, 抱元・抱一).

The three origins of our lives are Original Essence (Yuan Jing, 元精), Original Qi (Yuan Qi, 元氣), and Original Spirit (Yuan Shen, 元神). Original spirit is the origin of the others, since it exists before physical life begins. Searching for the spiritual root is the most important cultivation in Chinese society. Daoists say, "Cultivate the Xin (emotional mind) to cultivate the natural being. Keep the center and embrace the origin."[26] Scholarly society says, "Pay attention to the Xin to cultivate the natural being. Maintain the center to fully comprehend the origin."[27]

By contrast, the Buddhist family says: "Understand the Xin clearly to grasp human nature. Millions of methods return to one."[28] The medical family says: "Void Xin (humble mind) to stabilize the human natural being, cherish the origin and keep it."[29] The "one" is explained in a classic entitled the *Classic of Great Peace* (太平經). It says, "Ponder to keep one, why? What is one? The beginning of the counting numbers. What is one? The Dao of begetting. What is one? The beginning of the raising of the Qi? What is one? The root principle of the universe."[30] The "one" means the very origin of all matter and energy. According to *The Book of Change* (Yi Jing, 易經), this "one" means the state of Wuji (無極), of no extremity. The Daoist book, *The Complete Book of Principal Contents of Life and Human Nature* (*Xing Ming Gui Zhi Quan Shu*, 性命圭旨全書) says, "What the scholar means by the one, is to use the original body to understand human nature."[31] It is also said in Daoist family that, "Dao, use the one to understand thoroughly."[32]

Even in secular meditation practice, the goals of meditation can be divided into levels ranging from beginner to profound. All of these spiritual regulation processes are also pursued by other Qigong groups such as martial artists.

## 2-5. Muscle/Tendon Changing and Marrow/Brain Washing Qigong
易筋經與洗髓經

We should be familiar with the Qigong practice of Muscle/Tendon Changing (Yi Jin Jing, 易筋經) and Marrow/Brain Washing (Xi Sui Jin, 洗髓經). Small Circulation meditation plays a major role in this practice.

Our two bodies are the physical (Yang) body and the energy (Yin) body. The physical body consists of skin, muscle, tendon, ligament, bone, and marrow. The energy body refers to the structure supplying Qi to the physical body and the brain.

Many Qigong practitioners consider the Yin (Qi) body to be some kind of mental or spiritual body. Qi is neutral, supplying energy to the physical body for movement, and to the brain to support thought and behavior. But since thought and mental behavior are so closely related to spiritual cultivation, Chinese religious society regards the spiritual body to be the same as the Yin body. The physical body is called Ming (命) which means life, while the spiritual body is called Xing (性), which means human nature, namely the natural spirit we are born with.

Muscle/Tendon Changing and Marrow/Brain Washing Qigong are religious Qigong training methods, created and passed down by an Indian monk, Da Mo, in a Chinese Buddhist monastery called the Shaolin Temple (少林寺)(Figures 2-33 and 2-34). In Da Mo's classic, he emphasizes that to achieve spiritual enlightenment, we need a long and healthy life, which will allow us more time for spiritual cultivation. Muscle/Tendon Changing Qigong describes how to condition the body, while Marrow/Brain Washing Qigong teaches how to build up an abundant supply of Qi with which to nourish the brain and promote its function to a higher level. Then, the final goal of spiritual enlightenment can be reached:

> *The Xi Sui Jing says a man's body is touched by love and desire, and formed with shape, contaminated by sediment and dirtiness. If you wish to cultivate the real meaning of Buddhism, (Spirit) moving and stopping at will, then the five viscera and six bowels, four limbs and hundreds of bones must be completely washed clean individually. (When you are) pure and can see calmness and peace, (you) can cultivate and enter the domain of Buddhahood. If you do not cultivate this way, (your cultivation) will not have foundation and origin. Read till here, then know that believers thought that "acquiring the marrow" was not just a comparison.*

洗髓經者，謂人之生，感於愛慾，一落有形，悉皆滓穢；
欲修佛諦，動障真如，五臟六腑，四肢百骸，必先一一
洗滌淨盡，純見清虛，方可進修，入佛智地，不由此經
進修，無基無有是處；讀至此，然後知向者所謂得髓者，
非譬喻也。

*The Yi Jin Jing says that outside of the bone and marrow, under the skin and meat (muscles), there is nothing but the tendons and vessels which connect the body and transport the blood and Qi. All these are post-birth body, and must be promoted (trained). Borrow them to cultivate the real (Dao). If you do not promote them, you see weakening and withering immediately. If you see this just as ordinary training, how could you reach the final goal? If you give up and do not train them, there is no strength for cultivation, and nothing can be achieved. (When I read till here, then I know that what were called skin, meat, and bones are also not a comparison and not a casual comment.*

易筋者，謂髓骨之外，皮肉之內，莫非筋聯絡周身，通
行血氣，凡屬後天，皆其提挈，借假修真，非所贊勤，
立見頹靡，視作泛常，曷臻極至？舍是不為，進修不力，
無有是處；讀至此，然後知所謂皮肉骨者，非譬喻，亦
非漫語也。

From these two paragraphs, you can see that Muscle/Tendon Changing is for developing the body, while Marrow/Brain Washing is for spiritual advancement. This concept was very important to religious Qigong meditators. The ultimate goal of both Buddhist and Daoist study is to reach Buddhahood or enlightenment. They believe it normally takes hundreds of lifetimes to cultivate the spirit, and that gradually lifetime after lifetime, you progress toward the final destination. If each lifetime is long, you have more time for spiritual cultivation. The physical conditioning is critical, especially as the most effective period for spiritual cultivation is after the age of forty. Normally, before then, the spirit of your new life is still maturing to be able to make contact with your pre-birth spirit. If you live a long and healthy life, you have enough time to develop your spirit to a higher level. The longer your life, the higher the level of cultivation, of maturity and wisdom your spirit can reach.

The importance of longevity to spiritual cultivation was well understood by

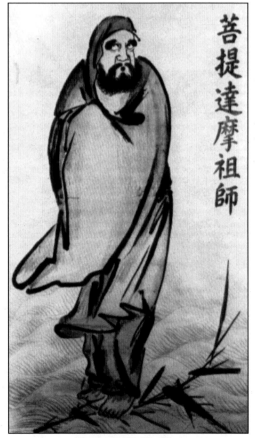

菩提達摩祖師

Figure 2-33. Da Mo

Daoists but was somewhat neglected by Buddhists. Daoists believe that both the physical body and spiritual body are of equal importance and should be cultivated together. It is called dual cultivation of spiritual virtues and physical life (Xing Ming Shuang Xiu, 性命雙修) in Daoist society. This was not the case in Buddhist society. Buddhists believe our physical body is only a temporary residence for the spirit, and spending time to build up physical strength is wasting precious time that could be spent on spiritual cultivation. Let us summarize the differences of approach to Muscle/Tendon Changing and Marrow/Brain Washing training in Buddhist and Daoist societies.

1. Although Buddhists developed these two training classics, they kept them strictly secret, without much opportunity to develop and evolve. Once Daoists learned them, they continued to research and develop them, and it seems the Daoist methods and theory are more complete and systematic than those of the Buddhists.

2. The Daoists have revealed more of their training to the public than the Buddhists have. Daoist training can produce health and longevity faster than the Buddhist training can, and can be practiced by seculars who do not wish to give up their normal existence for a life of seclusion. For this reason, more Daoist training documents have been found than Buddhist. However, the original theory, principles, and training methods were recorded in the Buddhist bibles.

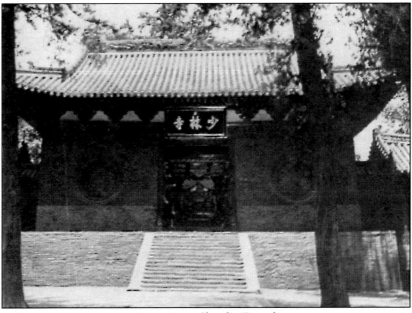

Figure 2-34. Shaolin Temple

3. Due to this constant research and development, many training techniques developed by the Daoists are more effective and efficient than the Buddhist alternatives, to improve health and increase longevity. However, when the training reaches the higher levels of spiritual cultivation found in the Xi Sui Jing, it seems the Buddhist methods of training are more effective. The Buddhists focus on training for the future instead of the present, while the Daoists to a certain extent pay more attention to the present.

4. Daoists have developed many techniques such as dual cultivation or Picking the Herb from Outside of the Dao to assist the Xi Sui Jing training. Some Daoists encourage gaining Qi balance through dual meditation or sexual practices. Sexual Qigong has always been forbidden in the Buddhist monasteries. This is probably the most significant difference between the two schools of training.

5. Daoist Xi Sui Jing training comprises both physical and spiritual practices, while the Buddhist approach is mainly spiritual. Daoist training begins with many physical exercises, such as massaging the testicles. The physical stimulation generates semen, which is converted into Qi either physically or mentally. The Daoist documents discuss many physical training techniques, while the Buddhist training emphasizes meditation.

6. Daoists have researched the use of herbs to assist Qigong training, while the Buddhists have never paid much attention to this. The Daoist documents have more herbal prescriptions than the Buddhist documents.

## Kan and Li in Yi Jin Jing and Xi Sui Jing

In any style of Qigong, you balance Yin and Yang by controlling Kan (坎, Water) and Li (離, Fire). Taijiquan trains slow meditative physical movements which are examples of Li, and may make your body too Yang. You balance this with still meditation, which is Kan and neutralizes excess Yang. In moving Taiji forms, there is also Kan and Li adjustment. While the moving is Li which causes Yang, the calm mind is Kan, which neutralizes the Yang. In still meditation, while the stillness of the physical body is Kan and causes Yin, the Qi must be actively led to circulate in the body, which is Li and results in Yang, which balances the Yin. In all Qigong practices, if there is Yin, there must be Yang to balance it, and vice versa.

It is the same with the Yi Jin Jing and Xi Sui Jing training. They are based on this Yin and Yang concept. *The Yi Jin Jing is Li because it generates Qi and causes Yang, while the Xi Sui Jing is Kan, utilizing and storing Qi, and causing Yin.* The Yi Jin Jing deals with the muscles, tendons, and skin, which are visible externally, while the Xi Sui Jing deals with the marrow and brain, which must be felt internally. While the Yi Jin Jing training emphasizes the physical body, the Xi Sui Jing training focuses on the spiritual. Thus Yin and Yang are balanced and coexist harmoniously.

In the Yi Jin Jing, the physical stimulation and exercises are considered Li, and cause the body to become Yang, while the still meditation for the Small Circulation is Kan, calming Li and makes the body more Yin. In the physical stimulation Li training, external strength is Li, while internal mental strength is Kan. In still meditation, the physical body is still and Kan, while the Qi led by the mind and moving internally is Li.

The same theory prevails in Xi Sui Jing training. The physical stimulation to increase the Original Essence production is Li, while the techniques of internal cultivation, which are used to lead Qi to the marrow and brain, are Kan.

The key to successful Qigong training is Yin and Yang balance, and the means to achieve this is adjustment of Kan and Li. This fundamental theory is the foundation of Qigong practice.

### The Role of Small Circulation in Yi Jin Jing and Xi Sui Jing

1. **To store and enhance Qi in the Real Lower Dan Tian to an abundant level.** To recondition the body from weak to strong, and to flood the brain with Qi for brain washing, you require abundant Qi, without which you cannot progress. The way to build up the Qi and store it in the Real Lower Dan Tian is through Embryonic Breathing (Tai Xi, 胎息) techniques, which are discussed later.

2. **To raise the level of Qi circulation in the Conception and Governing Vessels.** Once Qi is abundant in the Real Lower Dan Tian, the second goal of Small Circulation training is to lead it to the Conception and Governing Vessels (Ren Mai, Du Mai, 任脈・督脈). It circulates smoothly in these two vessels, which act as Qi reservoirs, and in the twelve channels, which function as rivers. With abundant Qi in the reservoirs, the Qi in the rivers can be regulated efficiently. The Conception Vessel regulates the Qi level of the six primary Yin channels, while the Governing Vessel regulates the six primary Yang channels. These twelve channels connect the Qi from the limbs to that of the internal organs. Once Qi is abundant and circulating smoothly in these twelve channels, your physical body will be stronger and healthier.

Small Circulation is actually a Muscle/Tendon Changing practice to recondition the body, while Embryonic Breathing helps establish the Qi storage necessary for the Marrow/Brain Washing practice.

## 2-6. WHAT IS SMALL CIRCULATION?

何謂小周天？

In this section, we discuss the three common Qi paths in Qigong meditation practice (Figure 2-35). From this we may define Small Circulation. Each of these three paths has its own training theory, purposes, and methods. Generally speaking, the Fire Path described below is recognized as Small Circulation.

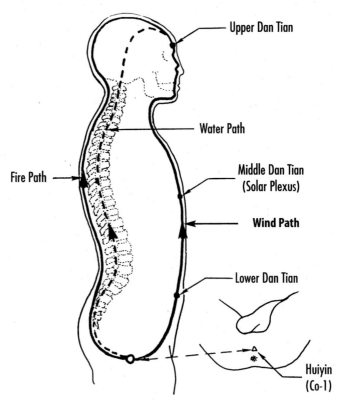

### Three Paths

**Fire Path (Small Circulation Meditation) (Huo Lu, 火路).** In Fire Path circulation, having built up abundant Qi in the Real Lower Dan Tian (Zhen Xia Dan Tian, 真下丹田)

Figure 2-35. The Fire, Water, and Wind Paths of Qi Circulation

through Embryonic Breathing, you then use your mind to lead Qi to the Conception and Governing Vessels (Ren Mai, Du Mai, 任脈 · 督脈). You enhance the Qi in these two Qi reservoirs and then circulate it up the Governing Vessel and down the Conception Vessel, thereby regulating Qi circulation in the Twelve Primary Qi Channels, linking the internal organs and the limbs. This strengthens and energizes the physical body and enhances the Guardian Qi (Wei Qi, 衛氣), making your body Yang. Thus the Fire Path meditation is Li (離, Fire) and generates fire in the body.

There are a few documents relating to the practice of Fire Path circulation. In the book, *Great Attainment of Acupuncture and Moxibustion* (針灸大成), it says, "Slowly swallow a mouthful of air and lead Qi into the Dan Tian. The impulse begins at the Mingmen (命門, navel or Qihai), lead it in the Governing Vessel, pass the Tailbone (Weilu, 尾閭), ascend up to the Niwan (泥丸, crown), to chase and move (initiate or awaken) the origin of human nature. Then lead it down the Conception Vessel, pass the Multi-Towers (Chong Lou, 重樓, throat) and down to return to Qihai (Co-6, 氣海). Two vessels revolving up and down. The front descends and the rear ascends, continuously and without stopping... After practicing for a long time, the tricky gates open automatically. The Qi circulates smoothly in hundreds of meridians and hundreds of sicknesses will not be initiated."[33] In the book, *Antithetic Writing of Regulating the Path* ( 理瀹駢文 ), it says, "Close the eyes and sit quietly. The nose inhales clean air. Expand the abdomen to enable internal Qi to descend to the Lower Dan Tian under the navel. Transport Qi past the perineum, along the Governing Vessel and past the Tailbone (Weilu, 尾閭 ), Squeezing Spine (Jiaji, 夾脊, between the shoulder blades) and Jade Pillow (Yuzhen, 玉枕 ), the three gates. Reach Baihui (Gv-20, 百會 ) cavity on top of the head, follow the face to the tongue and connect with the Conception Vessel, descend down along the front of the chest, to finally reach the Dan Tian and again circulate in the original path. Where there is Qi stagnation or pain, inhale and think of the place, and exhale to lead the Qi back to the Dan Tian. This can strengthen the body and repel sickness. It is also called San Mei Yin (Samadhi, 三昧印 )."[34]

From these two ancient documents, we may assume that Small Circulation Meditation is the same as Fire Path meditation.

**Water Path (Enlightenment Meditation)(Shui Lu, 水路 ).** The Water Path is the hardest but most effective method of using Kan ( 坎, Water) to neutralize the body's Yang. It is trained in Marrow/Brain Washing (Xi Sui Jing, 洗髓經 ). The mind directs Qi from the Real Lower Dan Tian via the Huiyin (Co-1, 會陰 ) up through the Thrusting Vessel (Chong Mai, 衝脈, spinal cord) to nourish the brain. When the brain is well nourished, the spirit can be raised for enlightenment. Water Path training calms the mind, but also helps lead Qi into the center of the body for marrow washing. Since bone marrow is where your body produces white and red blood cells, abundant Qi there promotes their production. Red blood cells carry oxygen and other nutrients required for cell replacement, slowing degeneration of your body. When white blood cells are abundant and healthy, the immune system is strong, preventing illness. Water Path Qigong meditation is for enlightenment or Buddhahood. We will discuss this in detail in future publications on the topics of Grand Circulation and Enlightenment Meditation.

**Wind Path (Kan Li Meditation)(Feng Lu, 風路 ).** The Wind Path is considered to be a reversed Small Circulation. In the Wind Path, the Water Qi accumulated in the Real Lower Dan Tian is led by the mind to circulate in the path which exactly reverses the path of the Fire Path Qi circulation. There are many reasons for this Wind Path Qi circulation. First, through reversing the natural Qi circulation, it is possible to cool down your overexcited mental and physical body. This is because when you practice the Wind Path Qi circulation, you are slowing down the natural Qi circulation. Second, through it you can lead the Water Qi from the Real Lower Dan Tian upward to cool down the Fire Qi accumulated in the Middle Dan Tian (Zhong Dan Tian, 中丹田 )(diaphragm). In this way, the mental and physical body can also be cooled down. This process is commonly called "Kan-Li." However, to Enlightenment Meditation practitioners, the Wind Path is crucial to conceive a

Spiritual Embryo (Ling Tai, 靈胎) at the Huang Ting (黃庭) cavity located between the Middle Dan Tian and Real Lower Dan Tian. In this practice, as mentioned earlier, the Water Qi is led upward to meet the Fire Qi which is led downward from the Middle Dan Tian and they meet each other at the Huang Ting. This process is also called "Kan-Li" (坎離) which causes the interaction of the Yin and Yang. From this Yin-Yang interaction, with the focussed attention of the Shen, a new Spiritual Embryo can be produced.

Small Circulation meditation is generally practiced as Fire Path Qigong meditation. Its two main purposes are to enhance the Qi (Chong Qi, 充氣) in the Real Lower Dan Tian (Zhen Xia Dan Tian, 真下丹田) and to lead the Qi (Yin Qi, 引氣) to circulate smoothly in the Conception and Governing Vessels.

In Daoist society, the name for Small Circulation is Yin-Yang Circulation Small Heavenly Cycle (Yin-Yang Xun Huan Yi Xiao Zhou Tian, 陰陽循環一小周天). In Buddhist society it is called San Mei Yin (三昧印) or San Mo Di (三摩地), adopted from the Sanskrit word Samhadi. Since both societies have very different names for the same practice it indicates that Small Circulation has been practiced intensely by both Daoist and Buddhist societies.

In *Anthology of Daoist Village* (道鄉集), it says, "The Cycling Heaven (Small Circulation) of the Daoist family is the same as Turning the Wheel of Law (Zhuan Fa Lun, 轉法輪) of the Buddhist family. The principles are the same though the approaches are different. It was the descendant people themselves that separated them."[35] Small Circulation is called Xiao Zhou Tian (小周天) which means Small Heavenly Cycle. Since humans are an integral part of nature, Qi circulation in the human body should resemble and be influenced by the Qi circulation between heaven and earth. Therefore, the head is referred to as Tian Liang Gai (天靈蓋), which means Heavenly Spiritual Cover, while the perinium is called Hai Di (海底) which means sea bottom. The Qi circulation between Heaven and Earth is called Da Zhou Tian (大周天), or Grand Heavenly Cycle. Qi circulating within the human body between the head and the perinium is called Xiao Zhou Tian (小周天), or Small Heavenly Cycle. Qi circulation through the Conception and Governing Vessels is closely related to and influenced by that of Heaven and Earth in 24-hour cycles.

Buddhist society also referred to Small Circulation meditation as Zhuan Fa Lun (轉法論) which means Turning the Wheel of Natural Law. Fa Lun (法輪) was translated from the Indian word Dharmachakra which is a common name for Buddhism.[36] In the book, *The Complete Book of Principal Contents of Life and Human Nature* (性命圭旨全書), it says, "The Buddhist family call it Ruling Wheel (Fa Lun, 法輪), the Daoist family call it Heavenly Cycle (Zhou Tian, 周天), and Confucians call it Circulating the Heavenly Court (Xing Ting, 行庭). But all have the same basis."[37] This document also describes the methods of practice in turning the Ruling Wheels. The interaction of Yin and Yang governs nature, and comprises the natural Ruling Wheels which influence the variations of the Qi circulation in Heaven and Earth.

Li, Shi-Zhen (李時珍)(1518-1593 A.D.) wrote in his book, *The Study of Strange Meridians and Eight Vessels* (奇經八脈考), "The Conception and Governing Vessels are the body's Zi (midnight) and Wu (noon). It is the Dao (Natural Way) of increasing the Yang fire and decreasing the Yin water. It is also the place where Kan and Li interact."[38] When one circulates Qi smoothly in these two vessels, it flows smoothly throughout the rest of the body, without stagnation. This is the basis for longevity.

There were a few points in particular that he emphasized.

1. The flow of Qi in the Conception and Governing Vessels is closely related to the time of day.

2. We adjust Yin and Yang through constant practice of Kan and Li.

3. Kan and Li interact on the path of the Conception and Governing Vessels.

4. The smooth flow of Qi in these two vessels affects the flow in the twelve primary channels (rivers, Jing, 經) and countless secondary Qi channels (streams, Luo, 絡).

5. Smooth Qi flow in these two vessels is the foundation of longevity.

**Summary**

1. The are many different schools of meditation practice. Normally, Small Circulation refers to the circulation of Qi in the Conception and Governing Vessels.

2. Small Circulation likens the Qi flow in the Yin Conception and Yang Governing Vessels with the Qi flow between Heaven and Earth, in nature as a whole.

3. Small Circulation is to some extent a process which occurs naturally. It just uses the mind to enhance the process through meditation.

4. The natural flow of the Conception and Governing Qi follows the time of day, which will be discussed in more detail later.

5. The full name of Small Circulation is Yin-Yang Circulation Small Heavenly Cycle (Yin-Yang Xun Huan Yi Xiao Zhou Tian, 陰陽循環一小周天) in Daoist society. In Buddhist society it is called San Mei Yin (三昧印) or San Mo Di (三摩地), from the Sanskrit Samadhi, meaning steadiness. Buddhists refer to it as Zhuan Fa Lun (轉法論), or Turning the Wheel of Natural Law.

## 2-7. WHAT IS GRAND CIRCULATION? 何謂大周天？

### Internal Grand Circulation Meditation 自我大周天靜坐

Through Internal Grand Circulation meditation your mind leads Qi to any part of the body. You first develop the sensitivity to feel each part of your body internally, from the skin to the bone marrow. The deeper your mind reaches in meditation, the more profound and effective this practice will be.

With practice, you lead the Qi to the remotest places within the body for healing. If your Qi is strong, you may also use it to heal and nourish other people, commonly referred to as Qi Massage (Qi An Mo, 氣按摩) or External Qi Healing (Wai Qi Liao Fa, 外氣療法). Martial artists use Grand Circulation to energize the body.

**Primary Qi Channel Circulation Meditation** (十二經大周天靜坐). The main purpose of this meditation is to enhance circulation in the Twelve Primary Qi Channels, so the internal organs grow strong and healthy. Qi distribution to the arms and legs also improves, which strengthens the physical body.

There is a specific natural order of Qi circulation from one channel to another, with certain times of day in which a channel's Qi is strongest. This cycle is called Zi Wu Liu Zhu (子午流注), or midnight to noon major Qi flow. If you understand this natural Qi flow timing, you can adopt the correct path and timing for your practice.

**Joint Grand Circulation Meditation** (關節大周天靜坐). The purpose here is to circulate Qi in the bone marrow and within the joints, as well as in the primary channels. This is especially important for Qi healers, enabling them to project Qi outside the body.

**Four Gates Breathing Circulation** (四心呼吸大周天靜坐). The purpose of Four Gates Breathing is to lead Qi from the Real Lower Dan Tian to the four gates. Two of these gates, called Laogong (P-8, 勞宮), which means Labor's Palace, belong to the Pericardium Channel and are located at the center of the palms (Figure 2-36). The other two gates are called Yongquan (K-1, 湧泉), which means Gushing Spring. They belong to the Kidney Channel and are located at the front center of the soles (Figure 2-37).

These four cavities are the main gates which regulate the Qi level of the heart and kidneys. When Qi flows smoothly to them, the body is healthy, and great power is generated in the limbs. Four Gates Meditation is emphasized in Chinese martial arts, especially in the internal arts. It has been discussed at length in the YMAA books, *The Essence of Taiji Qigong, The Essence of Shaolin White Crane.*

**Skin/Marrow Breathing Circulation** (膚髓息大周天靜坐). Again, this leads Qi to the skin surface to enhance your Guardian Qi (Wei Qi, 衛氣), and store Qi in the bone marrow as Marrow Qi (Sui Qi, 髓氣). When Guardian Qi is strong, your immune system functions efficiently. When Marrow Qi is strong, the bone marrow produces a regular supply of healthy blood cells.

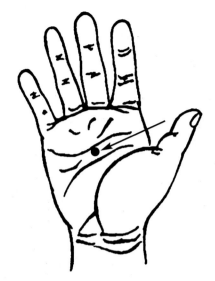
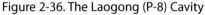

Figure 2-36. The Laogong (P-8) Cavity

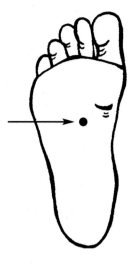

Figure 2-37. The Yongquan (K-1) Cavity

**Grand Circulation Meditation with a Partner** 雙修大周天靜坐

Once abundant Qi is stored in your Real Lower Dan Tian, and you circulate it smoothly throughout your body, you can heal and nourish other people. Double cultivation (Shuang Xiu, 雙修) as it is called, is the foundation of Qi healing. It is the most effective method for Qigong healers to train to exchange Qi with other people. Through this practice, two healthy people can nourish one another and elevate their training spirit significantly. Double cultivation is one of the most effective ways of accelerating spiritual enlightenment. We will discuss this subject in future publications.

**Grand Circulation Meditation with Great Nature** 天人合一大周天靜坐

**Grand Circulation Meditation with the Earth** (地人大周天靜坐). In this meditation you project your Qi beyond the body and exchange it with your environment, such as with the earth, trees, animals, and the air, all of which have their own Qi fields. It is possible to absorb Qi from around you, enhancing your own Qi level. In China, trees are regularly used for Qi regulation purposes. The difference between this Qi exchange and that involving a human partner is that these objects do not have a mind that we are able to recognize, so they cannot use their mind to lead their Qi as they exchange it with you.

**Grand Circulation Meditation with Heaven** (天人大周天靜坐). Grand Circulation Meditation with Heaven is also called Fifth Gate Meditation. Its purpose is to achieve spiritual unification with the universe, Tian Ren He Yi (天人合一). You lead Qi up through the Thrusting Vessel (Chong Mai, 衝脈) to the brain, nourish and energize it to a high energy state. The spirit grows and gradually the third eye opens. This is called enlightenment (Wu Zhen, 悟真). Having opened the third eye, there are no obstacles to communication between you and the surrounding environment, and you comprehend many things which cannot be understood by others. You communicate with others without speaking, as your telepathic capabilities develop. You comprehend the meaning of life and of nature.

## 2-8. WHAT IS ENLIGHTENMENT MEDITATION? 何謂仙道悟真靜坐？

To grasp the meaning of the universe, we combine our Qi with that of nature. Animals still have this spiritual connection, but humans lost it long ago. Due to the development of the human intellect and emotions, our spirit separated from that of nature, and our thoughts are contaminated by emotions and desires. Animals have not developed as we have, so they are still connected with nature, and their behavior is in line with the natural way of life. At birth we have a similar connection with the natural Qi and spirit. But as we grow, our minds are molded by the masked environment created by human minds. To survive in society we mask our faces, suppressing our natural spiritual instincts. Many people retire to the mountains for spiritual cultivation, to free themselves from this emotional bondage, attain a neutral state of mind, and sense the natural spirit more clearly.

To achieve unification with the natural spirit, one must open the third eye (Upper Dan Tian, Shang Dan Tian, 上丹田) by concentrating Qi inside it. First build up Qi in the Real Lower Dan Tian (Zhen Xia Dan Tian, 真下丹田), then lead it up to nourish the brain. Build up Qi there, using Embryonic Breathing (Tai Xi, 胎息). Only when the Qi stored in the Real Lower Dan Tian has reached an abundant level, is there enough Qi to open the third eye.

To reach the enlightenment, Daoists and Buddhists say you pass through four stages. The first is *Self-Recognition*, in which you remove the mask you wear. You see yourself clearly, recognizing and understanding your thought processes, and acknowledging what kind of person you really are. The second stage is *Self-Awareness*, in which you analyze past events and become aware of your interaction with your environment. The third stage, *Self-Awakening*, involves searching for freedom from emotional bondage. Finally, you attain the stage of *Freedom from Spiritual Bondage*, in which your ego and desires disappear. Your spirit establishes contact with the natural spirit, and you gain the Truth of Nature, or the Dao.

Daoists further classify these four stages of cultivation into sixteen steps, described in the document, *The Golden Elixir Methods of Regulating the Inner Mind— Procedures of Training Internal Elixir* (金丹心法 • 練內丹步驟).[39]

1. **A strong will** (Li Zhi, 立志). The first step towards enlightenment is to establish a strong will, without which you will not finish the training.

2. **Maintain good morality** (Duan Pin, 端品), including both the mental and the physical. Although you know right from wrong, you might ignore it and wander the path of sin. When wrong thought manifests, you harm yourself and others. Thoughts and behavior which cause harm to others is considered immoral in Buddhist and Daoist societies.

3. **Confession** (Hui Guo, 悔過). Once you have corrected your lines of thought and action, you contemplate bad deeds you committed in the past. Buddhists and Daoists believe past transgressions leave a stain on your conscience. Unless you recognize and admit your past mistakes, you continue to repeat them. At this stage you discard the mask you have been wearing.

4. **Transform into goodness** (Qian Shan, 遷善). You now recognize your good and bad personality traits, as you accentuate the positive and discard the negative ones. Once your mind is ready, you open your third eye. If you still have things to hide, you will be unable to open it, lest you let other people see into your mind.

5. **Build a firm spiritual foundation** (Zhu Ji, 築基), where your wisdom mind (Yi) gains ascendancy over your emotional mind (Xin). Your judgment becomes clear, guided by wisdom instead of by emotion.

6. **Cultivate yourself** (Lian Ji, 煉己). The next stage is to refine your thinking, as you comprehend the meaning of your spiritual life, and your spiritual body develops rapidly. Your thinking diverges from mainstream society, and you may decide to separate from secular society to avoid distractions. When you meditate, it is as though your physical body disappears, and you feel transparent and light. This is called "getting rid of the view of the body" in Buddhism.

7. **Establish the furnace** (An Lu, 安爐), and strengthen your spirit to survive separation from your physical body. Otherwise, once your body dies, your spirit must find a replacement in which to reincarnate, to prevent it gradually deteriorating and ceasing to exist. Buddhists and Daoists seek to develop their spiritual bodies to have independent eternal life without returning to the path of reincarnation.

8. **Picking the herb** (Cai Yao, 采藥) involves conversion of essence, both Original Essence (Yuan Jing, 元精) and Post-Birth Essence, into Qi. Original Essence is comprised of genetically determined hormones. Post-

Birth Essence is derived from our air and food. To enhance the conversion process, practice methods of increasing hormone production in the body, take herbs which can easily be converted into Qi, and ensure that you are consuming good quality food and fresh air.

9. **Starting the fire** (Qi Huo, 起火) involves building up Qi in the Lower Dan Tian through abdominal breathing. There are two alternative methods of abdominal breathing. The first is called Normal Abdominal Breathing (Zheng Fu Hu Xi, 正腹呼吸) or Buddhist Breathing (Fo Jia Hu Xi, 佛家呼吸). The second is called Reverse Abdominal Breathing (Fan Fu Hu Xi or Ni Fu Hu Xi, 反腹呼吸·逆腹呼吸), or Daoist Breathing (Dao Jia Hu Xi, 道家呼吸).

10. **Ceasing the fire** (Xi Huo, 熄火) involves storing the Qi you have built up, instead of manifesting it in the physical body. Only then will you be able to control the body's Qi and maintain its Yin-Yang balance. You store the Qi in the Real Dan Tian (Zhen Xia Dan Tian, 真下丹田), the human biobattery, through Embryonic Breathing (Tai Xi, 胎息).

11. **Generate the Embryo** (Jie Tai, 結胎). Original Essence is called Original Qi (Yuan Qi, 元氣), or Water Qi (Shui Qi, 水氣). It is pure and calming. However, Qi at the Middle Dan Tian, or sternum, originates from Post-Birth Essence, namely air and food. It is called Post-Heaven Qi (Hou Tian Qi, 後天氣) and considered to be Fire Qi (Huo Qi, 火氣), which is contaminate and liable to disturb and excite your emotional mind. So the Water Qi, or Kan (坎), can make you more Yin, while the Fire Qi, or Li (離) can make you more Yang.
To generate new life, in the form of a Spiritual Embryo (Shen Tai, 神胎), Yin and Yang must interact, through the method of Kan and Li (坎離). Lead the Water Qi up from the Lower Dan Tian or Real Lower Dan Tian, and the fire Qi down from the sternum, to meet at the Huang Ting (黃庭) cavity between sternum and navel. With continued practice, a Spiritual Embryo is generated. This converts Qi into spirit, and is called Ten Months of Pregnancy (Shi Yue Huai Tai, 十月懷胎).

12. **Nursing the baby** (Yang Ying, 養嬰). After ten months of pregnancy, the Spiritual Embryo is born, meaning the third eye has opened, and the spirit can leave the body and return to it at will. This is known as Refining Spirit and Returning it to Nothingness (Lian Shen Fan Xu, 練神返虛), or Three Years of Nursing (San Nian Bu Ru, 三年哺乳).

13. **Accumulation of good deeds** (Ji Xing, 積行). You now train your spirit in the finer differences between good and evil. By this stage, you have promoted your spirit to a very high level.

14. **Train Gong** (Xing Gong, 行功) to establish a connection between your new spirit and the natural spirit. By training your spirit to separate from the physical body for longer intervals and traveling greater distances, it will gradually become independent.

15. **Facing the wall** (Mian Bi, 面壁). This is called Crushing the Nothingness (Fen Sui Xu Kong, 粉碎虛空), or Nine Years of Facing the Wall (Jiu Nian Mian Bi, 九年面壁). You prepare to separate your spiritual body from your physical body permanently. You face the wall and ponder your life once more, to ensure you really wish to free yourself from all human bondage.

16. **Flying to ascend** (Fei Sheng, 飛升). Now that you are ready to separate your spiritual and physical bodies, you choose the day to separate them permanently. This is the final stage of cultivation, Unification of Heaven and Man (Tian Ren He Yi, 天人合一).

It should now be easier to understand the first few steps of spiritual cultivation, although the training methods and the meaning of cultivation may remain hidden until one reaches a more profound stage. It is similar to how our perspective of the world changes as we mature.

## Summary of Spiritual Enlightenment Cultivation

1. The first step is Small Circulation Meditation, the foundation of Internal Elixir (Nei Dan, 內丹) Qigong practice. By training it, you build up Qi and store it in the Real Lower Dan Tian, the human bioelectric battery. You also use the mind's ability to generate EMF to circulate Qi in the two main vessels which supply Qi to the Twelve Primary Qi Channels. This leads to an abundant Qi supply for the physical body and is the key to strengthening the body for health and longevity.

2. After Small Circulation, you train Grand Circulation Meditation, with methods of improving Qi circulation throughout the entire body, and exchanging Qi with others and with your environment. From this Qi communication, you start to understand the natural spirit, which is the initial step in understanding nature for the purpose of unification with the spirit of heaven.

   You use the mind's EMF, leading Qi to the surface of the skin to strengthen Guardian Qi, including the immune system. You also lead Qi to the marrow to maintain its health and proper function, which is vital to longevity.

   You lead Qi to the four gates, two Laogongs and two Yongquans. These are four of the five gates used to establish a connection with the environment. The fifth gate is your third eye which is related to the practice of enlightenment.

Finally, you exchange Qi with animals and other people or natural objects. You may adjust other people's Qi into a more harmonious and balanced state, which is the key to Qigong healing.

3. The final goal of meditation is spiritual enlightenment, achieved by opening the third eye. The spirit can leave and enter the body at will, and survive without the support of the physical body. Finally, the physical body is left behind and the practitioner gains eternal spiritual life.

## References

1. 《易》曰：〝一陰一陽之謂道。〞

2. 《道德經・四十二章》：〝道生一，一生二，二生三，三生萬物。〞

3. 《道德經・二十五章》：〝有物混成，先天地生。寂兮寥兮，獨立而不改，周行而不殆，可以為天下母。吾不知其名，強字之曰道。〞

4. 《道德經・一章》：〝玄之又玄，眾妙之門。〞

5. 《道德經・五十一章》：〝道生之，德畜之，物形之，勢成之。〞指萬物變化。

6. 《道德經・二十五章》：〝人法地，地法天，天法道，道法自然。〞指以自然為法。

7. 《淮南子・天文訓》：〝道始于一，一而不生，故分為陰陽，陰陽和合而萬物生。〞

8. 《道德經・一章》：〝無，名先天之始；有，名萬物之母。常無，欲以觀其妙；常有，欲以觀其徼。〞指事物正在變化之中。

9. 《朱子語類》：〝謂之太極者，所以指天地萬物之根。〞

10. 李時珍《奇經八脈考》：〝陽維主一身之表，陰維主一身之里，陽蹻主一身左右之陽，陰蹻主一身左右之陰，督主身後之陽，任、沖主身前之陰，帶脈橫束諸脈以總約之。〞

11. "Life's Invisible Current," by Albert L. Huebner, *East West Journal*, June 1986.

12. *The Body Electric*, by Robert O. Becker, M.D. and Gary Selden, Quill, William Morrow, New York, 1985.

13. "Healing with Nature's Energy," by Richard Leviton, *East West Journal*, June 1986.

14. *A Child is Born*, by Lennart Nilsson, A DTP/Seymour Lawrence Book, 1990.

15. 解剖生理學 (*A Study of Anatomic Physiology*) 李文森編著。華杏出版股份有限公司, Taipei, 1986.

16. *Grant's Atlas of Anatomy*, James E. Anderson, 7th Edition, Williams & Wilkins Co., 9-92, 1978.

17. "Complex and Hidden Brain in the Gut Makes Stomachaches and Butterflies," by Sandra Blakeslee, *The New York Times*, Science, January 23, 1996.

18. *The Second Brain: The Scientific Basis of Gut Instinct and a Groundbreaking New Understanding of Nervous Disorders of the Stomach and Intestine*, Michael D. Gershon, New York: Harper Collins Publications, 1998.

19. *Fundamentals of Physics*, Holliday and Resnick, pp. 512-514. John Wiley & Sons, Inc., 1972.

20. *Bioenergetics*, by Albert L. Lehninger, pp. 5-6, W. A, Benjamin, Inc. Menlo Park, California, 1971.

21. *Photographic Anatomy of the Human Body*, by J. W. Rohen, 邯鄲出版社 Taipei, Taiwan, 1984.

22. "Restoring Ebbing Hormones May Slow Aging," by Jane E. Brody, *The New York Times*, July 18, 1995.

23. 《阿含經》：〝坐禪思惟，莫有懈怠。〞

24. *The New Encyclopedia Brittanica*, Vol. 4, Encyclopedia Brittanica Inc., 1993.

25. *Fundamentals of Physics*, David Holliday and Robert Resnick, p. 308, John Wiley & Sons, Inc. New York, NY, 1970.

26. 道家：修心養性，守中抱一。

27. 儒家：存心養性，執中貫一。

28. 佛家：明心見性，萬法歸一。

29. 醫家：虛心定性，抱元守一。

30. 《太平經》：〝以思守一，何也？一者，數之始也；一者，生之道也；一者，元氣所起也；一者，天地之綱紀也。〞

31. 《性命圭旨全書‧大道說》：〝儒之一貫者，以此本體之一而貫之也。〞

32. 道，一以貫之。

33. 《針灸大成》：〝徐徐咽氣一口，緩緩納入丹田，沖起命門，引督脈過尾閭，而上升泥丸；追動性元，引任脈降重樓，而下返氣海。兩脈上下，旋轉如圓，前降後升，絡繹不絕。‧‧‧‧‧‧久而行之，關竅自開，脈絡流通，百病不作。〞

34. 《理瀹駢文》：〝閉目靜坐，鼻吸清氣，鼓腹使內氣下降臍下丹田，運氣過肛門，沿督脈尾閭、夾脊、玉枕三關，到頭頂百會穴，順面部至舌與任脈接，沿前胸而下，至丹田復順原徑路循行。患在何處，收氣即存想其處，放氣則歸于丹田。可強身卻病。又名三昧印。〞

35. 《道鄉集》：〝仙家之周天，即佛家轉法輪，理同各異，而後人便自分開。〞

36. 法輪，原是佛教用語，為梵文 Dharmachakra 的意譯，是對佛教的喻稱。

37. 《性命圭旨》：〝釋家謂之法輪，道家謂之周天，儒家謂之行庭，都是同一內容。〞

38. 李時珍《奇經八脈考》：〝任督兩脈，乃身之子午也，乃丹家陽火陰符升降之道，坎水離火交媾之鄉。〞人能通此兩脈，則百脈皆通，自然周身流轉無有停壅之患，而長生久視之道斷在此矣。

39. 金丹心法‧練內丹步驟：〝立志、端品、悔過、遷善、築基、煉己、安爐、采藥、起火、熄火、結胎、養嬰、積行、行功、面壁、飛升。〞

# Meditation Training Procedures

靜坐訓練步驟

## Chapter 3

# Four Refinements
# 四化

## 3-1. Introduction 介紹

First we compare the concepts of Jing (精, essence), Qi (氣, bioelectricity), and Shen (神, spirit). A clear understanding of Jing, Qi, and Shen is critical for effective Qigong training. They are the root of your life and your Qigong practice. Jing, Qi, and Shen are called San Bao (三寶, Three Treasures), San Yuan (三元, Three Origins) or San Ben (三本, Three Foundations). A Qigong practitioner firms his Jing (Gu Jing, 固精, Gu means to firm, solidify, retain, and conserve), and then converts it into Qi. This is Lian Jing Hua Qi (練精化氣), which means to refine the Jing and convert it into Qi. He leads Qi to the head to nourish Shen. This is Lian Qi Hua Shen (練氣化神), which means to refine the Qi and convert it into Shen. Finally, he uses his energized Shen to end (govern) his temperament. This is Lian Shen Liao Xing (練神了性), namely to refine the Shen to end human nature.

This conversion process enables you to gain health and longevity. During the course of your training you must pay a great deal of attention to these three elements. If you keep these three elements strong and healthy, you will live a long and healthy life. If you neglect or abuse them, you will be sick frequently and age rapidly. Each one of these three elements or treasures has its own root, which you must strengthen and protect.

**Jing** (精). The Chinese word Jing (精) can mean various things depending on context. It can be used as a verb, adjective, or noun. As a verb, it means to refine. For example, to refine or purify a liquid to a high quality is called Jing Lian (精煉). As an adjective, it denotes something refined, polished, and pure without mixture. People say Jing Xi (精細) for a work of art, which means delicate and painstaking. Jing Liang (精良) means of excellent quality. When Jing describes wisdom or personality, it means keen and sharp, e.g., Jing Ming (精明), which means keen and clever. Jing can describe a plan or idea as profound, astute, and carefully considered.

Used as a noun, Jing means the essence. It can mean spirit or ghost. Chinese believe semen is a man's refined essence, so Jing also means sperm or semen.

Jing, as essence, exists in everything, as the primal substance or original source from which anything is made and which exhibits the true nature of that thing. In animals or humans, it means the very original and essential source of life and growth. This Jing is the origin of the Shen (Spirit), which makes an animal different from a tree. In humans, Jing is passed down from the parents. Sperm is called Jing Zi (精子), which means the sons of essence. When this essence is mixed with the mother's Jing (egg), a new life is generated which is, in certain fundamental respects, an intertwinement of the Jings of both parents. The child is formed, the Qi circulates, and the Shen grows. The Jing which has been carried over from the parents is called Yuan Jing (元精), or Original Essence.

Original Essence is the fountainhead and root of your life. As you absorb the Jing of food and air, you convert their Jings into Qi to supply your body's needs. In Qigong society, Jing usually refers to Yuan Jing (元精). Yuan Jing differs in quantity and quality from person to person and is affected significantly by your parents' health and living habits while they conceived you. Generally speaking, it does not matter how much Yuan Jing you have carried over from your parents, if you know how to conserve it, you will have more than enough for your lifetime. Although you probably cannot increase the quantity of your Jing, it is possible to improve its quality through Qigong training.

Conserving and firming your Yuan Jing is of primary importance. To conserve means to refrain from abuse and excess sexual activity, through which you would lose Yuan Jing faster and your body would degenerate more rapidly. To firm your Jing means to store and maintain it, and keep your kidneys strong. Kidneys are the residence of Yuan Jing, and when they are strong, Yuan Jing will be firm and not lost without reason. The firming of Yuan Jing is called Gu Jing (固精). This is the first step in training before you can improve its quality. To conserve and firm your Jing, you must first know its root, where it resides, and how to convert it into Qi.

Before birth, your Yuan Jing is rooted in your parents. After birth, it resides in the kidneys, which now become its root. When you keep this root strong, you will have plenty of Yuan Jing to supply to your body. The kidneys encompass both Internal Kidneys (Nei Shen, 內腎) and External Kidneys (Wai Shen, 外腎). The kidneys along with the adrenal glands are the Internal Kidneys, while the gonads are the External Kidneys. Internal and external kidneys are closely connected and interrelated, and weak Qi in one will weaken the other.

You were created from the union of one egg and one sperm, which managed to reach and penetrate the egg before any of the other millions of sperm. From this, one human cell formed which started to divide, from one to two, from two to four, and so on, to form the embryo. Its health is determined by the original sperm and egg generated from the parents' Jing. It remains immersed in liquid, receiving all its nutrition and oxygen from the mother through the umbilical cord, which connects at the navel, close to the Lower Dan Tian and to the body's center of gravity. The umbilical cord is long, and the baby draws nutrients in with a pumping motion of its abdomen.

Once you are born, you breathe in oxygen through your nose and receive food through your mouth. You no longer need the abdominal motion to pump in nutrients through the umbilical cord, so it gradually stops, and you forget to use it. The Lower Dan Tian (Xia Dan Tian, 下丹田), or abdomen, is the source of Original Qi converted from the Yuan Jing continuously. The Lower Dan Tian is located on the Conception Vessel, one of the eight Qi reservoirs in the body which regulate the Qi flow in the other Qi channels. Qi in the Lower Dan Tian is Water Qi (Shui Qi, 水氣), able to cool down the Fire Qi (Huo Qi, 火氣) generated from the Jing of food and air, which resides at the Middle Dan Tian, or sternum.

To be strong and healthy, conserve your Yuan Jing. This is like the principal in your savings account, an original investment which will continue to return interest as long as it is conserved. Jing produces Qi, and by preserving it, you will continue to have Jing and Qi. An unhealthy lifestyle may damage and reduce your Yuan Jing.

To conserve Yuan Jing, control your sexual activity. The gonads are called External Kidneys (Wai Shen, 外腎), as sperm is a product of Yuan Jing and the Jing from food and air. Ejaculations exhaust your Yuan Jing and shorten your life. You need not stop sexual activity altogether. The proper amount of sexual activity is encouraged, to energize and activate the Jing, and convert Jing to Qi more efficiently. Jing is like fuel, and Qi is like energy generated from this fuel. The more efficiently you convert fuel into energy, the more energy you have.

Appropriate sexual activity energizes the Qi to nourish the Shen, balance your mind, and enhance your courage and morale. The proper amount depends on one's age and state of health. The Jing in the External Kidneys is the main source of Qi in the four major Yin Qi vessels in the legs (Yin Heel and Yin Linking Vessels on each leg). These four Qi reservoirs keep the legs strong and healthy. If your legs are weakened by sexual activity, you are losing too much Jing.

**Qi** (氣). Qigong describes the close relationship between Qi and blood circulation. Where Qi goes, blood follows. This is called Qi Xue (氣血, Qi Blood). Qi provides the energy the blood cells need for life and movement. Blood stores Qi, and helps to transport air Qi to every cell of the body.

The cells and tissues are like machines, each with its own unique function, and without current they die. The routes of the blood circulatory system, the nervous system, and the lymphatic system correspond with the course of the Qi channels, because Qi is the energy they need to function. The organs process raw materials into the finished product. Some raw materials are brought in for the energy with which other raw materials are converted into finished goods. The raw materials for your body are food and air, and the finished product is life.

The Qi in your body is like the electric current which the factory obtains from coal or oil. The factory has many wires connecting the power plant to the machines, and other wires connecting telephones, intercoms, and computers. There are also many conveyer belts, elevators, wagons, and trucks to move material from one place to another. It is no different in your body, where there are systems of intestines, blood vessels, complex networks of nerves, and Qi channels to distribute blood, sensory information, and energy. Unlike the digestive, circulatory, and central nervous systems, all of whose supportive vessels can be observed as material structures in the body, Qi channels cannot be observed as physical objects. These systems all have similar configurations throughout the body.

In a factory, different machines require different levels of current. It is the same for your organs, which require different levels of Qi. If a machine is supplied with an improper level of power, it will not function normally and may even be damaged. In the same way, when the Qi level is either too positive or too negative in your organs, they will be damaged and will degenerate more rapidly. In order for a factory to function smoothly and productively, it not only needs high quality machines, but also a reliable power supply. The same goes for your body. The quality of your organs is largely dependent upon what you inherited from your parents. To maintain them in a healthy state and to insure that they function well for a long time, you must have an appropriate Qi supply.

Qi is affected by the quality of air you inhale, the food you eat, your lifestyle, and also your emotions and personality. Food and air are the fuel source, your lifestyle is how you run the machines, and your personality is the management of the factory.

This clarifies the role Qi plays in your body. However, the metaphor used is an oversimplification. The behavior and function of Qi is much more complex than the power supply in a factory. You are neither a factory nor a robot, but a human being with feelings and emotions, which influence your Qi circulation. For example, when you pinch yourself, the Qi in that area is disturbed. This is sensed through the nervous system and interpreted by your brain as pain. No machine can do this. Moreover, after you have felt pain, unlike a machine, you react either through instinct or conscious thought. Human feelings and thought affect Qi circulation in the body, whereas a machine cannot influence its power supply. To understand and control your Qi, you must feel its flow, rather than just use the intellect.

The body has two general types of Qi. The first is called Pre-birth Qi, Original Qi (Yuan Qi, 元氣), or Xian Tian Qi (先天氣, Pre-Heavenly Qi). It is converted from Yuan Jing, which you received at conception, which is why Original Qi is also called Pre-birth Qi.

The second type is Post-birth Qi or Hou Tian Qi (後天氣, Post-heaven Qi). This is drawn from the Jing (essence) of the food and air we take in. Its residence is the Middle Dan Tian, the diaphragm. It circulates and mixes with the Pre-birth Original

Qi. Together, they circulate through the Governing Vessel (Du Mai, 督脈) and Conception Vessel (Ren Mai, 任脈), from where they are distributed to the entire body.

Pre-birth Qi is Water Qi (Shui Qi, 水氣) because it can cool down the Post-birth Qi, which is Fire Qi (Huo Qi, 火氣). Fire Qi brings the body to a positive Yang state, stimulating the emotions, and scattering and confusing the mind. Water Qi cools your body down, and helps the mind become clear, neutral, and centered. Fire Qi supports the emotional body, while Water Qi supports the wisdom part.

As Fire and Water Qi mix, they not only circulate to the Governing Vessel and Conception Vessel, but also to the Thrusting Vessel (Chong Mai, 衝脈), leading Qi directly up through the spinal cord to nourish the brain and energize the Shen and soul. These are very important in Qigong practice.

According to its function, Qi is divided into two major categories. The first is Ying Qi (營氣, Managing Qi), because it manages and controls body functions. This includes the functions of the brain and organs, and also body movement. Ying Qi is also divided into two types. The first circulates in the channels and is responsible for organ function. The circulation of Qi to the organs and the extremities continues automatically as long as you have enough Qi in your reservoirs and you maintain your body in good condition. The second type of Ying Qi is linked to your Yi (mind, intention). When your Yi decides to do something, for example to lift a box, this type of Ying Qi automatically flows to the muscles needed to do the job. This Qi is directed by your thoughts, and closely related to your feelings and emotions.

The second major category of Qi is Wei Qi (衛氣, Guardian Qi). This forms a shield on the surface of the body to protect you from negative external influences. It is also involved in the growth of hair, the repair of skin injuries, and many other functions of the skin. It is led through millions of tiny channels to the surface of the skin, and can even reach beyond the body. When your body is Yang, Wei Qi is strong and your pores open. When your body is Yin, Wei Qi is weak and your pores close to prevent Qi from being lost.

In summertime, your body is Yang and your Qi is strong, so your Qi shield may extend well beyond your physical body, with the pores wide open. In wintertime, your body is relatively Yin, and you conserve Qi to stay warm and keep pathogens out. The Qi shield shrinks to be close to the skin surface.

Wei Qi functions automatically in response to environmental changes, but is also influenced significantly by your feelings and emotions. For example, when you feel happy or angry, the Qi shield will be more open than when you are sad or scared. To maintain health, Ying Qi must function smoothly, while strong Wei Qi protects you from negative outside influences such as cold.

The key is training and raising the Shen (spirit), which directs and controls the Qi. When ill or facing death, those with strong Shen, indicative of a strong will to live, often survive. Those who are apathetic or depressed generally do not last long. A strong will to live raises the Shen, energizing Qi and keeping you alive and healthy. To raise Shen, first energize your brain with Qi, to concentrate more effectively. Your mind will be steady, your will strong, and your Shen raised.

It is important to generate Water Qi and learn to use it effectively. It can cool down Fire Qi, slowing the degeneration of the body. It also helps to calm the mind and keep it centered, allowing you to judge things objectively. Qigong practice will help you sense and direct it effectively. Water Qi comes from conversion of Yuan Jing, and they both have the kidneys as their root. Once generated, it resides in the Lower Dan Tian below the navel. To conserve it, keep your kidneys firm and strong.

**Shen** (神). It is very difficult to find an English word to precisely express Shen. As in so many other cases, the context determines the translation. Shen can be translated as spirit, god, immortal, soul, mind, divine, and supernatural.

When you are alive, Shen is the spirit which is directed by your mind. When your mind is not steady, it is said Xin Shen Bu Ning (心神不寧), which means the emotional mind and spirit are not at peace. The emotional mind (Xin) can energize and stimulate one's Shen to a higher state, but at the same time one must restrain the emotional mind with the wisdom mind (Yi). If the Yi can control the Xin, the mind as a whole will be concentrated, and the Yi will be able to govern the Shen. When one's Shen is excited, however, it is not being controlled by the Yi, so we say Shen Zhi Bu Qing (神志不清), which means the spirit and the will (generated from Yi) are not clear. In Qigong it is very important for you to train your wisdom Yi to control your emotional Xin effectively. To achieve this, Buddhists and Daoists train themselves to be free of emotions and attachments, as only in this way can they build a strong Shen completely under their control.

When healthy, you use your Yi to protect your Shen and keep it at its residence, the Upper Dan Tian. Even when energized, it is still controlled by your Yi. However, when you are very sick or near death, your Yi weakens, and your Shen leaves its residence to wander around. When you are dead, your Shen separates completely from the physical body. It is then called a Hun (魂) or soul. Often the term Shen Hun (神魂) is used, since the Hun originated with the Shen. Sometimes Shen Hun also refers to the spirit of a dying person, since his spirit is between Shen and Hun.

When your Shen is stronger and reaches a higher state, you can sense more sharply, and your mind is more clever and inspired. The world of living human beings is usually considered a Yang world (Yang Jian, 陽間), and the spirit world after death is considered a Yin world (Yin Jian, 陰間). When your Shen reaches this higher, more sensitive state, your mind transcends its normal capacity. Ideas beyond your usual grasp can be understood and controlled, and you may develop the ability to sense or even communicate with the Yin world. This supernatural Shen is called Ling (靈), describing one who is sharp, clever, nimble, and able to quickly empathize with people and things. When you die, this supernatural Shen (Ling Shen, 靈神) does not die with your body right away, but still holds your energy together as a ghost (Gui, 鬼). Therefore, a ghost is also called Ling Gui (靈鬼), meaning spiritual ghost, or Ling Hun (靈魂), meaning spiritual soul.

Ling is the supernatural part of the spirit. If strong enough, it lives long after physical death and has plenty of opportunity to reincarnate. However, once one reaches the stage of enlightenment or Buddhahood when alive, after death the spirit leaves the cycle of reincarnation to live forever. These spirits are called Shen Ming (神明), which means spiritually enlightened beings, or simply Shen (神), which here implies this spirit has become divine. Normally, if you die and your supernatural spiritual is not strong, it has only a short time to search for a new residence in which to be reborn before its energy disperses. In this case, the spirit is called Gui (鬼, ghost).

Your Jing and Qi may nourish Shen (Yang Shen, 養神) and strengthen Ling. When this Ling Shen (靈神) is strong enough, you may separate from the physical body at will. Having reached this stage, your body may live for hundreds of years. People who can do this are called Xian (仙), which means god, or immortal fairy. Since Xian originated with the Shen, it is sometimes called Shen Xian (神仙), or immortal spirit. The Xian is a living person whose Shen has reached enlightenment or Buddhahood. After death, his spirit is called Shen Ming (神明).

The foundation of Qigong training is to firm your Shen, nourish, and grow it until it is mature enough to separate from your physical body. To do this, you must know where the Shen resides, and how to keep, protect, nourish and train it. It is also essential to know the root or origin of your Shen.

Your Shen resides in the Upper Dan Tian, namely the brain. When you concentrate on the third eye, the Shen can be firmed. Firm here means to keep and to protect. When someone's mind is scattered and confused, his Shen wanders. This is called Shen Bu Shou She (神不守舍), which means the spirit is not kept at its residence.

According to Qigong theory, though your Xin (emotional mind, 心) can raise up the spirit, it can also confuse your Shen, so that it leaves its residence. Your Yi (wisdom mind) must constantly restrain and control Shen at its residence.

When Shen is highly energized, it conducts the Qi effectively. It is the force which keeps you alive, and the control tower for Qi. When it is strong, your Qi is strong and you can lead it efficiently. When it is weak, your Qi is weak and the body degenerates rapidly. Likewise, Qi supports the Shen, energizing it and keeping it sharp, clear, and strong.

You must understand the root of your Shen and how to nourish its growth. Original Essence (Yuan Jing, 元精) is the essential life inherited from your parents, your most important source of energy. Your Original Qi (Yuan Qi, 元氣) is created from Original Essence, and it mixes with Qi from food and the air to supply energy for growth and activity. This mixed Qi nourishes Shen as well. While Fire Qi energizes your Shen, Water Qi strengthens the wisdom mind to control the energized Shen. The Shen kept in its residence by Yi and nourished by Original Qi, is called Original Shen (Yuan Shen, 元神). So the root of your Original Shen is your Original Essence. When your Shen is energized but restrained by your Yi, it is called Jing Shen (精神), which means Essence Shen, or spirit of vitality.

Original Shen is the center of your being, making you calm, clearing your mind, and firming your will. When you concentrate on doing something, it is called Ju Jing Hui Shen (聚精會神, gathering Jing to meet Shen). Use Original Essence to raise up Original Shen. Since this Shen is nourished by Original Qi, which is Water Qi, it is considered Water Shen.

At a higher level of practice, cultivating Shen becomes most important. The final goal is to generate a Holy Embryo (Xian Tai, 仙胎), nourishing it until it is born and becomes independent. For the average practitioner, however, the final goal of cultivating Shen is to raise it up through Qi nourishment, while maintaining control with the Yi. This raised Shen directs and governs Qi efficiently and helps achieve health and longevity.

Shen and brain cannot be separated. Shen is the spiritual aspect of your being, generated and controlled by your mind. The mind generates the will which keeps the Shen firm. The Chinese commonly use Shen (Spirit) and Zhi (Will) together as Shen Zhi (神志) because they are so closely related. When Shen is raised and firm, this raised spirit strengthens the will. They are mutually related and assist each other. So the material foundation of your spirit is your brain. Nourish your Shen means to nourish your brain. The original source of nourishment is your Jing, which is converted into Qi, and led to the brain to nourish and energize it. In Qigong practice, this process is called Fan Jing Bu Nao (返精補腦), meaning to return the Jing to nourish the brain.

Now with a clear understanding of Jing, Qi, and Shen, you may grasp the interplay of these three treasures in Qigong practice, and how to use them to reach spiritual enlightenment. There are four necessary steps in training:

- **Refining the Essence and converting it into Qi** (Lian Jin Hua Qi) 練精化氣
  - One hundred days of building the foundation (Bai Ri Zhu Ji, 百日築基)
- **Purifying Qi and converting it into Spirit** (Lian Qi Hua Shen) 練氣化神
  - Ten months of pregnancy (Shi Yue Huai Tai, 十月懷胎)
- **Refining Spirit and returning it to Nothingness** (Lian Shen Fan Xu) 練神返虛
  - Three years of nursing (San Nian Bu Ru, 三年哺乳)
- **Crushing the Nothingness (Fen Sui Xu Kong)** 粉碎虛空
  - Nine years of facing the wall (Jiu Nian Mian Bi, 九年面壁)

The Dao of reaching enlightenment, or becoming a Buddha, requires years of training. One hundred days of building the foundation refers to the formation of the embryo of a spirit baby, commonly called Sheng Tai (聖胎, Holy Embryo) or Ling Tai (靈胎, Spiritual Embryo). This is followed by ten months of nourishing and growing, three years of nursing, and finally educating this spirit as it grows stronger and becomes independent. This builds up an independent spiritual body. After physical death, this spiritual body lives on, not needing to return to the path of reincarnation.

After this Xi Sui Jing training secret was revealed to seculars, a change took place in the training. Because the final goal of enlightenment or Buddhahood was not their main reason to practice and is so hard to attain, many secular practitioners looking only for longevity trained only the first three steps of training and ignored the final step. So there are very few documents describing this final step.

## 3-2. Refining the Essence and Converting It into Qi 練精化氣

One hundred days of building the foundation (Bai Ri Zhu Ji, 百日築基) is the first step in forming a Spiritual Embryo (Ling Tai, 靈胎), or Holy Embryo (Sheng Tai, 聖胎). Many secular practitioners looking only for longevity consider this spiritual baby as an elixir of longevity. Healthy harmonious interaction of Yin and Yang Qi is necessary to form it. Yin is the mother, while Yang is the father. Yin and Yang Qi must be abundant, each strong enough to balance the other. To build abundant Yin and Yang Qi in your body, you must practice the correct methods. For Yin and Yang to interact harmoniously, you must also adjust Kan and Li (坎離)(Figure 3-1). You lead Yin and Yang Qi to the Huang Ting (黃庭, yellow yard) to interact harmoniously.

What is the Holy Embryo, or Spiritual Embryo? "Baby Embryo, means golden elixir. To produce the golden elixir is to carry the baby embryo."[1] Elixir is the Qi which extends your life. Since it is as precious as gold, it is commonly called golden elixir. To establish an Embryonic Baby means to build up and to store Qi at the Huang Ting cavity. The Daoist Xue, Dao-Guang (薛道光) wrote, "What is the baby? It is the elixir. The elixir is unique and is the real sole Qi. It is the mother's Qi of heaven and earth. Mother swallows air, belonging to the five internal organs, yielding the baby's Qi. It is just like a cat keeping a mouse which cannot escape. The Qi of mother and son mutually love each other in the womb and finally combine and generate a baby. Therefore, it is said: 'The sole Grand Ultimate contains the real Qi. The way of containing the real sole Qi is like a human carrying an embryo, giving birth when ten months have completed.'"[2]

So to generate spiritual life, you need heaven Qi (Yang Qi) and earth Qi (Yin Qi). When these two combine and interact, life is formed. To produce the golden elixir, you absorb Qi from food and air (Yang Qi) and also from Original Essence

(Yin Qi). Then Qi can be stored to a high level and the foundation of longevity established.

From the scientific point of view, what you are doing is storing electric charge in the Huang Ting, the second human brain.[3,4] This second brain connects to the brain via the spinal cord, which is central to the human nervous system and is highly conductive tissue. So the two brains, though viewed as being separate, function as one. The upper brain generates thought (EMF), while the lower brain acts as a battery, supplying charge to the entire body. Whenever EMF is generated, the charge is led to the required area to activate the physical body, manifesting the mind and Qi into physical action.

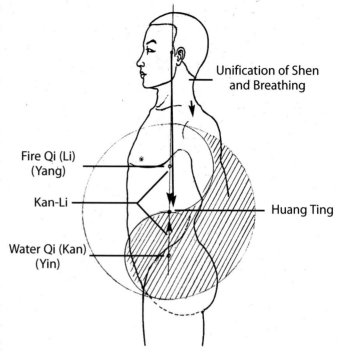

Unification of Shen and Breathing

Fire Qi (Li) (Yang)

Kan-Li

Water Qi (Kan) (Yin)

Huang Ting

Figure 3-1. Conceiving the Spiritual Embryo

For strong and abundant Qi, you need a powerful concentrated mind (high EMF) and a good battery able to store Qi in abundance. When both brains are healthy and functioning harmoniously, your immune system is rebuilt, extending life significantly.

The abundant Qi stored in the Huang Ting is led to the brain to nourish and activate its cells to a high enough functional level to raise up the spirit. This describes what happens when the Holy Embryo is formed and matured in the Huang Ting and then led to the brain to grow up, in the second stage of training.

What is the Huang Ting, and how can it store Qi and give birth to the Spiritual Embryo? This cavity was first called Yu Huan Xue (玉環穴, Jade Ring Cavity) in the book, *Illustration of Brass Acupuncture and Moxibustion* (*Tong Ren Yu Xue Zhen Jiu Tu*, 銅人俞穴針灸圖), by Dr. Wang, Wei-Yi (王唯一). Afterwards, the Daoist book *Wang Lu Shi Yu* (王錄識餘) said, "In the *Illustration of Brass Acupuncture and Moxibustion* it was recorded that within the body's cavities of viscera and bowels, there is a Jade Ring (Yu Huan). But I do not know what the Jade Ring is."[5] Later, the Daoist Zhang, Zi-Yang (張紫陽) explained the place which the immortals use to form the elixir,

"The heart is on top, the kidneys are underneath, spleen is to the left, and the liver is to the right. The life door is in front, the closed door to the rear, they are connected like a ring, it is white like cotton, an inch in diameter. It encompasses the Essence and refinement of the whole body. This is the Jade Ring."[6] The life door in front means the Qi door opens to the front and is closed in the rear. To lead Yin and Yang Qi there, you should access this cavity from the front.

The Huang Ting connects with the Conception and Thrusting Vessels through Yinjiao (Co-7, 陰交). Through the Thrusting Vessel, it connects with the upper brain and with the Governing Vessel at the Huiyin (Co-1, 會陰). The gut is the second brain, with a similar structure to the brain in the head, and able to store a great amount of Qi.[3,4] The Huang Ting (黃庭, Yellow Yard) is located between the sternum (Middle Dan Tian), where Yang Fire Qi is stored, and the Lower Dan Tian, where Yin Water Qi is stored. The fasciae in the Huang Ting area stores an abundance of Qi, increasing the amount available to the Holy Embryo.

Given that the gut is widely accepted as being a second brain with a similar structure to the upper brain, how can it create a spiritual embryo? Though scientists believe the second brain has the capability of memory, they are not sure whether it can think. If not, then no EMF can be generated, and the spirit cannot be grown here. Therefore, this place could only be used for the purpose of Yang and Yin Qi interaction and raising them up to a high level.

In Yi Jin Jing training you generate Qi by converting Original Essence in the Internal Kidneys. However, this does not provide enough Qi for the Xi Sui Jing training. To remedy this shortfall, more Essence must be drawn from the External Kidneys (testicles) by stimulating them and converting the essence they produce into Qi. From the standpoint of modern medicine, part of the health benefit of Xi Sui Jing Qigong comes from its use of stimulation to increase the production of hormones. These are secreted by the endocrine glands, including the testicles. They are complex chemical compounds transported by the blood or lymph, with powerful and specific effects on the functions of the body.

Hormones can stimulate activity, thinking, and growth. They are directly related to the strength of your life force, determining the length of your life and your state of health. They can stimulate your emotions and lift your mood, or depress you physically and emotionally. Traced back far enough, they are the very original source of one's thinking and ideas, even generating the enthusiasm for energetic activity. If you generate these hormones and use them properly, you can energize yourself to a degree quite impossible for the ordinary person.

Many important hormones can now be produced synthetically, but taking synthetic hormones is an unnatural and discontinuous process, unlike generating them within your body. When you produce the hormones yourself, your body adjusts to the gradual increase in production. However, if they come from outside, your body is subject to abrupt changes which produce unwanted side effects. Many hormones are obtained from certain foods, but without providing enough Qi to fill up the vessels. The Daoists say, "Food is better than medicine for increasing health. Using Qi to improve health is better than eating food."[7] Xi Sui Jing stimulates the production and secretion of hormones. These are used to increase the Qi, which in turn nourishes the brain and raises the spirit of vitality.

You can only develop a healthy spiritual baby when you have sufficient Qi. To form the embryo, you need at least one hundred days of proper diet, accurate Kan and Li adjustment, correct stimulation of the sexual organ to increase the Essence (semen), and abstinence from sex, to build up a strong Qi body combining Yin and Yang. In Xi Sui Qigong, the process of refining Essence and converting it into Qi during the first one hundred days lays the foundation (Bai Ri Zhu Ji, 百日築基). The spiritual Embryo will only be healthy if it has this firm foundation.

The testicle Essence is one of the main sources of a man's energy. When it is abundant, his vital energy is high and his life force strong. When he loses the balance between production and expenditure of semen, his emotions also lose their balance. This leads to depression and speedy degeneration of the body. Part of this Essence is needed by the brain, to stimulate thought and to energize the body for activity. When semen production is insufficient, the brain does not obtain enough Qi, and the spirit's control of Qi circulation weakens. This results in sickness.

So the first step in Xi Sui Jing training is to increase semen production and convert it into Qi faster and more effectively than the body normally does. With the average mature man, the supply of semen fills up naturally without stimulation. It usually takes two to three weeks to replenish the supply of semen once it is lost. When a man's semen is full, hormones stimulate the brain and generate sexual desire, energizing him and making him impatient and inclined to lose his temper.

The time needed for the semen to replenish itself varies from one man to another. If one has sex frequently, semen is replenished faster. However, if one abstains for a period of time, the testicles start to function more slowly. If one has sex too often, the semen level will be low most of the time, affecting the conversion of hormones into Qi. The four Qi vessels in the legs receive most of their Qi from the conversion of semen. If you have too much sex you will find your legs weaken through Qi deficiency in these vessels.

The body produces semen during sleep from midnight until morning, because Qi circulation starts in the head (Baihui, Gv-20, 百會) and circulates down the front of the body, following the Conception Vessel and then Governing Vessel, reaching Baihui again. The Huiyin and Baihui, which are connected by the Thrusting Vessel, are both major points of Qi flow at midnight. When Qi circulation reaches the Huiyin, it stimulates the genitals and interacts with Original Qi from the Dan Tian to generate semen Qi (Jing Qi, 精氣).

Healthy males usually have erections when they wake in the morning. This starts quite soon after birth. Of course, at this age boys cannot generate sperm, and they do not have sexual urges. Chinese medical society believes that once a boy is formed, his testicles continuously generate semen. This interacts with the Original Qi (Yuan Qi, 元氣) at the Dan Tian and generates Semen Qi (Jing Qi, 精氣), which is transported to the brain, including the pituitary gland, to stimulate growth. When a boy's Yuan Qi is healthy and strong, the interaction of semen and Yuan Qi is also effective, and the boy grows normally. Once he reaches his teens, his testicles will also start to generate sperm. Normally, more is produced than is needed for growth, so Qi is full and abundant, making him healthy and strong.

Starting at midnight when you are sleeping and your body is relaxed, the Semen Qi from the testicles nourishes the brain and rebalances its energy. It is this rebalancing which generates dreams.

In Xi Sui Jing training, there are two general methods for stimulating semen production. One is Wai Dan, using physical stimulation, and the other is Nei Dan, using mental stimulation. The more the groin is stimulated, the more semen will be produced and the longer this organ will function normally. You must convert this semen into Qi more efficiently than is normally done by your body. If you do not effectively convert the excess semen into Qi, lead it to the brain, and spread it out among the twelve channels, the abundant semen will cause your sexual desire to increase and your emotions to lose their balance.

Theoretically, the method of Essence-Qi conversion is very simple. You lead the Qi from the four vessels in the legs upward to the Huang Ting cavity and also to the brain. This causes the Qi in these four vessels to become deficient, and more Essence must be converted to replenish the supply. In this case, you are consuming the extra Essence being generated. The process of leading the Qi upward is called Lian Qi Sheng Hua (練氣昇華), which means train the Qi to sublimate. When the Qi is led up to nourish the brain, it is called Huan Jing Bu Nao (還精補腦), which means to return the Essence to nourish the brain.

The more you practice, the more efficiently you convert semen into Qi. There are two major styles of semen conversion, Buddhist and Daoist. Buddhists emphasize Nei Dan conversion, which is generally much slower than the Daoists, who, in addition to Nei Dan, also train Wai Dan conversion. In Nei Dan conversion, Yi and breathing are the keys to leading the Qi up. Coordinating posture and movements at the Huiyin, the Qi is led up to the Huang Ting and brain.

Wai Dan conversion also leads the Qi in the legs up to the Huang Ting and brain. Daoist methods of testicle stimulation are faster, because they increase semen production and Wai Dan Essence-Qi conversion. They are called Gao Wan Yun Dong (睪丸運動, Testicle Exercises) or Chi Lao Huan Ji Yun Dong (遲老還機運動, slowing aging and returning the functioning exercises). The more semen you have, the more Qi you can convert it into, and the more efficiently you can do so.

### 3-3. Purifying Qi and Converting It into Spirit 練氣化神

**Ten months of pregnancy** (Shi Yue Huai Tai, 十月懷胎)

During the first stage, the Spiritual Embryo is formed in the Huang Ting. This is the seed from which the baby grows. The second stage is ten months of pregnancy (28 days for each Chinese lunar month), during which you provide it with purified Qi, just as a mother supplies nutrition and oxygen to the embryo. You train converting semen efficiently into Qi as the Spiritual Embryo grows and develops. If this process is insufficient, the baby's development will be deficient, and it may die. You are developing it into an entity with its own life.

You lead Yin and Yang Qi to the Huang Ting, where they interact harmoniously, forming the Spirit Embryo. In the second stage, you accumulate more Qi in your Huang Ting. It takes ten months of intensive practice to accumulate enough for the third stage of training, in which you activate extra brain cells and improve their function. This raises up your spirit to a high level.

As the embryo grows, its spirit also develops to become a healthy, complete being. You nourish it with Qi and also with spirit, like a mother who focuses her spirit and concentration on her embryo to obtain a spiritually healthy baby. The mother's thoughts and habits are passed on to the baby. In the same way, the Spirit Embryo develops its spirit, and this stage of training is called Purifying the Qi and converting it into Shen. The Daoist Li, Qing-An (李清菴) said, "Shen and Qi combine to create the super spiritual quality. Xin (心) and breath depend on one another to generate the Holy Embryo."[8] To endow the Embryo with spirit, you combine your Shen and Qi in the Huang Ting, giving the holy Embryo a supernatural, spiritual quality. Xin is your emotional mind, and the breathing is the training strategy. Coordinate your emotions and breathing, and focus on this holy Embryo, so its spirit can grow and mature.

Some practitioners believe that once the Embryo is formed, it should be moved to the Upper Dan Tian to grow, but this is a matter of choice. First you need plenty of Qi, then you use it to nourish the Embryo, and finally, you establish its spirit. With abundant Qi to activate and energize your brain cells and raise up your spirit, where the Embryo grows is not important. "When the elixir is accomplished in ten months, the holy Embryo is completed, and the real person appears."[9] After meditating for ten months, the Qi is abundantly stored in the Huang Ting. Then you lead it up to nourish your brain. You can now discard the mask you have been wearing, as this is the stage of self-recognition.

### 3-4. Refine Spirit and Return It to Nothingness 練神返虛

**Three Years of Nursing** (San Nian Bu Ru, 三年哺乳)

Having carried the spiritual Embryo for ten months, it is ready to be born. Qi has been stored in abundance at the Huang Ting, and the Embryo's Shen has been established. You now lead the Embryo up to the Upper Dan Tian to be born. The Upper Dan Tian, with the Yintang cavity (M-HN-3, 印堂, third eye), is where you sense and communicate with Nature's energy, and with the spirit world. This place is called Shen Gu (神谷, Spiritual Valley), as its physical structure looks like the entrance to a deep valley formed by the two lobes of the brain. When you communicate with the natural energy, it seems to be happening in a deep valley which reaches the center of your thinking and also far beyond what you can see.

The brain holds many mysteries which today's science still cannot explain. I believe the valley formed by the two brain lobes is the key to the length of brainwaves. Energy resonates in this valley and is transmitted outward like waves from the antenna of a radio station. The Upper Dan Tian is the gate which allows us to communicate with Nature and for our thoughts to be passed to others.

If one can activate more brain cells through Qigong, one may increase the brain's sensitivity to a wider range of wavelengths. One may perceive things more clearly, and have a heightened sensitivity to natural energy. One might even intuitively sense the thoughts of others without oral communication. With abundant Qi and strong concentration, it is also possible to cure others using your mind and Qi. This is the stage of self-awareness and awakening.

Having led the Qi to activate the brain, the next obstacle is opening the gate of the third eye. This is obstructed by the skin, the skullbone, and the frontal sinus. They block much of the energy emitted or received by the brain, which is why this gate is considered closed. However, bones are semi-conductors. Through concentrated meditation, we can generate significant potential difference, or EMF, between the brain and the outside of the head. Once this potential difference reaches the threshold level, the bone becomes a conductor. Then you can communicate with the outside world without obstruction. The gate is called Xuan Guan (玄關, Tricky Gate). When concentrated Qi opens, the process is called Kai Qiao (開竅, opening the tricky gate). Once this gate is opened, it stays open.

Another gate is located on top of the head, called Baihui (Gv-20, 百會) in acupuncture or Ni Wan Gong (泥丸宮) in Qigong, where your brain can communicate with natural energy. It is not the spiritual center, but simply a gate able to exchange Qi with nature. This gate is commonly used to absorb heaven Qi from the sun and stars, and earth Qi from the earth's magnetic field.

In this third stage of enlightenment meditation, you lead the abundant Qi to the brain to activate unused brain cells and thereby increase brain capacity. Then you concentrate the abundant Qi to open the gate. This means the spirit baby is born in the Upper Dan Tian, which you now nurse. This means to protect, care for, and nourish it as it develops, and is called Yang Shen (養神, nurse the Shen). By increasing the brain's Qi level, you can sense and communicate with nature more effectively. As your spirit communes with nature, it becomes accustomed to staying with the natural energy and gradually forgets the physical body. Since the natural spirit cannot be seen, it is nothingness, which also refers to the absence of emotions and desires. So this stage of training is called Refining Shen and returning it to Nothingness. Since your spirit body originated from physical and emotional nothingness, in this training, you are returning to nothingness. The Buddhists call this Si Da Jie Kong (四大皆空), or Four Large are Empty. This means the four elements (earth, fire, water, and air) are absent from the mind, so that you are completely indifferent to worldly temptations.

You nurse your spirit baby for at least three years. Just like a real baby, it needs to be protected and nurtured until it can be self-sufficient. If it travels, it cannot go too far, like a small child gradually familiarizing itself with its new environment. This is the first stage of enlightenment or Buddhahood.

I would like to translate a Daoist song about this stage of cultivation.

### The Song of Great Dao
### 大道歌
### 《遵身八箋・清修妙論箋》

大道不遠在身中，萬物皆空性不空。性若不空和氣住，
氣歸元海壽無窮。欲得身中神不出，莫向靈台留一物。
物在心中神不清，耗散真精損筋骨。神御氣兮氣留形，
不須藥物自長生。術則易知訣難遇，總然易了不專行。
所以千人萬人學，畢竟終無一個存。神若出兮便收來，
神返身中氣自回。如此朝朝並暮暮，自然赤子產靈胎。

*The Great Dao is not far but in the body. Ten thousand material objects are empty, but human nature is not empty. If human nature is not empty, and can stay together in harmony with Qi, the Qi will return to the original ocean (Real Lower Dan Tian), and longevity is unlimited. To keep the spirit staying in the body, do not leave even one object in Lingtai (spiritual platform). If any object remains in the heart, the spirit will not be clear. This wastes the real essence and damages the tendons and bones (physical body). The spirit directs the Qi, and through Qi, the shape endures. Then you will live long without needing herbs. The techniques are easy, but the secrets are hard to meet. The correct way has always been changed and separated from the path. So even though a thousand or ten thousand people learn, not even one accomplishes the training. When the spirit leaves the body, immediately bring it back. When the spirit returns, the Qi will also return automatically. Practice thus every morning and evening, and the spiritual Embryo will be born naturally and automatically.*

The great Dao of longevity and enlightenment is within us, to be reached through cultivation. The mind should not be engaged in material objects which, after all, are empty and impermanent. Train to overcome the influence of objects generated from earth, fire, water, and air. Cultivate your true nature,, and raise up your spirit. Once you harmonize with the Qi, it can be kept at the Real Lower Dan Tian. You live for a long time, since you do not waste your Qi.

Keep your mind pure, free from material objects around you and from emotional bondage. Keep your spirit in its spiritual center. If it wanders away, it leads Qi away and wastes it. When the spirit is kept firmly inside the body, the Qi will stay. When the Qi is abundant and stays, the body will be strong and healthy. This is the key to longevity. The key to producing the spiritual Embryo is to keep the spirit inside the body.

To develop the Spiritual Embryo, cultivate and raise your spirit, with the abundant Qi stored in the Real Lower Dan Tian. But if your mind is swayed by material attractions, you cannot store enough Qi to generate the Spiritual Embryo. This is the stage of cultivating your true nature to be free from physical and emotional bondage.

## 3-5. CRUSHING THE NOTHINGNESS 粉碎虛空

**Nine Years of Facing the Wall** (Jiu Nian Mian Bi, 九年面壁)

At this stage, you see the spiritual world as more real than the physical. Crushing nothingness means destroying the illusion which connects the physical world with the spiritual plane. According to Buddhism, your spirit cannot separate from your physical body completely, because it is still connected to the human world by emotions and desires. Only if you free yourself from these bonds can your spirit separate and be independent. Nine years of meditation gives your spirit the time to experience the natural energy world and to learn to live independently. Then it can separate from your physical body and continue living without it. It lives in the natural energy and continues even when the physical body is dead.

The highest goal of a Buddhist monk is to reach enlightenment or Buddhahood. He develops his Shen to be independent and exist even after the body dies. His Qi energizes his brain so strongly that it interacts with the electrical charge in the air and generates a glow around his head. This may even occur in earlier stages. It is frequently shown in pictures of Buddha, especially when he is shown meditating in the dark. It is identical to the halo in pictures of Western saints.

This stage is called Lian Shen (練神), or train the spirit. Your spirit receives its education from the natural energy. This generally takes more than twelve years, in fact, usually many lifetimes. You strengthen your Baby Shen in every lifetime, and one day you reach enlightenment. However, many Buddhists and Daoists believe the entire training depends on one's understanding. If one could really understand it, one could reach enlightenment in virtually no time at all. I am inclined to agree with them. In virtually every field of endeavor, if one ponders and understands the principles, he finds ways to reach the goal far sooner than expected.

I would like to point out that there are many documents about the first two stages, but very little written about the last two stages of enlightenment training. However, if your desire is sincere and your mind focuses on the goal, you will understand what you need to do to reach the next level. No one can understand you better than yourself.

## References

1. 胎指金丹，產金丹喻為懷胎。

2. 薛道光《悟真篇》註：〝嬰兒者，即丹也。丹是一，一是真一之氣，天地之母氣也。以母咽氣歸五內，以伏子氣，猶貓伏鼠而不走也。子母之氣相戀于胞胎之中，結成嬰兒之一。故曰：太一含真氣。言含真一之氣。如人懷胎，十月滿足，然後降生。〞

3. "Complex and Hidden Brain in the Gut Makes Stomachaches and Butterflies," by Sandra Blakeslee, *The New York Times,* Science, January 23, 1996.

4. *The Second Brain: The Scientific Basis of Gut Instinct and a Groundbreaking New Understanding of Nervous Disorders of the Stomach and Intestine,* Michael D. Gershon, New York: Harper Collins Publications, 1998.

5. 王錄識餘云：〝銅人針灸圖，載臟腑一身俞穴有玉環，余不知玉環是何物。〞

6. 張紫陽玉清金華祕文，論神仙結丹處曰：〝心上腎下，脾左肝右，生門在前，密戶居後，其連如環，其白如綿，方圓徑寸，密裹一身之精粹，此即玉環。〞

7. 藥補不如食補，食補不如氣補。

8. 李清菴詩云：〝神氣和合生靈質，心息相依結聖胎。〞

9. 《金丹真傳・溫養》：〝丹成十月聖胎完，自有真人出現。〞

## CHAPTER 4

# Five Regulatings
五調

## 4-1. INTRODUCTION 介紹

Whether you practice Internal Elixir (Nei Dan, 內丹) or External Elixir (Wai Dan, 外丹) Qigong, there are five regulating processes to reach the final goal of practice. These are: regulating the body (Tiao Shen, 調身), regulating the breathing (Tiao Xi, 調息), regulating the emotional mind (Tiao Xin, 調心), regulating Qi (Tiao Qi, 調氣), and regulating the spirit (Tiao Shen, 調神). These five are commonly called Wu Tiao (五調, Five Regulatings).

The Chinese word Tiao (調), which I translate as "regulating", consists of two words, namely Yan (言), which means speaking or negotiating, and Zhou (周), which means to be complete, perfect, or round. Tiao means to adjust or to fine tune until it is complete and harmonious with others. It is like tuning the notes of a piano to be in harmony with one another. Tiao means to coordinate, cooperate, and harmonize by ongoing adjustment. All five aspects, body, breathing, mind, Qi, and spirit, need to be regulated until harmony is achieved.

The key to regulating is through *feeling, which is the language of the mind and body*. The deeper and more sensitively you feel, the more profoundly you can regulate, and vice versa. It requires significant effort to reach the finest stage of feeling and regulating. This training of inner feeling is called Gongfu of self-internal-observation (Nei Shi Gongfu, 內視功夫, internal feeling or awareness). The more refined your Gongfu, the deeper you harmonize with others.

At the beginning, your mind is focused on regulating and on making it happen, so it is not natural or smooth. Later it becomes regulating without regulating. "The real regulating is without regulating."[1] It is like learning to drive, with your mind on the road and the controls of the car. This is the stage of regulating. Once you are experienced, your mind does not have to regulate. You drive without driving, and everything happens naturally and smoothly. With the five Qigong regulatings, you practice until regulating is unnecessary. Then your feeling is profound, and regulating is achieved naturally and automatically.

Next we will discuss these five regulatings, and the importance of mutually coordinating them, as they pertain to meditation.

## 4-2. REGULATING THE BODY (TIAO SHEN) 調身

A tense posture in meditation affects Qi circulation, and disturbs the mind. "When shape (posture) is incorrect, Qi will not be smooth. When Qi is not smooth, the Yi (wisdom mind) is not at peace. When Yi is not at peace, then Qi is disordered."[2]

The purposes of regulating the body are to:

1. **Find the most natural and comfortable posture for meditation.** This allows the Qi and breathing to flow smoothly, so the mind relaxes and focuses on the raising the Spirit.

2. **Provide the best conditions for self-internal-feeling.** When your body is well regulated, your feeling can reach a profound level. When mind and body communicate, your judgment will be accurate, and your mind circulates Qi effectively.

3. **Coordinate body and mind,** using Yi (意, wisdom mind) and correct feeling.

**Three Stages of Relaxation.** Relaxation is a major key to success in Qigong practice. It opens your Qi channels, and allows Qi to circulate smoothly and easily.

Each stage has two aspects, mental and physical. Mental relaxation precedes physical relaxation. There are two minds, the emotional (Xin, 心) and the wisdom mind (Yi, 意). The Xin affects your feelings and the condition of your body. The Yi leads you to a calm and peaceful state, which allows you to exercise sound judgment. Your wisdom mind must first relax, so it can control the emotional mind and let it relax too. When the peaceful wisdom mind and emotional mind coordinate with your breathing, the physical body also relaxes.

There are three stages of relaxation. The first is superficial physical relaxation, which most people can achieve. Adopt a comfortable posture and avoid unnecessary strain. You may *look* relaxed, but you are still tense inside. Your mind does not have to reach a very deep level to achieve this stage.

The second stage involves relaxing the muscles, tendons, and ligaments. Your meditative mind *feels* deep inside the muscles, tendons, and ligaments. From this feeling you can gauge the level of your relaxation. This level opens your Qi channels to allow Qi to accumulate in the Real Lower Dan Tian.

The final stage is relaxation which reaches the internal organs, the bone marrow, and every pore of your skin. Your mind must achieve profound calmness and peace to *sense* the organs and marrow, and to lead the Qi to any point in your body. You will feel light and transparent, as though your body has disappeared. You can also lead the Qi to strengthen your Guardian Qi (Wei Qi, 衛氣) to protect you from outside influences. You can adjust Qi in your organs to regulate Qi disorders, protecting them and slowing their degeneration.

An important aspect of Qigong training is leading the five Qi's toward their origins (Wu Qi Chao Yuan, 五氣朝元). This involves adjusting Qi in the five Yin organs, namely lungs, heart, kidneys, liver, and spleen. One can generally feel the lungs more easily, because they move when you inhale and exhale. Once you have relaxed them, you can feel your heartbeat. After that, the kidneys can be sensed more easily than the liver and spleen because liquid flows constantly through them. The liver will be next, and then the spleen. Because the liver is much larger than the spleen, it is easier to feel the blood move inside it.

**Yin and Yang in Regulating the Body.** To regulate the body into a desired state, you apply the concept of Yin and Yang in your practice, adjusting them using Kan (坎, Water) and Li (離, Fire). When your mind is calm, and breathing long and smooth, your body relaxes deeper and Qi can circulate smoothly. The deep calm mind and long breath are Kan (Water), making your physical body more Yin, and your Qi body more Yang. The physical body is cooler, while the Qi body is more assertive.

By contrast, when you are excited, with short and heavy breathing, your physical body will also be tense, hot, and energized. Qi stagnates so it can manifest into physical form. The excited mind and heavy breathing is Li (Fire), making your physical body Yang, and the Qi body more Yin. The physical body is excited and the Qi circulation is slow and stagnant. Depending on your purpose, you regulate your body accordingly. To make your body more Yang and build up external strength, use Li. To internalize and make your Qi body more Yang, use Kan to make it happen.

When you practice Small Circulation meditation, since you are focusing on the Qi body instead of the physical, bring your physical body to the most relaxed Yin state so Qi can be directed to circulate smoothly and abundantly.

**Regulating the Body and the Spirit.** When you meditate, relax your body as much as possible, so your mind can be calm, the Qi can circulate smoothly, and your feeling can be centered and balanced. Harmonize your mind and body, and build up a firm root. Then the spirit can be raised. Relaxing the body is the first step in raising the spirit.

## 4-3. REGULATING THE BREATHING (TIAO XI) 調息

Once regulating your body reaches the stage of *regulating without regulating*, you focus on the breathing. The body can be regarded as a battlefield, with Qi as soldiers, the mind as the general, and the spirit as fighting morale. *Breathing is regarded as the strategy.* When breathing methods are correct, Qi is led effectively. Since ancient times, Qigong breathing methods have been studied and practiced, and kept top secret by only being passed down orally in each style. Embryonic Breathing (Tai Xi, 胎息) is the crucial key to storing Qi at the Real Lower Dan Tian (Zhen Xia Dan Tian, 真下丹田) and for cultivating spiritual enlightenment. Embryonic Breathing is so important in Internal Elixir Qigong (Nei Dan Qigong, 內丹氣功), that it is discussed in great detail in the first book of this series, *Qigong Meditation—Embryonic Breathing*. It is briefly reviewed in Chapter 6 of this book. In this section, we will only summarize the general concepts of regulating breathing, its purpose, theory, and some techniques.

### Purposes of Regulating the Breathing

1. **To convert nutrition, or food essence, into Qi efficiently.** The source of post-birth Qi is mainly from food. According to the biochemical formula, the more oxygen we inhale, the more efficient the biochemical reaction, and the more energy generated. The body converts this energy into heat, light, and bioelectricity (Qi).

$$glucose + 6O_2 \longrightarrow 6CO_2 + 6H_2O$$

$$\Delta G^{O'} = -686 \text{ Kcal}$$

2. **To improve metabolism, which is the efficiency of cell replacement.** Approximately one trillion cells die every day in a healthy person.[3] To slow the aging process, they must be replaced each day, for which oxygen is one of the elements required. Without it, the new cells will be deformed and unhealthy. Dead cells (carbon) must also be disposed of. The respiratory system supplies the oxygen and removes the dead cells. Inhaling and exhaling deeply allows cell replacement to proceed smoothly.

3. **To serve the strategic purpose of regulating Yin and Yang.** Breathing is a Kan and Li method with which you may adjust the body's Yin and Yang. Inhalation makes the body more Yin, while exhalation makes it more Yang.

4. **To coordinate and harmonize the body, mind, Qi, and spirit.** Breathing, as one of the five important regulatings, plays the important role of coordinating and harmonizing the others. Concentrating in a deep, profound inhalation can calm you and condense your spirit. Focusing in exhalation can raise the body's energy, excite the mind, and raise up the spirit. Correct breathing assists in leading Qi more efficiently.

**Breathing and Qigong.** There are Eight Qi Vessels (Mai, 脈), which function like reservoirs, and Twelve Primary Qi Channels (Jing, 經), which function like rivers in your body. In addition, there are millions of tiny channels called Luo (絡) branching out from the twelve channels to the surface of the skin, to generate a shield of Guardian Qi (Wei Qi, 衛氣). This Qi is responsible for hair growth and for defending against negative outside influences. These tiny channels also enter the bone marrow (Sui Qi, 髓氣) to keep it healthy and producing blood cells. They also establish pathways for Qi exchange and communication between internal organs.

Qi circulates naturally and automatically without Qigong training. Qigong practice coordinates the mind and breathing to generate electromotive force, to control the Qi circulation more efficiently. As one exhales, one expands the Qi and leads it from the primary channels to the skin, and the body becomes more Yang. When one inhales, one draws in Qi and leads it from the primary channels to the bone marrow, and the body becomes more Yin (Figure 4-1). When inhalation and exhalation are balanced, Yin and Yang are balanced.

As you get older, your breath becomes shorter, and less Qi is led to the skin and bone marrow. Qi stagnates there, and the skin starts to wrinkle, while the hair turns gray or falls out. Fewer blood cells are produced, and they are not as healthy as before. Because they carry less nutrition and oxygen through the body, you get sick more often and age faster. The first key to maintaining youth is regulating your breathing to control Kan and Li, and thus the Yin and Yang of your body.

Table 4-1. General Rules of Breathing's Kan-Li and Yin-Yang

| Kan-Li | Method | Consequence | |
|--------|--------|-------------|---|
| Kan | Inhalation | Yin* | |
| Li | Exhalation | Yang* | |
| Kan | Inhale then hold the breath | | Yin |
| Li | Exhale then hold the breath | Yang | |
| Kan | Soft, slow, calm, and long breath | Yin | |
| Li | Heavy, fast and short breath | Yang | |
| Kan | Normal Abdominal Breathing (Buddhist Breathing) | Yin | |
| Li | Reverse Abdominal Breathing (Daoist Breathing) | Yang | |

*Yin and Yang are relative, not absolute. After defining a reference standard or level, compare them with each other.

Yin*: Cold, calm, body relaxed, and Qi body energized

Yang*: Hot, excited, physical body tense, and energized

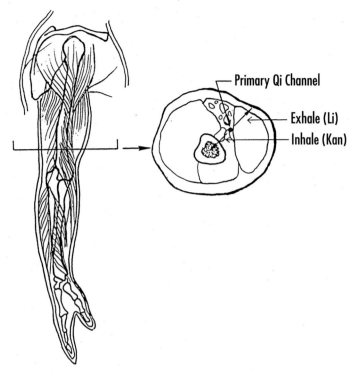

Figure 4-1. The Expansion and Condensing
of Qi during Breathing

## Breathing Methods

### 1. Normal Breathing (Pin Chang Hu Xi, 平常呼吸)

Normal Breathing is also called Chest Breathing (Xiong Bu Hu Xi, 胸部呼吸), in which the breath is controlled by emotion. Regulate it by relaxing the lungs. Concentrate until the practice is neutral, calm, and peaceful. The breathing can be long and deep while the body relaxes, and the heartbeat slows down. You may practice in any comfortable position, ten minutes each morning and evening until one day you notice that your mind does not have to pay attention to the chest. Then concentrate on feeling the result of the training. When you exhale, you feel the pores of the skin open, and when you inhale, the pores close. It seems that all the pores are breathing with you. This is a low level of skin or body breathing. The feeling is very comfortable. When you can do this comfortably and automatically, you have regulated your Chest Breathing.

You should practice until you reach a level of regulating without regulating (Wu Tiao Er Tiao, 無調而調), which is known as "the real regulating". Then you will be practicing all the time since you have built up a natural habit for your breathing. The most powerful Qigong practice is one which you have integrated into your lifestyle, including your breathing behavior.

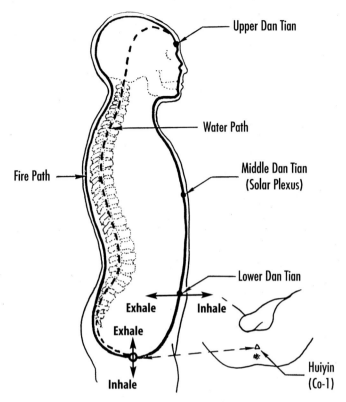

Figure 4-2. Normal Abdominal Breathing

## 2. Normal Abdominal Breathing (Zheng Fu Hu Xi, 正腹呼吸 )

Normal Abdominal Breathing is called Buddhist Breathing (Fo Jia Hu Xi, 佛家呼吸). Control your abdominal muscles and coordinate them with the breathing. When you inhale, the abdomen expands, and when you exhale, it withdraws. Practice until the process becomes smooth, with the body relaxed. Concentrate on your abdomen initially to control the abdominal muscles. Afterwards the process becomes natural and smooth, and you are ready to build up Qi at the False Lower Dan Tian (Jia Xia Dan Tian, 假下丹田, Qihai, Co-6, 氣海).

Then coordinate your breathing with the movements of your Huiyin (Co-1, 會陰, perineum). When you inhale, gently push the Huiyin down, and when you exhale hold it up (Figure 4-2). You gently hold up the Huiyin without tensing, and it remains relaxed. Tensing impedes Qi circulation and causes tension in the abdomen, which can generate other problems. Initially, use your mind to control the muscles of the abdomen and perineum. Later, your mind does not need to be there to make it happen, and you regulate without regulating. You feel a wonderful comfortable feeling at the Huiyin, and the Qi is led more strongly to the skin than when you did "Chest Breathing." It will feel as though your whole body is breathing with you.

Table 4-2. Normal Abdominal Breathing

Body Neutral (inhalation and exhalation are equal length)
    Yin   —Inhalation (Abdomen Expands, Huiyin **Pushed Out Gently**)
    Yang —Exhalation (Abdomen Withdraws, Huiyin **Held Up Gently**)
Body Yin
        —Inhalation longer (Abdomen Expands, Huiyin **Pushed Out Gently**)

        —Exhalation (Abdomen Withdraws, Huiyin **Relaxed**)
Body Yang
        —Inhalation (Abdomen Expands, Huiyin **Pushed Out Gently**)
        —Exhalation longer (Abdomen Withdraws, Huiyin **Held Up Strongly**)

### 3. Reverse Abdominal Breathing (Fan Fu Hu Xi, Ni Fu Hu Xi, 反腹呼吸 · 逆腹呼吸)

Reverse Abdominal Breathing is called Daoist Breathing (Dao Jia Hu Xi, 道家呼吸), which you start training once you have mastered Buddhist Breathing. It is called Reverse Abdominal Breathing because the movement of the abdomen is the reverse of Buddhist Breathing. The abdomen withdraws when you inhale and expands when you exhale (Figure 4-3). Buddhist breathing is more relaxed, by contrast with Daoist breathing, which is more aggressive. Daoist breathing makes the body more Yang, while Buddhist breathing makes it more Yin.

Many people wrongly believe that reverse breathing is against the Dao, or nature's path. This is not true. It is simply used for different purposes. If you observe your breathing patterns, you notice we use reverse breathing in two types of situations.

First, when emotionally disturbed, we often use reverse breathing. When you laugh, you make the sound "Ha" (哈), using reverse breathing. Your abdomen expands, exhalation is longer than inhalation, Guardian Qi (Wei Qi, 衛氣) expands, and you get hot. This is the natural way of releasing excess energy from excitement or happiness. When you cry, you make the sound "Hen" (哼) while inhaling, your abdomen withdraws, and inhalation is longer than exhalation. Guardian Qi shrinks and you feel cold. This is the natural way of preventing energy loss from inside your body. When you are sad, your spirit and your body's energy are low.

The second occasion in which we use reverse breathing is to energize the body, such as when pushing or lifting something heavy. You inhale deeply to take in more oxygen and then exhale while pushing the object, which is reverse breathing. When we are disturbed emotionally or have aggressive or strong intentions, we use reverse breathing naturally.

With practice, you can lead the Qi to the skin more efficiently than with Buddhist breathing. You can also lead it to the bone marrow to enhance the marrow

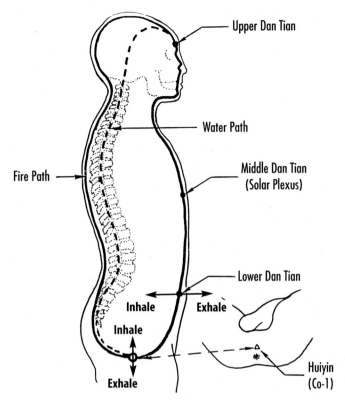

Figure 4-3. Reverse Abdominal Breathing

Qi (Sui Qi, 髓氣). Compare Normal Abdominal Breathing with Reverse Abdominal Breathing to see how Qi is led in these two different breathing strategies.

In Normal Abdominal Breathing, Qi circulates mainly in the primary Qi channels (Jing, 經) connecting the internal organs to the extremities. Some also spread out through the secondary Qi channels (Luo, 絡) to reach the skin and bone marrow (Figure 4-4). Since most Qi remains in the primary Qi channels, the body is not energized and stays relaxed, enabling a state of deep relaxation. Normal Abdominal Breathing (Kan, 坎) makes the body Yin, while Reverse Abdominal Breathing (Li, 離) makes it Yang.

In Reverse Abdominal Breathing, most Qi is led sideways through the Luo to the skin and bone marrow, while much less circulates in the primary Qi channels (Figure

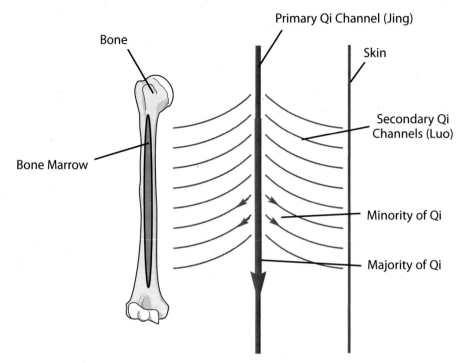

Figure 4-4. In Normal Abdominal Breathing, a Majority of
the Qi Circulates in the Primary Qi Channels

4-5). Skin breathing (Ti Xi, Fu Xi, 體息・膚息) and marrow breathing (Sui Xi, 髓息)
can be achieved more aggressively through Reverse Abdominal Breathing.

Table 4-3. Reverse Abdominal Breathing
(Emotionally unsettled, the mind has Intention of Yin or Yang)

Body Neutral*
    Yin    —Inhalation (Abdomen Withdraws, Huiyin **Held Up Gently**)
    Yang  —Exhalation (Abdomen Expands, Huiyin **Pushed Out Gently**)
        *Inhalation and exhalation are of equal length.

Body Yin
        —Inhalation Longer (Abdomen Withdraws, Huiyin **Held Up Firmly**)
        —Exhalation (Abdomen Expands, Huiyin **Relaxed**)
    *Hen sound can enhance the body's Yin.

Body Yang
        —Inhalation (Abdomen Withdraws, Huiyin **Held Up Gently**)
        —Exhalation (Abdomen Expands, Huiyin **Pushed Out Firmly**)
    *Ha sound can enhance the body's Yang.

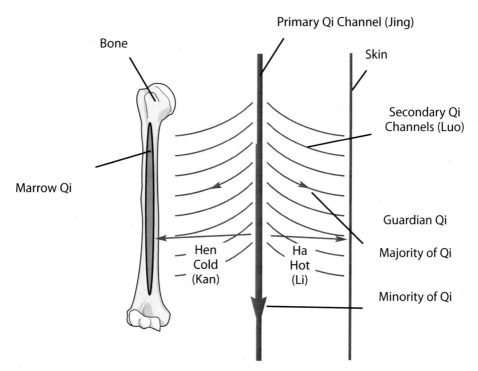

Figure 4-5. In Reverse Abdominal Breathing, a Majority of
the Qi is Led to the Skin Surface and Bone Marrow

In Reverse Abdominal Breathing, when you inhale, you withdraw your abdomen and hold up your Huiyin, while moving the diaphragm downward. Tension generated at the stomach area may cause pain, like when you laugh loudly or cry. So before practicing it, first practice Normal Abdominal Breathing for a while to relax and control the abdominal muscles. Use small movements at the beginning, before increasing the scale of abdominal movement.

### 4. Embryonic Breathing (Tai Xi, 胎息)

Embryonic Breathing has always been a huge subject in Internal Elixir Qigong practice. It is the breathing method which allows you to store Qi in the Real Lower Dan Tian (Zhen Xia Dan Tian, 真下丹田) and charge your biobattery to a high level. Your vital energy is raised, the immune system strengthened, and the body reconditioned. More importantly, once abundant Qi is stored, you can lead it upward through the spinal cord (Chong Mai, 衝脈) to nourish the brain and raise the spirit. This is the crucial key of spiritual enlightenment. Embryonic Breathing is also crucial in skin breathing and marrow breathing, which is closely related to our immune system and longevity.

Since Embryonic Breathing is also vital for Small Circulation, we discuss it separate-

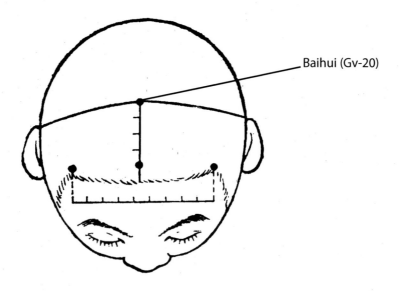

Figure 4-6. The Baihui (Gv-20) Cavity

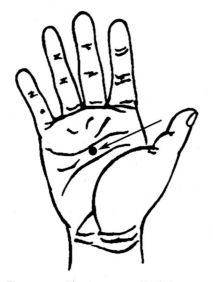

Figure 4-7. The Laogong (P-8) Cavity

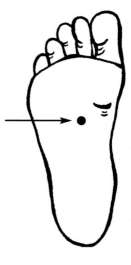

Figure 4-8. The Yongquan
(K-1) Cavity

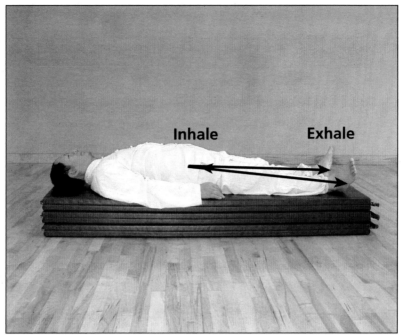

Figure 4-9. Yongquan Breathing with Normal Abdominal Breathing

ly in Chapter 6, together with skin breathing and marrow breathing. Again, for more detail, please refer to the previous book, *Qigong Meditation—Embryonic Breathing*.

### 5. Skin—Marrow Breathing (Fu Sui Xi, 膚髓息)

Skin Breathing (Fu Xi, 膚息) is sometimes called Body Breathing (Ti Xi, 體息) Actually, body breathing involves breathing with the whole body, not just the skin. When you exhale, you lead Qi to the muscles and skin, and when you inhale, you lead Qi to the marrow and internal organs. You feel your whole body transparent to Qi, as though it had disappeared. Skin-Marrow Breathing is closely related to Embryonic Breathing. When Qi is led to the Real Lower Dan Tian, you are also leading it to the bone marrow, and when it is led to the Girdle Vessel (Dai Mai, 帶脈), you are also leading it to the skin.

### 6. Five Gates Breathing (Wu Xin Hu Xi, 五心呼吸)

The five gates are: the head (Upper Dan Tian and Baihui, Gv-20, 百會), the two Laogong (P-8, 勞宮) cavities on the palms, and the two Yongquan (K-1, 湧泉) cavities on the soles of the feet (Figures 4-6 to 4-8). Beginners use the Baihui gate in the top of the head because there, it is easier to communicate with natural Qi. Later, the third eye (Tian Yan, 天眼) is used instead.

Having built up Qi at the Real Lower Dan Tian, you harmonize your breathing and lead the Qi to the Yongquan cavities. For Yongquan breathing (Yongquan Hu Xi, 湧泉呼吸) you may adopt any posture, even lying down and using Normal

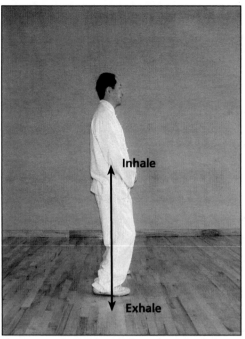

Figure 4-10. Yongquan Breathing with Reverse Abdominal Breathing

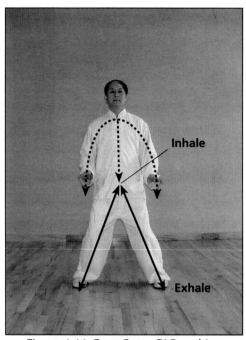

Figure 4-11. Four Gates Qi Breathing

Abdominal Breathing. Inhale leading Qi from Yongquan to the Real Lower Dan Tian, and exhale leading it back to Yongquan (Figure 4-9). When you inhale, the abdomen and Huiyin (Co-1, 會陰) expand, and when you exhale, they withdraw. Even though the mind is involved, it does not aggressively lead the Qi, and relaxation is paramount.

To lead Qi to the Yongquan aggressively, Reverse Abdominal Breathing is more effective, and the best posture is standing. Inhale, leading Qi from the Yongquan cavities to the Real Lower Dan Tian, and when you exhale, your mind leads the Qi back to the Yongquan, while you slightly squat down and imagine pushing your feet down into the ground (Figure 4-10). When you inhale, the abdomen withdraws while the Huiyin is held up, and when you exhale, they expand.

Yongquan cavity breathing is also called Sole Breathing (Zhong Xi, 踵息) described by the well known Daoist scholar, Zhuang Zi (莊子), during the Chinese Warring States Period (403-222 B.C., 戰國). He said, "The breathing of the ancient truthful persons (Zhen Ren, 真人, Daoists) was deep and profound. They used the soles to breathe, while seculars use the throat."[4] So Yongquan breathing has been trained for more than two thousand years. For medical Qigong, Yongquan breathing is one of the most effective methods to regulate abnormal Qi in three of the Yin organs, namely liver, kidneys, and spleen.

With Yongquan breathing well established, and having reached the real regulating of no regulating, add the Laogong breathing at the center of your palms. These two gates regulate the heart and lungs. Use either Normal Abdominal Breathing or Reverse Abdominal Breathing. Inhale leading Qi from the four gates to the Real Lower Dan Tian, and exhale leading it back again (Figure 4-11).

Four gates breathing is a common method of Grand Qi Circulation (Da Zhou Tian, 大周天). Once you reach a profound level, add the fifth gate, which elevates the practice into Spiritual Breathing (Shen Xi, 神息).

### 7. Spiritual Breathing (Shen Xi, 神息)

Spiritual Breathing is also called Fifth Gate Breathing (Di Wu Xin Hu Xi, 第五心呼吸), Baihui Breathing (Baihui Hu Xi, 百會呼吸), or Upper Dan Tian Breathing (Shang Dan Tian Hu Xi, 上丹田呼吸). It means to breathe through the third eye, and is crucial in opening the third eye for enlightenment.

Reaching the level of spiritual breathing presupposes regulating your body, breathing, mind, and Qi, and now the spirit. Your Qigong practice and the search for spiritual enlightenment has reached the final stage and is approaching maturity. According to *The Complete Book of Principal Contents of Life and Human Nature* (性命圭旨全書): "What is spiritual breathing? It means the maturity of cultivation."[5] That means cultivating the interaction of Kan and Li has reached the stage of regulating without regulating, and all the cultivations have become natural. We will discuss this subject further in the forthcoming books on the subjects of Qigong Meditation and Spiritual Enlightenment.

There are some other breathing methods trained in the Daoist Qigong such as Turtle Breathing (Gui Xi, 龜息) and Hibernation Breathing (Dong Mian Xi, 冬眠息). Since they are not related to Small Circulation, and I do not have profound understanding of their practice, they are not discussed here.

**Final goals of regulating the breathing.** *The Complete Book of Principal Contents of Life and Human Nature* (性命圭旨全書) says, "Regulate the breathing, you must regulate until the real regulating ceases. Train the spirit, you must train until the spirit of being without spirit."[6] Practice Embryonic Breathing until you achieve regulating without regulating. It is the same in cultivating your spirit. First aim for spiritual neutrality and enlightenment. Afterwards, no further enlightenment is necessary.

*The Correct Theory of Becoming a Heavenly Fairy, A Frank Discussion of Taming the Breathing* (天仙正理・伏氣直論) states, "When ancient people talked about the way of regulating the breathing, it is to follow the rules of nature's to and fro (circulation) without stubbornly keeping the shape of to and fro. This means to match the breathing as if there were no breathing."[7] The goal of regulating the breath is to follow nature without stagnation and practicing until regulating becomes unnecessary.

## Some Ancient Documents About Regulating the Breath

### 1. The question from a Buddhist guest about listening to the heart
《聽心齋客問》

*Expanding the bellows means to regulate the real breathing. When exhaling, the air exits, and when inhaling, the air enters. When exiting, then it is like the earth Qi's ascending, and when entering, it is like the heaven Qi's descending. This breathing is the same as the heaven and the earth. Isn't the space between the heaven and the earth just like the wind bellows?*

鼓橐籥，曰調真息。呼則氣出，吸則氣入，出則如地氣
上升，入則如天氣下降，與天地同。故天地間，其猶橐
籥乎？

Tuo Yue (橐籥) means the bellows, used to assist air circulation. We know that breathing is a strategy in Qigong practice, able to make Qi circulate smoothly in the body. The lungs are the air bellows, while the Lower Dan Tian is the Qi bellows. When the lungs take in air, the Qi sinks to the Lower Dan Tian like the Qi descending in nature. When air is expelled by the lungs, the Qi in the Lower Dan Tian rises up through the body like Qi ascending in nature. The human body is a small microcosm of heaven and earth. The tricky key to taking in the air and expelling it is the nose, while the piston of the Qi bellows in the Lower Dan Tian is at the Huiyin (Co-1, 會陰, perineum). Once you regulate your breathing to be natural (regulating without regulating), it is called Real Breathing (Zhen Xi, 真息).

### 2. An essay about regulating the breath
### (The Complete Book of Zhu-Zi, Song Dynasty)
《調息箴》
（朱子全書・宋・朱熹撰）

*The tip of the nose has white, I observe it all the time and at all places. Allow it to be soft, gentle, and supple. When extreme calmness has been reached, it hisses like a spring fish in the pond. When action has reached its extremity, it is harmonized like the torpor of a hundred insects. Open and close harmoniously, and its marvelousness is unlimited. What else can preside? It is achieved by not presiding. The clouds in the sky and the heaven cycling as it is. Who dares to question it? Keeping in one place harmoniously. Then, can live one thousand two hundred years.*

鼻端有白，我其觀之，隨時隨處，容與猗猗。靜極而嘘，
如春沼魚，動極而翕，如百蟲蟄。氤氳開闔，其妙無窮，
誰其尸之？不宰之功。雲臥天行，非予敢議，守一處和，
千二百歲。

The white at the tip of the nose means the air. Regulate the breath until it is soft, gentle, and supple. When I am extremely calm, inhaling deeply, then I exhale like a fish in the spring time. When I am extremely active, exhaling efficiently, then I retain it calmly and harmoniously like the torpor of insects. Breathing harmoniously this way, what else can compare? Success depends on regulating without regulating. Then it is like the clouds in the sky, and nature repeating its cycles; who else dares to contest with you? Keep the mind at the Real Lower Dan Tian (Zhen Xia Dan Tian, 真下丹田) harmoniously, and you may live to be one thousand two hundred years old.

To obtain longevity, first, regulate your breathing until no regulating is necessary. Second, keep Qi at its residence at the Real Lower Dan Tian. This is Embryonic Breathing (Tai Xi, 胎息).

### 3. Regulating the breath[8]
### (Original Truth of Using No Herbs, Qing Dynasty)
《調息》
（勿藥元詮·清·汪昂輯）

*Regulating the breath has been thoroughly studied by three groups: Buddhism, Daoism, and Confucianism. Upon reaching the great achievement, one may enter the Dao, and reaching the small achievement preserves health. Sanskrit documents from India teach looking at the tip of the nose, counting the breaths in and out internally. This is the beginning practice of Stopping Vision (Zhi Guan, attraction of visual objects). Zhuang Zi in his book Nan Hua Jing said, "A sage breathes through the soles." Great Yi (Yi Jing, The Book of Change) explains in its trigram, "When it gets dark, gentlemen enter Yan Xi (meditation or profound breathing)." Wang, Long-Xi said, "The ancient sages had deep breathing without sleeping. Therefore, it is said, when getting dark, enter the Yan Xi." The method of Yan Xi is, when it is getting dark, the ears do not hear, the eyes do not see, the four limbs are not moving, and the heart has no thoughts or cares. It is like a seed fire. Pre-Heaven Original Shen and Original Qi gather to nourish each other mutually. The real Yi is soft as cotton, opening and closing naturally. The self-being exists in the same body (space or dimension) as insubstantial emptiness, so it can live as long as insubstantial emptiness. Those worldly people (seculars) are bothered with daily management, the spirit is bound and tired. They depend on the single night's sleep to be used during the day. A point of spiritual light (self-subconscious spiritual being) all covered by the Post-Heaven's dirty Qi. This is, the Yang falls into the Yin.*

調息一法，貫徹三教，大之可以入道，小用可以養生。
故迦文垂教，以視鼻端，自數出入息，為止觀初門。莊
子《南華經》曰：「聖人之息以踵。」大易隨卦曰：「君
子以向晦入晏息。」王龍溪曰：「古之聖人，有息無睡，
故曰向晦入晏息。」晏息之法，當向晦時，耳無聞，目
無見，四體無動，心無思慮，如種火相似，先天元神元
氣，停育相抱，真意綿綿，開闔自然，與虛空同體，故
能與虛空同壽也。世人終日營擾，精神困憊，夜間靠此
一睡，始夠一日之用。一點靈光，盡為后天濁氣所淹，
是謂陽陷于陰也。

The Qigong techniques of regulating breathing have been studied and practiced in three major philosophic schools, namely Buddhism, Daoism, and Confucianism. If you practice breathing correctly, you gain good health and longevity. In Buddhist and Daoist societies, through correct breathing practice, the Qi is stored and led up to the brain to nourish the Shen (神) for enlightenment. Entering the Dao (Ru Dao, 入道) means to enter the path of searching for the truth. The Daoists who comprehend the truth of nature are called Truthful Persons (Zhen Ren, 真人).

Regulating the breathing in Buddhist society is considered crucial to regulating the mind. To stop the mind from continuous distraction and wandering in meditation, concentrate your breathing (look at the tip of the nose, Yan Guan Bi, 眼觀鼻) and count the breaths. Make the breathing deeper and calmer. Slowly, the thoughts connecting with the surroundings and with the past, present, and future, are stopped. In Buddhist meditation, this is called Stopping Vision (Zhi Guan, 止觀). "Use the eyes to look at the tip of the nose" does not mean to physically look at the nose. It simply means to gather your attention and to concentrate on your breathing.

As Zhuang Zi (莊子) said, "A sage breathes through the soles," namely Two Gates breathing through the Yongquan (K-1, 湧泉) cavities. Later it developed into Four Gates breathing, and finally reached the practice of Five Gates breathing (Wu Xin Hu Xi, 五心呼吸). *Yi Jing* (易經) said, "When it gets dark, gentlemen enter the Yan Xi (晏息, deep breathing meditation)." The best times for regulating the breath is after sunset. Then, nature and the body turn from Yang to Yin. If you practice regulating the breathing at this time, you can easily calm your body and mind to reach a profound level of meditation. This is also mentioned by Daoist Wang, Long-Xi (王龍溪). He implies that ancient sages, through regulating the breathing, did not need more than a little sleep, since they obtained a deep level of rest from meditation.

The way of Yan Xi (晏息) is to, after sunset, close the ears to the noises around you. Partially close your eyes to stop the vision and enhance your feeling. Keep the body extremely calm and relaxed. The mind should be without worries or cares. It is just like a tiny fire, little Yang within Yin, in the darkness. The subconscious Yin mind awakens while the conscious Yang mind is calm. Original Spirit (Yuan Shen, 元神) is raised and harmonized with Original Qi (Yuan Qi, 元氣). In this profound meditative state, your Shen unifies with natural Shen. Ordinary people must rely on their night's sleep to overcome tiredness. Even during sleep, their minds are confused by dreams generated from emotions and desires, so mind and body degenerate quickly. In this way, the Yang falls into the Yin.

### 4. The method of regulating the breathing[8]
### (Original Truth of Using No Herbs, Qing Dynasty)
### 《調息法》
### （勿藥元詮・清・汪昂輯）

*The method of regulating the breathing is, do not be restricted by the timing, sit anywhere and anytime you wish. The body is balanced and upright, allow it to be comfortable and natural. Do not lean and bend forward. Loosen the clothes and ease the belt to regulate the body properly. Circle the tongue in the mouth several times. Gently and slowly breathe out dirty air, then gently and slowly breathe in through the nose. Repeat this, and when saliva is generated, swallow it. After biting the teeth a few times, the tongue touches the palate of the mouth. The lips and teeth are closed, and the eyes are closed like the new moon. Then gradually begin regulating the breathing. Do not pant and do not be coarse. Either count the exhalation or the inhalation, from one to ten, from ten to a hundred. Restrain your mind in counting and do not be disordered. If the mind and the breathing are in harmony, and random thoughts are no longer generated, stop counting and allow it to be natural. The longer you can sit, the more marvelous it will be. When you raise up the body, slowly and comfortably extend your arms and legs, not suddenly. If you practice this intelligently, various peculiar visions appear in the calmness. This can direct you to enlighten your mind and comprehend the Dao. It is not just for preserving health and extending life.*

調息之法，不拘時候，隨便而坐，平直其身，縱任其體，不倚不曲，解衣緩帶，務令調適。口中舌攪數遍，微微呵出濁氣，鼻中微微納之，或三、五遍，或一、二遍，有津咽下；叩齒數通，舌抵上齶，唇齒相著，兩目垂帘，令朧朧然；漸次調息，不喘不粗，或數息出，或數息入，從一至十，從十至百，攝心在數，勿令散亂，如心息相依，雜念不生，則止勿數，任其自然，坐久愈妙。若欲起身，須徐徐舒放手足，勿得遽起。能勤行之，靜中光景，種種奇特，直可明心悟道，不但養身全生而已也。

From the same source as the previous one, this paragraph describes regulating the breathing. There are many methods, though the principles and theory remain the same. It is important to keep the body relaxed (regulating the body), keep the mind calm (regulating the mind), and breathe softly, deeply, and naturally (regulating the breathing). To regulate your breathing to a profound level, you must also regulate your body and mind. They must harmonize and coordinate with each other. The key to regulating the breathing is not to hold it, but to regulate it, until it can be natural, smooth, and slender.

## 5. Four demeanors of regulating the breathing[8]
## (Original interpretation of using no herbs, Qing Dynasty)
### 《調息四相》
### （勿藥元詮・清・汪昂輯）

*There are four demeanors in regulating the breathing. Those when they breathe, there is a sound, it is classified as wind breathing. If the wind persists, then Qi and mind are dispersed. Those when they breathe, there is no sound but the nose is obstructed, it is classified as panting breathing. If the panting persists, then Qi and mind are stagnant. Those when they breathe, there is no sound and no stagnation but to and fro has shape, it is classified as Qi breathing. If the mind focuses on Qi, then it is fatigued. Those when they breathe, have neither sound nor stagnation, the air exits and enters softly, as though it existed and as though it does not exist. Shen and breathing mutually rely on each other. This is the demeanor of real regulating of the breathing. When the breathing is truly regulated, then the mind is steady, and real Qi can circulate naturally. This allows you to capture the variations of nature. Every breath returns to its origin. This is the root of life.*

調息有四相：呼吸有聲者風也，守風則散；雖無聲而鼻
中澀滯者喘也，守喘則結；不聲不滯而往來有形者氣也，
守氣則勞；不聲不滯，出入綿綿，若存若亡，神氣相依，
是息相也。息調則心定，真氣往來，自能奪天地之造化，
息息歸根，命之蒂也。

This paragraph explains how, from the demeanors of a meditator, we can tell how correct is his breathing. Those who breathe heavily make noise, indicating that Qi is dispersed. Those who breathe without smoothness and uniformity, their Qi circulation is stagnant. Those who pay too much attention to their breathing are fatigued. Only in those whose breathing is soft, slender, uniform, deep, natural, and smooth, is their Shen peacefully harmonized with Qi circulation. Original Spirit awakens, allowing you to return to the origin of your life.

### 6. Li Zhen Ren's sixteen marvelous secret words of longevity
### (Eight notes on Longevity, Ming Dynasty)

《李真人長生一十六字妙訣 》
（遵生八箋 · 明 · 高濂撰 ）

*Once inhaling, immediately lift up (the perineum) to return Qi to the navel (Lower Dan Tian). Once lifting, immediately swallow the saliva, to allow the water and fire to blend.*

一吸便提，氣氣歸臍；一提便咽，水火相見。

Kan (坎) means water Qi produced from Original Essence (Yuan Jing, 元精), while Li (離) means fire Qi generated from Post-Birth Essence, namely food and air. When these two blend, Shen can be raised to a higher level.

These words reveal the secret of how to cause fire Qi and water Qi to blend and interact. This secret is at the Huiyin (Co-1, 會陰), or perineum. When you inhale, gently lift up your perineum, and lead Qi to the Lower Dan Tian. Immediately after inhaling, swallow the saliva to lead Qi down to the Lower Dan Tian. Reverse Abdominal Breathing should be used for this practice.

The above documents offer you some references. In Chapter 6, we discuss breathing techniques, especially Embryonic Breathing (Tai Xi, 胎息), in more detail.

## 4-4. REGULATING THE MIND (TIAO XIN) 調心

Regulate the emotional mind (Xin, 心) until it is under control. This is the most difficult subject to train in Nei Dan Qigong. It sets your mind to deal with itself, and since everyone has his own way of thinking, it is also the most difficult subject to explain.

The methods of regulating the mind have been widely studied, discussed, and practiced in all Chinese Qigong societies, which include scholar, medical, religious, and martial arts groups. First we define the mind and then the purposes of regulating it. We discuss the Buddhist and Daoist point of view, and finally we analyze methods of practice.

**Two Minds, Xin and Yi** 心 · 意. Chinese society describes two minds. Xin, the emotional mind (心, heart), is Yang, making you confused, scattered, depressed, or excited. Yi, the other mind (意, intention), relates to rational and logical thought. It is Yin, making you calm, concentrated, and able to feel and ponder deeply. The word Yi (意) consists of three words. Li (立) on top means to establish, Yue (曰) in the middle means to speak, and Xin (心) at the bottom means the heart. So Yi means to establish communication while the emotional mind is under control.

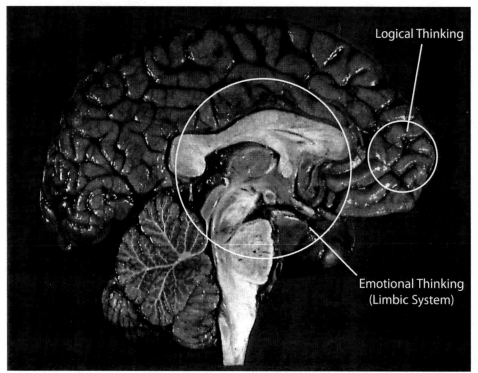

Figure 4-12. Brain and Emotions

Xin and Yi are directed by different parts of the brain.[9,10] Magnetic resonance imaging (MRI) has determined that the prefrontal cortex of the brain controls logic and judgment, while the limbic system near the center of the brain governs emotional thinking (Figure 4-12). According to the Director of the Center for Brain Research and Informational Sciences at Radford University in Virginia, the prefrontal cortex controls executive functions, and is the seat of civilization.

By the age of twenty, the limbic system is fully functional, while the prefrontal cortex is still being formed. In adults, emotional responses are modulated by the prefrontal cortex, the part of the brain just behind the forehead that acts as a mental traffic cop, keeping tabs on many other parts of the brain, including the limbic system."

The Yi generated by the prefrontal cortex determines wise, clear thought and judgment, and calm, logical behavior, while the Xin from the limbic system leads to confusion and emotional behavior. The key to making the prefrontal cortex mature earlier and faster than normal, is to use it as early as possible. Learning mathematics, physics, philosophy, or listening to classical music, leads Qi to the front of the brain for faster development. Those who meditate to open the third eye focus their minds at the front of the brain and become wiser.

We use Yi to control, coordinate, and harmonize the Xin. In scientific terms, we develop the prefrontal cortex to a powerful level, to control and direct the thinking generated by the limbic system of the brain.

**Purposes of Regulating the Mind** 調心之目的. The purposes of regulating the mind vary from one school to another. Qigong practitioners in scholar and medical societies aim for a calm, peaceful, and harmonious mind so emotions do not disturb Qi circulation. Thoughts affect Qi circulation in the organs. Happiness and excitement affect the heart, while anger affects the liver. The kidneys are affected by fear and the lungs by sadness. (Table 4-4) Regulating your emotional mind to harmony and peace benefits your health.

According to the ancient medical book, *Thousand Golden Prescriptions for Emergencies* (備急千金要方), "Contemplate too much, then the spirit is tired. Obsess too much, then aspirations are dispersed. Too much desire, then the will is confused. Involved too much in affairs, then the body is fatigued. Talk too much, then Qi is deficient. Laugh too much, the internal organs can be injured. Worry too much, then the heart is fearful. Too much joy, then expectations stop. Too much happiness, then (one) makes mistakes and is disordered. Angry too often, then circulation in hundreds of vessels is unsteady. Too many favors, then bewitched and ignore regular affairs. Too much wickedness, then gaunt without happiness. Without getting rid of these twelve 'too much,' then the control of flourish and protection (spirit and health) are lost, and blood and Qi circulation disordered. This is the root of losing the life."[11] Wrong sentiments are the root of sickness. In medical and scholar Qigong, regulating the mind to be calm, neutral, and not disturbed by emotions, is the main task of practice.

Daoist and Buddhist religious groups, having regulated the emotional mind to a peaceful state, also aim for Buddhahood and enlightenment. Having controlled the emotional mind and developed their wisdom mind to a profound stage, they search for the meaning of life and nature.

|  | WOOD 木 | FIRE 火 | EARTH 土 | METAL 金 | WATER 水 |
|---|---|---|---|---|---|
| **Direction** | East | South | Center | West | North |
| **Season** | Spring | Summer | Long Summer | Autumn | Winter |
| **Climactic Condition** | Wind | Summer Heat | Dampness | Dryness | Cold |
| **Process** | Birth | Growth | Transformation | Harvest | Storage |
| **Color** | Green | Red | Yellow | White | Black |
| **Taste** | Sour | Bitter | Sweet | Pungent | Salty |
| **Smell** | Goatish | Burning | Fragrant | Rank | Rotten |
| **Yin Organ** | Liver | Heart | Spleen | Lungs | Kidneys |
| **Yang Organ** | Gall Bladder | Small Intestine | Stomach | Large Intestine | Bladder |
| **Opening** | Eyes | Tongue | Mouth | Nose | Ears |
| **Tissue** | Sinews | Blood Vessels | Flesh | Skin/Hair | Bones |
| **Emotion** | Anger | Happiness | Pensiveness | Sadness | Fear |
| **Human Sound** | Shout | Laughter | Song | Weeping | Groan |

Table 4-4. Emotion and Internal Organs

Finally, martial arts Qigong practitioners raise up the spirit of vitality and build a highly concentrated mind to lead Qi efficiently and to develop the sense of enemy, which is critical in battle. While your mind is calm and clear, your spirit is raised to a state of high alert.

Whatever the goals of each school, the principles of training are the same.

*1. To Harmonize Body and Mind.*

To achieve a calm meditative mind, first attend to the condition of your body. When it is tensed and energized, breathing is rapid and your mind excited. Body and mind must coordinate and harmonize with each other. This is called the balance of the body and the Xin (Shen Xin Ping Heng, 身心平衡). *The Complete Book of Principal Contents of Life and Human Nature* (性命圭旨全書) said, "When the body is not moving, the Xin is peaceful. When Xin is not moving, the spirit abides by itself."[12] The first step in regulating the mind is to calm the body, so the mind can be calm. When the emotions are calm, the wisdom mind can function efficiently, and the spirit of vitality can be raised.

*2. To Harmonize the Breathing and the Mind.*

Regulating the emotional mind (Xin) is done by the wisdom mind (Yi). Xin is compared to a monkey or ape while Yi is compared to a horse (Xin Yuan Yi Ma, 心猿意馬). A monkey is weak, unsteady, and disturbing, generating confusion and excitement. A horse, though powerful, can be calm, steady, and controlled.

Thousands of years of experience in meditation have discovered that, in order to 'tame the monkey mind', and lead it into a cage, one needs a banana. This banana is the breathing. As you focus on your breathing, your emotional mind becomes restrained and calm. When your breathing becomes long, slender, soft, and calm, your mind becomes calm, and vice versa. Mind and breathing mutually affect each other, working harmoniously to reach a high level of meditation. This is called Xin and breathing mutually rely on each other (Xin Xi Xiang Yi, 心息相依).

*The Complete Book of Principal Contents of Life and Human Nature* (性命圭旨全書) said, "To conform with the Daoist's deep profound breathing, Xin and breathing rely on each other mutually. When breathing is regulated, Xin can be calm."[13] To have a calm emotional mind, first regulate your breathing through Daoist breathing methods.

*Questions From A Buddhist Guest About Listening to the Heart* (聽心齋客問) explains, "The Xin has been relying on affairs and objects for a long time; separated from its residence, it cannot be independent. Therefore, use Gongfu of regulating the breath to restrain Xin. Xin and breathing can then mutually rely on each other. Regulating does not mean to use Yi, but only a thought of one inhalation and one exhalation. Once Xin separates from its residence, it is without others and without self, and breathing cannot be regulated. Keep the breathing soft and continuous as though existing, yet not existing (regulating without regulating). After a long time, it will be become proficient naturally."[14] This paragraph explains that our emotional mind concerns itself with human affairs and objects around us and is influenced by them. Then it is confused and cannot be independent. The way to restrain it is to regulate the breathing, until the emotional mind and the breathing are mutually dependent on each other. You should not have an intention (Yi), but simply pay attention to the breathing. After you have practiced for a period of time, you will be able to breathe softly, naturally, smoothly, and continuously. The Xin will stay at its residence without disturbance.

*3. Use the Mind to Build Up, Store, and Lead Qi Circulation.*

In religious and martial Qigong, one of the main goals is using the mind to build up Qi, store it, and lead its circulation. To build up and store Qi in the Real Lower Dan Tian (Zhen Xia Dan Tian, 真下丹田), practice Embryonic Breathing (Tai Xi, 胎息), and keep your mind in this Qi residence. If your mind is away from this center, Qi is led away from it and consumed, without being stored and built up to a higher level. "Keep the Yi at the Dan Tian" (Yi Shou Dan Tian, 意守丹田).

After building up abundant Qi, use your mind to lead it. "Use the Yi to lead the Qi" (Yi Yi Yin Qi, 以意引氣). In Nei Dan practice, first lead Qi to circulate in the Conception (Ren Mai, 任脈) and Governing Vessels (Du Mai, 督脈) to complete Small Circulation (Xiao Zhou Tian, 小周天). Then lead the Qi to the extremities, skin, bone marrow, and brain for Grand Circulation (Da Zhou Tian, 大周天).

*4. Raise the Spirit of Vitality for Enlightenment.*

Again, the final goal of Buddhist and Daoist Qigong is enlightenment or Buddhahood. To this end, build up and store Qi at the Real Lower Dan Tian, then lead it up through the Thrusting Vessel (Chong Mai, 衝脈, Spinal Cord) to the brain, to nourish the brain and raise the spirit. The goal is to open the third eye. Having lied and cheated to conceal our secrets behind a mask through thousands of years, humans have closed our third eye. By doing so, we lost the power of telepathy and communion with the spirit of nature. To reopen this third eye, we must be truthful, not hiding anything, and then accumulate Qi in the front of the brain.

To raise the spirit to enlightenment, regulate your Xin to an extremely calm, clear, and steady state. *Dao Scriptures* (道藏) said, "Xin is the master of the whole body, the commander of hundred spirits. When calm, wisdom is generated; when acting, confusion originates. Its steadiness and confusion are within the movement and the calmness."[15]

Let us summarize the Qigong methods practiced in Buddhist and Daoist society, first discussing the origin of thoughts. By recognizing the root of emotional disturbance and confusion, we can find ways to stop it.

**The Origin of Thoughts** 起念之源. Buddhists cultivate a neutral and empty state of mind, separate from the Four Greatnesses (Si Da, 四大), the earth (Di, 地), water

(Shui, 水), fire (Huo, 火), and wind (Feng, 風)(Si Da Jie Kong, 四大皆空). They believe this renders their spirits independent, so they can escape from the recurring cycle of reincarnation.

Most thought is generated from emotions, by the seven passions and six desires. After thoughts pass through the wisdom mind, then action is taken. When a person's wisdom mind is strong, the action will be rational and reasonable. But if one's emotional mind is so strong that the wisdom mind cannot interpret the emotional thought before initiating action, the action will be emotional and irrational. For example, when you encounter a traffic jam, initially you feel no problem. If the jam lasts for an hour, your emotional mind becomes uneasy and impatient, turning into anger and frustration. Your emotional mind has been agitated and excited. But if your wisdom mind steps in and asks whether traffic will improve if you lose your temper, the answer is no. In this case your wisdom mind takes over to control your emotional mind.

**Observing Thoughts** 觀念. To prevent emotional thought from initiating, keep your mind in a neutral state, which is not the usual way of human nature. Old thoughts commonly linger in one's mind, and one keeps thinking about them, being constantly disturbed and agitated. This kind of thought is called Nian (念), which means "the old thought always borne in mind." To stop this disturbing thought, first recognize it. Many people fear to face it and simply hide behind a mask, but sooner or later, it reappears to disturb them.

To keep the old thought from lingering in your mind, first be awakened. This step is called observing the thoughts (Guan Nian, 觀念). From this observation, you awaken. Zhi You Zi (至游子) said, "Do not fear initiation of a thought, but be afraid of awakening too late."[16] Often, if emotional action has already taken place before your awakening, the mistake will have been committed. When you regret at this time, it is already too late to undo your action.

To reach a profound level of observing thoughts and understanding them is no easy task. There are three extents (San Jie, 三界) of this mental cultivation. *Dao Scriptures* (道藏) said, "The extent of desire, extent of color, and extent of colorlessness. When Xin forgets worry and thoughts, it transcends desire. When it forgets the surrounding environment, it transcends color. When it sees nothing, it transcends colorlessness."[17] This is equivalent to the Buddhist saying that the mind should be separated from the Four Greatnesses: earth (Di, 地), water (Shui, 水), fire (Huo, 火), and wind (Feng, 風)(Si Da Jie Kong, 四大皆空). This means the free thought, unbounded by surrounding objects.

Buddhists have three ways of observing thoughts, called "three observations" (San Guan, 三觀). These are: observation of emptiness (Kong Guan, 空觀), observation of falsehood (illusion, Jia Guan, 假觀), and observation of the neutral (neither empty nor illusory, Zhong Guan, 中觀).[18]

In Kong Guan (空觀, observation of emptiness), you observe and then comprehend the meaning of events. After long pondering, you see everything bothering us emotionally is only temporary and small compared with our lifetime or with the age of the universe. All emotional disturbances are empty and meaningless. Our lives come from emptiness and end with it. What really matters is how truthful we are, so our spirit can grow. Every physical lifetime serves the education and growth of our spirit. Any disturbance is only empty thought. Once you grasp this, you can analyze the event from the truthful subconscious point of view.

A story may inspire your thinking about this. In ancient China, two monks walked down a muddy road when they came upon a large puddle completely blocking the road. A very beautiful lady in a lovely gown stood at the edge of the puddle, unable to go farther without spoiling her clothes.

Without hesitation, one of the monks picked her up and carried her across the puddle, set her down on the other side, and continued on his way. Hours later, when the two monks were preparing to camp for the night, the second monk turned to the first and said: "I can no longer hold this back. I'm quite angry at you! We are not supposed to look at women, particularly pretty ones, never mind touching them. Why did you do that?" The first monk replied, "I left her at the mud puddle, why are you still carrying her?" Emptiness in your mind depends on how you think.

In Jia Guan (假觀, observation of falseness), you pay attention to tracing back the root of each event. You realize we fight for glory, dignity, love, wealth, and power, created from the illusion of the mind. We humans created all these emotions as a matrix and entered it. Afterwards, most of us do not enjoy it and constantly bear the pain of illusion. Each lifetime is like a show on stage, with everyone wearing a mask, playing their allotted role, and hiding their true spiritual identity. We lie, cheat, smile, and cry, without involvement of our real spiritual identity, which is truthful and pure. Events and problems are false, not real, being only an illusion of life. Once you comprehend this, all thoughts generated by the emotional mind become meaningless.

Ponder a story from Japanese Zen society, about a bold and handsome young Samurai warrior standing before an aged Zen master, asking, "Master, I have reached a high level of Zen theory and practice, but would like to ask a serious question."

The master humbly replied, "May I ask what question you would like to ask?"

"Please teach me about heaven and hell?" The Samurai replied.

The master froze motionless for just a moment and then suddenly snapped his head in disgust and seethed, "Teach you about heaven and hell? I doubt you could even keep your own sword from rusting, you ignorant fool. How dare you suppose you could understand anything I might have to say?"

The old man went on, becoming more insulting, while the young swordsman's surprise turned first to confusion, then to dismay and hot anger. Master or no master, who insults a Samurai and lives? At last, teeth clenched and blood boiling in blind fury, the warrior drew his sword to end the old man's tirade and life.

The master looked straight into his eyes and said gently, "That is hell."

At the peak of his rage, the Samurai realized this was indeed his teaching, that the master had driven him into a living hell of uncontrollable anger and ego. The young man, profoundly humbled, sheathed his sword and bowed to this great spiritual teacher. Looking into the wise man's aged, beaming face, he felt more love and compassion than he had ever felt in his life. The master, sensing the changed demeanor, raised his index finger and said, "And that is heaven."

Emotional disturbances are created from false illusion in the mind. Do we create heaven and hell in our minds, and keep ourselves trapped in this matrix, or do heaven and hell really exist? Do we create God in our imagination or does God create man in His? What proof is there, and how truthful would it be?

In Zhong Guan (中觀, observation of neutral), you neither deny the emptiness of the matter, nor its illusory existence. You may, through observation, lead your thoughts into the neutral point that all things are empty and also false. It is the observation of double reflections (Shuang Zhao, 雙照), or relative comparison.

In a small village in southern China lived the hardest worker in his community. Day and night he toiled, and year by year his riches grew. As time passed, his hoard of money increased, as did his concern for failure or loss. He worried about how to make more money and how to keep both friends and enemies away from the massive wealth he had accumulated.

He raised the fence around his house and strengthened the walls, with strong locks on the doors and bars on the windows, until the house resembled a jail. He felt safe and believed himself the happiest man alive as he counted his money all day.

A curious passerby peered in and saw him sitting there smiling as he counted. He called out, "Why are you so happy? It seems you're in jail!"

The man answered, "No! It's not that I'm in jail, it's that you are outside of it."

Many of us dream of money, making it our obsession. Invisible walls are built and personal jails created in which we enjoy ourselves, yet friendships are held at bay. What does it really mean to be happy, to be rich both materially and spiritually? The truly rich are those who know how to make money yet also know how to share with others. This sets you free from the bondage of material obsession.

A wealthy businessman from the north spotted a fisherman, relaxing against his canoe and smoking a pipe. The businessman was dismayed, "Why aren't you sailing for fish?

"I caught enough today already."

"The sun is still high in the sky, you could catch plenty more, couldn't you?" insisted the businessman.

"Why should I?" retorted the fisherman.

"Money! You would have more money!" the businessman exclaimed. "With a better engine on your boat, you could go to deeper water and catch more fish. Soon you could buy a better net and catch even more fish and make even more money. Finally, you may become rich enough to buy a fleet of new boats, even becoming as rich as me."

"And then what would I do?"

"Sit and enjoy your life."

"That is what I am doing now," said the fisherman.

When you desire something, know when to stop. Keep your mind neutral, and see two ends instead of only one direction. To free yourself from emotional bondage, practice these three observations until you comprehend the meaning of life from the depths of your heart. You will see the reason for everything that happens, in the spiritual learning process, without dwelling on events. After watching a stage show that touches you emotionally, if you dwell on it emotionally, you are in emotional bondage. Instead, learn from it about the meaning of life, so your mind looks far instead of near.

Since we are all on the stage of life, each one carries a mask which allows us to fit in the show. However, deep inside we all know that it is only a show and not our true identity. Without a mask in this masked society, we could not survive.

My grandmother told me a story about a king, who always wore a stern and solemn mask whenever he met his officers. Because of this, his officials respected, loved, feared, and obeyed him, so he could rule the country effectively. One day his wife told him that what the officials respected and loved was not him, but his mask. To prove his wife wrong, he removed it. From then on, his officials could see his real face and discern his thinking from his facial expression. They started to fight each other in front of him, and even to dispute his policies and decisions. In a short time, the country fell into disorder. The king realized the power of the mask. He gave the order to chop off the heads of all those officials who had seen his face. He replaced the mask on his face and could once again rule the country effectively.

You can see why it is hard for many spiritual people (truthful persons) to survive in this masked society and why they shun lay society to go to the mountains.

**Stopping Thoughts** 止念. "Stopping thoughts" means to stop old thoughts which hang around in your mind. These can be emotionally troubling, disturbing your state of calm. Stopping thoughts also means to stop a new thought from being initiated. The emotionally disturbed mind is the origin of the body's Yang fire. *The Complete Book of Principal Contents of Human Life and Temperament, Hen Anthology* (性命圭旨全書・亨集), said that, "If a thought is initiated, then everywhere is fire. In the quiet place where thoughts cease, Spring can blossom."[19] Spring blossoming means the harmonization of the mind, body, breathing, and spirit.

To stop thoughts, first stop your inner observation from observing, which is the stage of Zhi Guan (止觀). Awaken and comprehend the root of thoughts through observation to find the way to stop them. Then, observation becomes necessary, because it is regulated.

*Wei Mo Classic* (維摩經) said, "To restrain the Xin from emotional affinity is called stopping. To see deeply and reach far clearly, is called observation." It also said, "Every thought returns to its origin, is called stopping. Everything can be discriminated clearly, is called observation."[20]

The first phrase explains that to reach Zhi Guan, you first stop emotional affinity with the outside world. This is the meaning of "stopping" (Zhi, 止). When your mind is so clear and profound that you analyze the situation through observation, and can thus stop both the old thought and also the initiation of a new one, it is called observation (Guan, 觀).

The second phrase explains "stopping" (Zhi, 止) to be the bringing of all disturbing thoughts back to focus on the Dan Tian where they originate. Pay attention to the Dan Tian, either Upper Dan Tian for Shen or Real Lower Dan Tian for Qi, and coordinate with your deep breathing. Then all disturbing thoughts can be stopped and replaced with one thought. To see deeply to the root of reality is called observation (Guan, 觀).

**Methods of Stopping Thoughts** 止念法. Buddhist and Daoist societies developed many methods of regulating thought. The first step is to restrain the wandering emotional mind from the attraction of the outside world. Close your eyes and focus on regular, deep, and soft breathing, which calms the emotional mind. As mentioned earlier, it is said, "The eyes observe (Guan, 觀) the breathing, and the breathing observes the Xin."[21]

Once you have reached Zhi Guan, you prevent new thoughts from initiating. Pay attention to your breathing, and keep your mind at the Dan Tian. In *Zhuang Zi, Secular World* (莊子・人間世), it is said, "With a unified will, do not listen with the ears but with Xin. Do not listen with Xin, but with Qi. Listening ceases at the ears, and Xin stops when harmony (Fu) is reached. What is Qi? It is insubstantial and exists in all objects. Only by following the Dao can you gather this insubstantial Qi, which is obtained from the purification of Xin (Xin Zhai)."[22]

To regulate your emotional mind (Xin, 心), stop listening to the outside world, and pay attention to your emotional mind. Once you bring your thoughts from outside to inside your body, pay attention to Qi through breathing. Fu (符) means to match, harmonize, coordinate, or cooperate. Stopping the activity of Xin is achieved through the coordination of breathing.

To gather Qi at the Real Lower Dan Tian, first calm the Xin. Xin Zhai (心齋) means purified Xin and implies a calm and sincere mind. In this way Qi can be preserved at its residence. This is the way of Dao (道).

In the *Anthology of a Daoist Village* (道鄉集), it is said, "Today, I would like to teach you the method of ceasing thought. For example, when my Xin looks at the water, my thought will be on the water. When my Xin looks at the moon, my thought will be on the moon. If my eyes focus on looking at the Qi cavity (Qi Xue, Dan Tian), my Xin will be on the Qi cavity."[23] This defines the key to stopping thought as paying attention to the Qi Xue (氣穴). Qi Xue means Upper Dan Tian or Real Lower Dan Tian. Once you pay attention to the breathing and keep your mind at the Dan Tian, the thought disappears.

**Cease Activity of Xin 息心.** The final goal in regulating the mind is stabilizing it from emotional disturbance, and keeping it from wandering about, also called Ding Xin (定心). But first you must cease the activity of Xin (Xi Xin, 息心). *The Collection of Neutral Harmony* (中和集) states, "Carefully study the writings of those holy men in Three Teachings (San Jiao, Three Schools), the word of ceasing, Xi, is the simplest and most straightforward. If you put Gongfu in ceasing, you will not need much effort to reach Buddhahood and immortality. Cease the feeling of affinity (Xi Yuan) to reach the pivotal function of original Chan. Cease the Xin (Xi Xin) to comprehend and understand the theory of Confucianism profoundly. Cease the breathing (Xi Qi) to reach the marvelous Dao of condensing the Shen. These three ceasings are mutually required by each other without any conquest."[24]

San Jiao (三教) means Three Teachings or Three Schools, namely Buddhism, Daoism, and Confucianism. All of them describe methods of ceasing (Xi, 息). Xi means to stop or cease any action or prevent it from being initiated. Here it means regulating without regulating (Bu Tiao Er Tiao, 不調而調). When regulating is no longer necessary, all regulating processes cease.

The key practice of Buddhists is to cease the affinity (Xi Yuan, 息緣) which connects with secular affairs. Then the emotional mind will be calm and peaceful, the Shen of the subconscious mind will awaken, and Buddhahood can be achieved. This cultivation is called Chan. *The Transliteration of Wisdom Garden* (慧苑音義) said, "Chan, it means to calm down the Xin to ponder."[25] It is the meditation of stabilizing the activity of Xin.

The cultivation of "ceasing" in the Confucian school is to cease the Xin's activity, so the scholar philosophies can be comprehended. These include the relationships between humans, and between humans and nature. When these philosophies are understood, the mind can be peaceful and calm.

But to Daoists, "ceasing" means to cease regulating the breathing, by practicing Embryonic Breathing with the condensed mind. This is the necessary path to reach enlightenment.

**Stabilizing Xin** 定心. Regulating the mind to keep it calm and stable is called Ding (定), the stabilization of Xin. You bring mind and body into harmony, so you can ponder profoundly and finally comprehend the Dao. In *Four Books, Great Study* (四書 · 大學), Confucius said, "Only knowing how to cease, can you then have steadiness (Ding). When there is steadiness, your mind can be calm. Then you can be peaceful, and able to ponder. When you ponder, you will gain."[26] To Confucian scholar society, the final goal of meditation is to gain, or understand, the meaning of life and the laws of nature (Dao). To comprehend this deep philosophy, you go through necessary procedures. The first is to cease (Zhi, 止) the initiation of thought, so your mind becomes steady, controlled, calm, and peaceful, and clear for you to ponder. Through deep pondering, you comprehend the reasons for events.

How do we define Ding (定, stabilization). In *Theory of Evaluating Wisdom* (智度論), it is said, "Regulate the Xin to where it should be. Cease worry and condense (stabilize) the Xin. When Xin is steady at one place without moving, it is called steadiness (Ding). Regulate the Xin to accept the solution through observation. This is called acceptance (Shou, 受). To regulate the violence of the Xin, to straighten its curve (intricacy) and stabilize its dispersion, this is called regulating, straightening, and stabilizing. To regulate the actions of Xin and allow it to be as it should, is called regulate the Xin to where it should be. To cease the mind's affinity and worry, so as to condense and focus the thought of Xin, is called cease worry and condense the Xin."[27]

In Buddhist meditation, Ding (定, steadiness of the Xin and the body) is always emphasized. Entering this steadiness is called Ru Ding (入定). First cut off all emotional disturbance and keep your mind at the Upper and Real Lower Dan Tian. The Upper Dan Tian (brain) is the residence of the Shen, while the Real Lower Dan Tian (second brain) is the residence of Qi. When Qi is kept at its residence, the body can be calmed without stimulation or excitement. When Shen is condensed at its residence, the mind becomes calm and clear.

Learn to face your emotional mind, analyze and understand it, and remove the mask from your face. Only when these affinities of Xin can be removed, can your mind be kept steady at one place. This is the way to reach steadiness (Ding, 定).

The final goal is profound stabilization of Xin, called Great Steadiness (Da Ding, 大定). Da Ding means, "When Xin for Buddhism is clear and bright, it is called Da Ding."[28] The mind peaceful and calm, the body extremely relaxed, as Shen and body harmonize and coordinate with each other. This defines the steadiness and the calmness of both mental and physical bodies. Once you reach this stage, you have established a firm foundation for cultivation of spiritual enlightenment.

I would like to share a Samurai story with you.

A boy of ten was playing in his house when a Samurai swordsman entered and started killing people. He hid behind a large clothes cabinet. Through a gap he saw clearly what was happening. The swordsman was his father's political enemy, and the boy was the family's only survivor. The swordsman finished his killing, then left without searching the cabinet.

The boy traveled the country searching for the best Zen master. He swore he would become the most famous and skillful Samurai swordsman, so he could avenge the murder of his family. He found a master and practiced day and night, with vengeance in his heart.

By his early twenties, he became one of the best-known Samurai swordsmen in Japan. He traveled to every corner of Japan, searching for his enemy. But after twenty-five years of searching, all efforts were in vain, and his enemy seemed to have disappeared from society.

His disappointment great, one day he entered a deep valley where only a few tribesmen lived. He came to a small river, where an old man was rebuilding a bridge, slowly and strenuously moving wood piece by piece. The original bridge had been swept away by a torrent, and the villagers had to travel far downstream to cross the river.

Talking to the old man, he could not believe his eyes. The old man was the one who had killed his family more than thirty years before. Without hesitation, he drew his sword to cut off his head. Before doing so, he explained why. The old man freely admitted to killing his family, but had one final request.

"This bridge is the only hope for the village. Allow me to finish building it before killing me," the old man asked.

Since the old man's request was good, he agreed to permit him to finish the bridge. But he would watch him day and night, so he could not run away. The avenger built a tent next to the old man and watched him build the bridge. Progress was slow and time-consuming, and after six months, he joined in to help the old man finish the bridge, to hasten the day of his revenge.

Eating together, talking and helping each other, in time they became good friends. The bridge was completed in the third year. On completing the job, the old man came to the Samurai's tent. He had washed his body clean. He knelt before the avenger, and said, "It is time for you to take my life to avenge your family."

The Samurai found he could not draw his sword for revenge. He knelt in front of the old man and said: "My first life was hatefulness like hell. My second life is kindness and peace like heaven. I cannot kill you, otherwise I would also kill my second life." So they traveled together and treated each other like father and son.

## 4-5. REGULATING THE QI (TIAO QI) 調氣

The purposes of regulating Qi are 1. Producing Qi (Sheng Qi, 生氣); 2. Nourishing and protecting Qi (Yang Qi, 養氣); 3. Storing Qi (Xu Qi, 蓄氣); and 4. Transporting Qi (Xing Qi, 行氣). Next, we discuss the theory and key practices of these four.

### 1. Producing Qi (Sheng Qi, 生氣)

There are three ways to produce Qi, namely herbs, breathing, and massage.

**Herbs.** Qi originates primarily from the biochemical reaction of the food we eat and the oxygen we inhale, which releases energy. Different foods produce different quantity and quality of energy, so herbs have been thoroughly researched in Chinese medical science. Different herbs are used to regulate the body's energy status.

Qi from food and air is called Post-Heaven Qi (Hou Tian Qi, 後天氣) or Fire Qi (Huo Qi, 火氣), because food and air are not pure and clean. The Qi generated from them can cause emotional disturbance and physical problems. This is the main cause of fire in our mental and physical bodies.

**Abdominal Breathing.** Through deep abdominal breathing, oxygen and carbon dioxide are exchanged efficiently, promoting the body's metabolism. The energy from the biochemical reaction is stronger. Deep abdominal breathing also helps convert abdominal fat into Qi, increasing the quantity of Qi in the body.

This kind of breathing is called Pre-Heaven Breathing (Xian Tian Hu Xi, 先天呼吸) and the Qi produced is called Pre-Heaven Qi (Xian Tian Qi, 先天氣), which is clean and pure, able to calm down your mind and make your physical body healthy.

**Massaging the Abdomen.** The *Muscle/Tendon Changing and Marrow/Brain Washing classic* describes the correct way to massage the abdomen. Wrong techniques make the body, especially the intestines, too Yang, triggering constipation. If Qi is increased too rapidly, it can also go up and damage the heart. If you do not know the techniques, you should not attempt to increase Qi in this way. Abdominal breathing is much safer than massage. To know more about Muscle/Tendon Changing and Marrow/Brain Washing Qigong, please refer to the book, *Qigong—The Secret of Youth*, by YMAA.

Other than these three methods, you may also strive to maintain your hormone level (Original Essence, Yuan Jing, 元精). Hormones act as catalysts in regulating the body's metabolism and expediting biochemical reactions, so Qi can be produced smoothly and abundantly.

## 2. Protecting and Nourishing Qi (Yang Qi, 養氣)

Protecting means to preserve and keep, and nourishing means to cultivate and raise up. After generating Qi, then maintain it, and cultivate it to a stronger level. It is like raising a child. After you have generated life, you protect it and raise it so it can grow stronger.

**Protect Original Essence.** Protect Qi by protecting your Original Essence (Yuan Jing, 元精). A man regulates his sexual activities, abuse of which weakens the kidneys. According to Chinese medicine, this is the primary cause of losing Qi for men.

Also regulate your lifestyle. If you are fatigued mentally or physically, the consumption of Qi increases, so regulate your mental and physical activities. Gain enough sleep and rest, and have a regular daily schedule.

**Regulate the Breathing.** To keep the Qi in the body, breathe deeply and softly without holding your breath. Breathing too fast increases the heartbeat, tensing the body and mind, and consuming Qi.

But maintaining physical strength requires exercise, during which breathing and heartbeat speed up. The key is knowing when to stop and how much exercise is needed to maintain health. Yang exercise is necessary to maintain physical life, and Yin rest is also required to preserve and restore life, through conservation of Qi. Both are equally important, and you need both.

When you exercise, breathe properly without holding your breath. You need a large quantity of oxygen to convert the glucose into the energy required. Holding the breath too much consumes Qi.

**Regulate the Xin.** Mental fatigue, especially emotional disturbance, uses up Qi. To protect your Qi, the most important key is regulating your emotional mind. In a neutral state, Qi can stay at its residence without manifesting, so it is preserved and protected. There is a document which emphasizes regulating the mind to preserve Qi, which I translate next and offer some commentary.

## Steel with One Hundred Words
## (Lu, Yan)[8]
## 《百字碑》
### （古今圖書集成・博物匯編神異論；呂岩作）

*When cultivating Qi, do not just talk about preserving it. When calming down the mind, it should be doing without doing. If you know the origins of movement (Yang) and stillness (Yin), there is nothing for you to ask anyone else. Face the real reality, you must deal with daily affairs, but you should not be infatuated by them. Then your temperament can be steady and self-controlled, and Qi will naturally be preserved. Then the elixir can be conceived, and Kan and Li can interact under control within the kettle. Interaction of Yin and Yang initiates the repeated cycle, and this will bring a natural derivation of new life, enlightened like thunder. White clouds move upwards, and sweet dew sprinkles Xu Mi (fullness of human virtue). I drink the wine of longevity by myself, how can others know how free and unfettered I am? I sit down to listen to songs by the instrument without strings. I comprehend clearly the pivotal function of natural creation. These sentences offer the ladder to ascend to Heaven (enlightenment).*

養氣忘言守，降心為不為。動靜知宗祖，無事更尋誰？
真常須應物，應物要不迷。不迷性自住，性住氣自回。
氣回丹自結，壺中配坎離。陰陽生反復，普化一聲雷。
白雲朝頂上，甘露洒須彌。自飲長生酒，逍遙誰得知？
坐聽無弦曲，明通造化機。都來十二句，端的上天梯。

Cultivating Qi is not just about maintaining it. Most important is to regulate your Xin (emotional mind). This must be regulated until no more regulating is necessary and it becomes natural. Your mind becomes clear and your judgment neutral and accurate. Whether active or still, you know where the origins are. If you know clearly what is happening, why do you need to ask anyone else? To live in this human world, you deal with necessary affairs, but without being lured by money, glory, dignity, pride, jealousy, power, or other human desires and emotions. If your mind is separated from these temptations, it can be calm and steady. Qi returns to its origin (Real Lower Dan Tian), forming the elixir (Spiritual Embryo). You control life easily through adjusting Kan and Li. Through Kan and Li, the Yin and Yang of your spirit and body is regulated as you wish. Through cultivating Yin and Yang, when the time is ripe, you open your third eye for enlightenment like a clap of thunder. When this happens, you have no doubt about your life, which will be like pure white clouds floating in the sky and sweet dew upon Xu Mi (須彌). Xu Mi is the Daoist term for the spiritual being in the fullness of human virtue. You live long and enjoy life to the fullest. You communicate with nature like listening to songs without sound, understanding its pivotal functions.

**Gather and Exchange Qi with Nature and Partners.** Energy from the sun, moon, earth, trees, and any other source of natural energy can nourish the body. By meditating facing the sun at dawn, one absorbs solar energy to enhance the body's Qi. Practicing Qigong facing the moon a couple of days before full moon, is also a good way of absorbing Qi. Orienting a house by coordinating the sun's and the earth's magnetic fields is known as Feng Shui (風水, wind-water), which determines good energy for living. Using natural energy to nourish one's Qi is very important in Qigong practice.

To harmonize and balance Qi, and to nourish one another, many Daoists use partners to exchange Qi through meditation or special Qigong practices. This is known as dual cultivation (Shuang Xiu, 雙修), which is also described in *Qigong—The Secret of Youth*, and in future publications.

## 3. Storing Qi (Xu Qi, 蓄氣)

After conserving, protecting, and cultivating Qi, you must store it in the biobattery at the Real Lower Dan Tian. You lead the Qi there and keep it there.

To keep the Qi there, you keep your mind there. When your mind strays, you are leading Qi away and consuming it. Keeping the mind at this center is called Yi Shou Dan Tian (意守丹田), achieved through Embryonic Breathing (Tai Xi, 胎息). There is a document which explains the importance of Embryonic Breathing, which I translate here with commentary. For more on the subject, refer to my previous book, *Qigong Meditation—Embryonic Breathing*.

### Classic of Embryonic Breathing[8,29,30]
### 《胎息經》

*The embryo is conceived from the concealed Qi. Qi is developed through (regulating) the breath of the embryo. When Qi is present, the body may live. When Shen abandons the body and the shape disperses, death follows. Knowing the spirit and Qi makes long life possible. Firmly protect the insubstantial emptiness (Spiritual Embryo) to cultivate spirit and Qi. When spirit moves, the Qi moves. When spirit stops, the Qi stops. For a long life, spirit and Qi must coordinate harmoniously with each other. When Xin is not infatuated by thoughts coming or going, then Spirit and Qi will not exit and enter, and will thus remain naturally. To practice intelligently is the true way.*

胎從伏氣中結，氣從有胎中息。氣入身來為之生，神去離形為之死。知神氣可以長生，固守虛無以養神氣。神行則氣行，神住則氣住。若欲長生，神氣相住。心不動念，無來無去，不出不入，自然常住。勤而行之，是真道路。

Nobody knows when or by whom this classic was written, but it has been passed down for generations and is considered one of the most important documents about Embryonic Breathing.

The Holy Embryo (Sheng Tai, 聖胎) or Spiritual Embryo (Shen Tai, 神胎) is conceived from Qi stored at the Real Lower Dan Tian. To obtain this concealed Qi, practice Embryonic Breathing. Once you have stored it abundantly, your life force becomes strong, bringing you good health and longevity. But to manifest this Qi as physical life force, you need a strong spirit, to focus the circulation and manifestation of Qi. Without this living spirit, you lose your health and die. One who cultivates his spirit and Qi lives a long and healthy life. The first part of the classic explains how to regulate the relationship between physical life, Qi, and Shen.

Keep your mind firmly at the Real Lower Dan Tian, called Xu Wu (虛無), which means nothingness. Your mind remaining at the Real Lower Dan Tian, is the state of Wuji (無極, No Extremity), the state of no discrimination, or nothingness. Only here can you really be in a neutral state of mind. Clear out emotions and desires. This is described in *Dao De Jing* as, "Approach the nothingness to its extremity, and maintain calmness with sincerity."[31] The mind leads the Qi. When actively thinking, you are leading Qi away from its residence and consuming it. To store abundant Qi, you must conserve, protect and build it. These three important things are emphasized in Internal Elixir Qigong (Nei Dan Qigong, 內丹氣功).

To build up abundant Qi, you not only keep your mind at the Real Lower Dan Tian, but also practice Embryonic Breathing. To manifest Qi efficiently for daily life, you need a strong and highly controlled Shen. Qi consumption is limited and efficiency high. The key to longevity is to coordinate and harmonize Shen and Qi. To keep Shen pure and strong, calm the Xin. Xin is like a monkey, while Yi is like a horse (Xin Yuan Yi Ma, 心猿意馬). To keep the monkey steady, restrain it in 'its cage', the Wuji state. This is crucial to success.

## 4. Transporting Qi (Xing Qi, 行氣)

Having preserved, protected, cultivated, and stored Qi, you need to circulate it efficiently. "Use your mind to lead the Qi" (Yi Yi Yin Qi, 以意引氣). The key to this is "**leading**" (Yin, 引). The mind should not be in the Qi, but ahead of it. If your mind pays attention to the Qi, it stagnates. If you want to move from where you are standing, your mind must be on the spot you wish to move to. If your mind stays at the place where you are standing, no movement can take place. "The Yi should not be on the Qi, if on the Qi, then stagnant"[32]

The methods of leading and what you wish to accomplish depend on how extensively and profoundly you grasp the theory, the principles of Yin and Yang, and the goal of your training. There are five common goals for a Qigong practitioner, which vary according to the depth of the training.

**Connection of the Yi and Qi.** Before you can connect your Yi with the Qi, you must recognize the existence of the Qi, originating from the feeling of its existence. Qi is energy that cannot be seen but only felt. You train to establish a sensitive feeling for it. When this feeling focuses on the inner body, it is called Gongfu of Inner Vision (Nei Shi Gongfu, 內視功夫).

After this, you establish the connection between the Yi and the Qi. This feeling is like a piece of rope you hold connected to a cow's nose. Without this rope, you will not be able to lead the Qi.

Once you have established this connection, then you must also know how much effort and force you need to lead the cow. Too strong or too weak, the cow will either resist or stay still. This coordination is called Harmonization of the Yi and Qi (Yi Qi Xiang He, 意氣相合).

**Leading Qi To or Away From a Specific Spot of the Body.** Once you can lead the Qi, you lead it from one place to another in the body for different purposes. For healing, you may lead it to a deficient place for Qi nourishment (Bu, 補). You can also lead stagnant Qi away from a specific place for releasing (Xie, 洩). If your kidneys are deficient in winter time, you can lead Qi to them for nourishment. If you have a joint injury, you can lead Qi away to ease the pain and relax the joint, to expedite the healing process.

Qigong practitioners also lead Qi above the diaphragm to energize and excite the mind and body (Yang), and lead it below the diaphragm to cool down (Yin). One leads Qi to the Laogong (P-8, 勞宮) cavities and to the fingertips for healing, by exchanging Qi with a patient. Qigong martial artists lead Qi to the Yongquan (K-1, 湧泉) cavities to establish a firm root for combat.

There are many applications once you can efficiently lead the Qi with your Yi. The more you practice, the better the results will be. Success depends on your Yi, how strong it is and how much you focus in meditation.

**Small Cyclic Heaven Circulation.** For a healthy and resilient body, one builds up Qi, then circulates it in the Conception and Governing Vessels (Ren, Du Mai, 任・督脈). This is called Small Cyclic Heaven Circulation (Xiao Zhou Tian, 小周天) or simply Small Circulation. When Qi circulation is abundant in these two vessels, the Qi in the Twelve Primary Qi Channels can be regulated smoothly. This maintains abundant Qi supply to the whole body, making it strong and healthy.

**Grand Cyclic Heaven Circulation.** Once you have accomplished Small Cyclic Heaven, you have a firm foundation for Grand Cyclic Heaven (Da Zhou Tian, 大周天) practice. This includes: A. Twelve Primary Qi Channels Grand Circulation, B. Martial Arts Grand Circulation, C. Mutual Qi Exchange Grand Circulation and D. Spiritual Enlightenment Grand Circulation.

Since these are such large subjects, we introduce their theory and practice in separate books. Martial Arts Grand Circulation is discussed in the book, *The Essence of Shaolin White Crane*.

**Spiritual Enlightenment.** Even though Spiritual Enlightenment practice is part of Grand Cyclic Heaven Circulation, due to its profound theory and difficulty in practice, it is discussed separately. It is of more interest to Buddhists and Daoists aiming for Buddhahood or spiritual enlightenment.

In Spiritual Enlightenment Grand Cyclic Heaven Circulation, you practice Embryonic Breathing to store Qi at the Real Lower Dan Tian, and condition the bio-battery there. Then lead Qi up through the spinal cord (Chong Mai, 衝脈) to energize brain cells and activate their function. When the energy level of the brain reaches a certain level, the Qi moves along the Spiritual Valley (Shen Gu, 神谷) to reopen the third eye for enlightenment. We will discuss this in more detail in Spiritual Enlightenment Meditation.

### Jade Pendant Inscription of Transporting Qi[29,30]
### 《行氣玉佩銘》

*When transporting Qi, if deep, then accumulate. If Qi is accumulated, it can be extended. When extended, it can be sunk downward. If sunk downward, then steady. If steady, then firm. If firm, then able to germinate. Having germinated, it can grow. When growing, it retreats. When retreating, it returns to heaven. The foundation of heaven is the top (Upper Dan Tian) and the foundation of earth is the bottom (Real Lower Dan Tian). Following these rules, one may live, otherwise one dies.*

行氣，深則蓄，蓄則伸，伸則下，下則定，定則固，固
則萌，萌則長，長則退，退則天。天几舂在上，地几舂
在下，順則生，逆則死。

When circulating Qi in the body, deep breathing relaxes the body and calms the mind. Qi circulation can be deep and Qi storage abundant. Only then can Qi be strong enough to be distributed everywhere in the body. "Transport Qi as though through a pearl with a nine-curved hole, even the tiniest place will be reached."[33] The body's metabolism becomes smooth, natural, and healthy. Abundant Qi is led down and stored in the Real Lower Dan Tian to stabilize and strengthen the life.

Leading and storing Qi in the Real Lower Dan Tian is the process of Embryonic Breathing (Tai Xi, 胎息). It returns mental and physical life to its origin, in the Wuji state (無極). Then new life can germinate and grow. After fulfilling the purpose of Qi manifestation, retreat and return to the origin, the Real Lower Dan Tian. This process is the way of the heavenly cycle (Dao, 道). Conserving and storing Qi at the Real Lower Dan Tian, you manifest it efficiently in your life. Having completed the manifestation, you return the Qi and conserve it again at the Real Lower Dan Tian. Manifesting Qi to the maximum depends on how thoroughly you purify your spirit and raise it up to govern the Qi circulation. The head is the heaven (Tian, 天 ) while the abdomen is the earth (Di, 地 ) in Qigong practice. The Upper Dan Tian is the residence of the spirit while the Lower Dan Tian is the residence of Qi. Store Qi at the Real Lower Dan Tian and keep your spirit high and focused at the Upper Dan Tian to achieve longevity.

## 4-6. REGULATING THE SPIRIT (TIAO SHEN) 調神

Before you read this section, you are advised to re-read the definition of Shen in Chapter 3, to understand the profound meaning of ancient documents and the methods of cultivating Shen.

Here we discuss two important Qigong terminologies, Spiritual Valley (Shen Gu, 神谷 ) and Valley Spirit (Gu Shen, 谷神 ) which appear in many ancient documents. We then introduce the five keys of training to regulate the Shen, followed by two main training keys. Finally we summarize the goals of Shen training.

### Valley Spirit and Spirit Valley

In Chapter 6 of *Dao De Jing* (道德經 · 六章 ), it is said, "The Valley Spirit (Gu Shen) does not die, so it is called Xuan Pin. The key to reaching this Xuan Pin is the root of heaven and earth. It is very soft and continuous as if it were existing. When it is used, it will not be exhausted."[34]

The spirit (Shen, 神 ) resides at the space between the two hemispheres of the brain. It resembles a valley between mountains, trapping energy and generating resonant vibrations which correspond with the energy outside the valley. The Shen in this valley is called Valley Spirit (Gu Shen, 谷神 ) and the valley is called Spiritual Valley (Shen Gu, 神谷 ). The Shen residing in this valley governs the energy vibration of the whole body and thus the Qi status and its manifestation. When this Shen is strong, Qi manifesting in your life will be strong, and your life will be long and healthy.

Xuan (玄 ) means original (Yuan, 元 ). Pin (牝 ) refers to female animals and means mothers. Therefore, Xuan Pin means the Origin or Root of Lives. When the Valley Spirit is centered (condensed) and functions actively, the life force is strong. Xuan Pin (玄牝 ) is called Taiji (太極, Grand Ultimate) in *Yi Jing* (*The Book of Change*). This Taiji is the Dao (道 ) of lives in the great nature. Xuan Pin can be summarized as "The root of creation, variation, bearing, and raising of millions of lives. It is the mother of millions of objects in heaven and earth. It is another name for Dao."[35]

The door to reaching this Xuan Pin is through natural Shen (heaven and earth). This is very soft and continuous as though existing, and yet not existing. It cannot be seen, but is felt through cultivation. When used, it will not be exhausted.

To reach this natural Shen, you must open your third eye, called Tian Mu (天目,

heaven eye), or Yu Men (玉門, jade gate) by religious societies, and Yintang (M-HN-3, 印堂, seal hall) by medical society. *Wudang's Illustration of Cultivating Truth* (武當修真圖) said, "The place under the Mingtang (明堂, Ezhong (M-HN-2), 額中, center of forehead), above the midpoint of the line connecting the two eyebrows, where the spiritual light emits, is named heaven eye (Tian Mu, 天目)."[36] It is also mentioned in the document, *Seven Bamboo Slips of the Bamboo Bookcase* (云笈七簽), "The space between the two eyebrows is the Jade Gate (Yu Men, 玉門) of Ni Wan (泥丸)."[37] Ni Wan (泥丸) is a Daoist term, meaning Mud Pill, namely the brain, or Upper Dan Tian. The lower center of the Spiritual Valley (Shen Gu, 神谷) between the two hemispheres of the brain is called Ni Wan Gong (泥丸宮), or Mud Pill Palace (Figures 4-13 and 4-14).

To regulate Shen means to cultivate it until it reaches the supernatural divine state. In Daoist society, there is a song which says, "There is a Shen in every human body. There is a supernatural divine light (Ling Guang, 靈光) which can be developed in this Shen. This supernatural divine light alone can shine into thousands of valleys. Its Dao of variations is unlimited, spreading millions of ways."[38] Once you cultivate Shen to an enlightened level, it can reach everywhere in the universe.

There is a song in Buddhist society which says, "Do not search far for Buddha

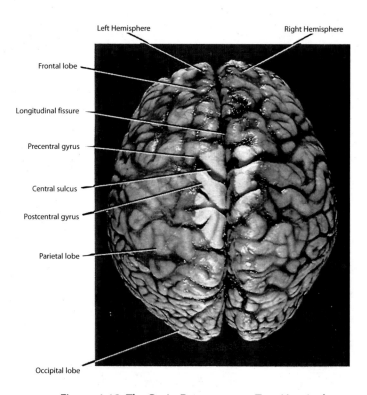

Figure 4-13. The Brain Encompasses Two Hemispheres

since he is in the Spiritual Mountain. Where is the Spiritual Mountain? It is actually in your mind. Everyone should have a pagoda at Spiritual Mountain, under which to cultivate his being."[39] Pagoda (Ta, 塔) implies good deeds you have done, and the comprehension of nature you have accumulated in spiritual cultivation.

To conclude this subsection, I translate a few ancient documents about Shen. Keep reading them repeatedly, and you will suddenly comprehend the meaning of spiritual cultivation.

## Observing Vessels
### 《脈望》

*The brain is the Upper Dan Tian, the palace where the Original Shen (Yuan Shen) resides. If one grasps this Original Shen and makes it stay at this Original Palace, then the golden Qi arises automatically, and the Real Breathing can be stabilized naturally. If one way is opened, then hundreds of ways will all be opened. When the big gate is opened, then hundreds of gates are all opened.*

腦為上田，元神所居之宮，人能握元神，棲于本宮，則
金氣自升，真息自定，所謂一竅開而百竅齊開，大關通
則百關盡通也。

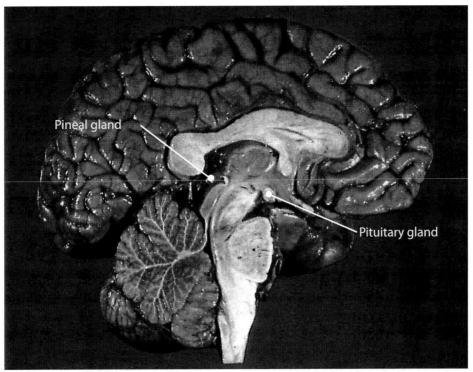

Figure 4-14. The Pituitary and Pineal Glands (Mud Pill Palace) in the Spiritual Valley

The brain is the Upper Dan Tian (Shang Dan Tian, 上丹田), the residence of the Shen. The Shen resides at the Upper Dan Tian since birth and is called Original Shen (Yuan Shen, 元神). The document, *Detailed Outline of Galenical* (本草綱目) said, "brain is the residence of Original Shen."[40] If you condense your Shen and contain it in its residence, the Qi in your body will be conserved. Keep your mind calm and peaceful, and avoid being distracted by human affairs and emotional disturbances. Then Qi storage at the Real Lower Dan Tian (Zhen Xia Dan Tian, 真下丹田) will be abundant and can be led up to nourish the brain and Shen. The breathing becomes slender, soft, and steady. This clears away obstacles to Qi in the entire body, and brings health and longevity.

## Concealed Secret of Fong's Family
### 《馮氏錦囊》

*There is a crux in the body named Xuan Pin, which enables life to live by receiving Qi. This is the residence of Shen, where the Three Origins (San Yuan) are gathered. It is the cavity where Jing (essence), Shen (spirit), Hun (soul) and Po (vigor) meet. It is the root where the Golden Elixir (Jin Dan, Qi) returns to, and where the immortals conceive their Holy Embryo.*

身中一竅，名曰玄牝，受氣以生，實為府神，三元所聚，
精神魂魄會于此穴，乃金丹還返之根，神仙凝結聖胎之
地也。

This document describes the Spiritual Valley (Shen Gu, 神谷), or Mud Pill Palace (Ni Wan Gong, 泥丸宮), where the Shen resides. Having Shen, and with the body nourished by Qi, there is physical life. When Shen departs from the body, there is death. To nourish this Shen, gather the Three Origins (San Yuan, 三元), namely Jing (精, Essence), Qi (氣), and Shen (神, Spirit) at this place. Then Shen can be raised up to a high level.

Po (魄) is the vital spirit supported by Qi while one is alive. When one dies, the Po becomes Hun (魂, Soul), meaning the spirit after death. Jin Dan (金丹) means Golden Elixir and implies precious Qi. When this precious Qi is led up to nourish the Shen, you can reach immortality. Remember the song which says, "There is a Shen in every human body. There is a supernatural divine light (Ling Guang, 靈光) which can be developed in this Shen. This supernatural divine light alone can shine into thousands of valleys. Its Dao of variations is unlimited, spreading millions of ways."[38] Once you cultivate Shen to an enlightened level, it can reach everywhere in the universe.

## Songs of Valley Spirit—1
### 谷神歌 - 一

*I have an interior insubstantial empty valley. When talking about it, it seems to be there, again it seems not to be there. When talking about it, even if it were not there, we could not ignore it. When talking about it, even if it were there, it could not be resided in.*

*Valley, valley, so marvelous. Shen, Shen, it is the real Great Dao. Keep it, protect it, you can be on the list of those without death. Cultivate and refine it, you can be called an immortal divine (Xian Ren).*

我有一腹空谷虛，言之道有又還無，言之無兮不可舍，
言之有兮不可居。
谷兮谷兮太玄妙，神兮神兮真大道，保之守之不死名，
修之煉之仙人號。

This song describes the importance of the Spiritual Valley (Shen Gu, 神谷) and how crucial it is for the cultivation of Valley Spirit (Gu Shen, 谷神). This Spiritual Valley is between the two lobes of the brain (Ni Wan Gong, 泥丸宮). It cannot be seen but only felt. In it, the Valley Spirit resides. To reach the Dao of enlightenment, you must feel the existence of the Spiritual Valley, keep the Shen there firmly, and cultivate it. This is the way to reach immortality. Xian Ren (仙人) are those who have attained spiritual immortality and enlightenment.

## Songs of Valley Spirit—2
### 谷神歌 - 二

*When the Valley Spirit obtains its Yi (one), the Ling (ingenuity) can be developed. When the Spiritual Valley obtains its Yi (center), fullness can be achieved. If one keeps this oneness, then from this alone one may achieve longevity.*

*It is not too difficult to obtain longevity. However, it cannot be achieved if one neglects the body. If trained and the accomplishment achieved, the ordinary bones are changed naturally.*

神得一以靈，谷得一以盈，若人能守一，只此自長生。
長生本不遠，離身還不見，煉之功若成，自然凡骨變。

Yi (一) here means one, singularity, or simplicity. If the Shen can condense into oneness at its residence without dispersing, the powerful spiritual vibration enables you to develop Ling (靈), which means ingenuity, intelligence, dexterity, cleverness, and comprehension.

When the Spiritual Valley obtains this concentrated Shen, the coherent resonant energy becomes full and strong, and the Qi is governed effectively by the Shen. To attain longevity, also heed your physical health and not just mental and spiritual cultivation. The key is both physical and mental. Only if these two balance each other and have a strong foundation, can you lead a long, healthy life. Daoists usually cultivate both body and mind. This dual cultivation is called Xing Ming Shuang Xiu (性命雙修) and means dual cultivation of temperament and life.

## Songs of Valley Spirit—3
## 谷神歌－三

*If Valley Spirit does not die, you have gained the gate to Xuan Pin. Exit and enter as softly as the Dao exists within. When cultivating Shen to return it to the insubstantial nothingness at midnight, use the river to transport the Qi to Kunlun.*

*The dragon is singing and the tiger is also shouting, the wind and the clouds meet and the old yellow lady is screaming. The fair lady in the fire is shy and charming. Look inward to see the baby in the water.*

谷神不死玄牝門，出入綿綿道若存，修煉還虛夜半子，
河車搬載上崑崙。
龍又吟、虎又嘯，風雲際會黃婆叫，火中妊女正含嬌，
回觀水底嬰兒俏。

Xuan (玄) means Original (Yuan, 元), and Pin (牝) means mothers. So Xuan Pin (玄牝) means the origin or root of lives, the key to longevity. To keep the Shen at its residence, follow the Dao, softly, gently, and persistently. Cut off external distractions and emotional disturbances, gradually and gently. If you try to force it, the emotional mind will be even more disturbed. To lead the Qi up through the Thrusting Vessel to nourish the brain, you must train at midnight, because Qi is strongest at that time.

Dragon (Long, 龍) and Tiger (Hu, 虎) means Yin and Yang Qi in the body. The Old Yellow Lady (Huang Po, 黃婆) is the matchmaker who brings Yin and Yang together. Through interaction of Yin and Yang, the spiritual baby embryo is conceived. Huang Po is the Shen and the breathing, which bring Yin and Yang together.

*The baby (Ying Er) and the shy lady (Cha Nu) meet the old yellow lady (Huang Po), and son and mother meet each other with the same Yi (mind). In the Golden Palace (Jin Dian) and Jade Hall (Yu Tang), there are twelve doors. Golden Male (Jin Gong) and Wooden Mother (Mu Mu) are just coming.*

*After passing layers of key doors, immediately lock the gate. Inspect cows in the Big Dipper (Dou Niu), and immediately start the fire. Advance the fire to eliminate Yin and initiate the sole Yang. Thousand years of peach have started to bear fruit.*

嬰兒妊女見黃婆，兒女相逢兩意合，金殿玉堂門十二，
金公木母正來過。
重門過后牢關鎖，點撿斗牛先下火，進火消陰始一陽，
千歲仙桃初結果。

The baby (Shen) and the shy lady (Qi) are now brought together by the old yellow lady (Huang Po, 黃婆, mind and breathing) in harmony with each other. They are led up from Huang Ting (黃庭) to the Upper Dan Tian, passing through twelve doors (throat area). Original Essence and Shen become one. Ying Er (嬰兒) means baby (son) and implies the Spiritual Embryo. Cha Nu (妊女, the shy lady, mother) implies Qi. This means the Xin has been calmed and unified with the Shen at Huang Ting (黃庭). The baby embryo is conceived and led to the Upper Dan Tian.

Jin Dian (金殿) is also called Jin Shi (金室), or Golden Palace, and implies the lungs. Yu Tang (玉堂) means Jade Hall, the palate of the mouth. Twelve doors means the throat area. Jin Gong (金公) means Golden Male, or Original Essence (Yuan Jing, 元精), and Mu Mu (木母) means Wooden Mother, or liver. Liver (Shen) belongs to wood in the Five Elements (Wuxing, 五行) and produces heart fire (Xin, 心). When Shen and Xin are harmonized, the mind is calm and the spirit condenses.

After passing the throat to the Upper Dan Tian, immediately confine the Spiritual Embryo there. Dou Niu (斗牛) means Big Dipper, which implies the process of condensing Shen at the Upper Dan Tian. After long practice, the Spiritual Embryo can be born.

*The Golden Bird (Jin Niao) flies on the east coast of the curved river (Qu Jiang). The Jade Rabbit (Yu Tu) shines with clear light on the west coast. The bird and the rabbit walk to the tip of the mountain. The fair lady in the furnace takes off her blue cloth.*

*After taking off the blue cloth, the pure clean body is exposed. The baby is then led to the layers of curtains. After ten months of strong and heavy emotion, a boy is born. Say he can live long and will not die.*

*I advise you to practice and cultivate. If the Valley Spirit does not die, the goal of immortality can be achieved. Comprehend the theory and carefully adopt those marvelous details. One day, I will reach the Immortal Land (Ying Zhou) with you.*

曲江東岸金烏飛，西岸清光玉兔輝，烏兔走歸峰頂上，
爐中妊女脫青衣。
脫卻青衣露素體，嬰兒引入重幃里，十月情濃產一男，
說道長生永不死。
勸君煉，勸君修，谷神不死此中求，此中悟取玄微處，
與君白日登瀛洲。

Qu Jiang (曲江) means Curved River (Intestines, Real Lower Dan Tian). Jin Niao (金烏) means Golden Bird (Original Spirit, Yuan Shen, 元神). Yu Tu (玉兔) means Jade Rabbit (Original Essence, Yuan Jing, 元精). The first sentence means Original Spirit and Original Essence become one, being led up to the furnace, or Upper Dan Tian. The lady takes off her blue clothes, to give birth to the baby. Blue clothes imply manifestation of Shen via the liver. The Liver's color is between blue and green in Chinese medicine. Shen is manifested through birth of the spiritual baby.

The baby is born after ten months of pregnancy and kept behind the curtain for nursing. It is the beginning of eternal spiritual life. Ying Zhou (瀛洲) is the holy mountain in the east sea where dwell the immortals of Chinese legend.

### Thesis of Valley Spirit's Immortality[29]
### 谷神不死論
### （紫清指玄集·宋·白玉蟾撰）

*What is the valley? It means Heavenly Valley (Tian Gu). What is Shen? It means the Original Spirit of the body. The Heavenly Valley has the capability of creation and variation, though it holds the insubstantial nihility. A valley on earth contains millions of objects and has mountains and rivers. Humans have the same natural disposition as heaven and earth, therefore we also have a valley. There is a real one-ness conceived in this valley where the Original Spirit (Yuan Shen) resides. There are nine palaces in the head which correspond with the nine heavens above. Among them, there is a palace at the center called Ni Wan (Mud Pill), or Huang Ting (Yellow Yard), also called Kunlun, or Tian Gu (Heavenly Valley). The names are numerous. It is where the Original Spirit resides. It is empty as a valley, and Shen lives in it. This Shen is called Gu Shen (Valley Spirit).*

谷者，天谷也。神者，一身之元神也。天之谷，含造化，
容虛空；地之谷，容萬物，載山川。人與天地同所稟也，
亦有谷焉。其谷藏真一，宅元神，是以頭有九宮，上應
九天，中間一宮，謂之泥丸，亦曰黃庭，又名崑崙，又
名天谷，其名頗多，乃元神所住之宮，其空如谷，而神
居之，故謂之谷神。

The space between the two hemispheres of the brain is called Heavenly Valley (Tian Gu, 天谷). The head is regarded as Heaven, while the perineum (Huiyin, Co-1, 會陰) is considered the Sea Bottom (Hai Di, 海底). This Heavenly Valley has many other names, such as Spiritual Valley (Shen Gu, 神谷), Yellow Yard (Huang Ting, 黃庭), Mud Pill (Ni Wan, 泥丸) or Kunlun (崑崙).

It is named Spiritual Valley because the Shen lives there. It is called Yellow Yard since it is an important place for cultivation. (The Huang Ting at the stomach area where the Spiritual Embryo is conceived is also called Yellow Yard). It is named Mud Pill due to the appearance of the pineal and pituitary glands. It is called Kunlun because that is one of the highest mountains in China.

Though the Spiritual Valley is empty and does not contain material objects like the valleys on the earth, which contain rivers, trees, and many other objects, it has the capability of creation and variation. Daoists believe there are nine layers of spiritual cultivation, with a palace in each. The brain also has nine palaces corresponding to the nine palaces of heaven. Among them, the center one is most important. This is where the Original Spirit (Yuan Shen, 元神) resides. This central palace is called Ni Wan Gong (泥丸宮, Mud Pill Palace). When you concentrate your mind there, the pineal and pituitary glands are activated by the abundant Qi. This significantly enhances production of melatonin and human growth hormone (HGH), two hormones crucial to longevity and vitality.

*When Shen exists, there is life. When Shen goes, there is death. Being attached to objects (human affairs) during daytime and to dreams at night, Shen cannot abide peacefully at home. Yellow corn unripened, the dream not yet awakened, the whole life's glory, splendor, wealth, and rank. A hundred years of sorrow, worry, happiness, and joy, isn't it happening just as in a dream? Once dead, life cannot reverse. Shen roams and cannot return. Life and death are parted, the path between life and death is cut off. Thus we see that if Shen does not live, one cannot live by oneself, and if the Shen is dead, one will also be dead naturally. If Shen abides in its valley without dying, how then can one die? The reason Valley Spirit (Gu Shen) does not die is because of Xuan Pin.*

神存則生，神去則死。日則接于物，夜則接于夢，神不
能安其居也。黃粱未熟，南柯未寤，一生之榮辱富貴，
百歲之悲憂悅樂，備嘗于一夢之間，使其去而不還，游
而不返，則生死路隔，幽明之途絕矣。由是觀之，人不
能自生而神生之，人不能自死而神死之。若神居其谷而
不死，人安得而死乎？然谷神所以不死者，由玄牝也。

If your mind is always distracted by human affairs and emotions, your Shen cannot stay at its residence. Human life is short and passes like a dream. If you waste time longing for glory, dignity, power, and wealth, neglecting to cultivate your Shen and keep it steady at its residence, you wake up one day to the realization that everything you have longed for is only a dream. To have immortal Shen, keep the Valley Spirit at the Spiritual Valley. Lao Zi said, "If the Valley Spirit (Gu Shen) does not die, it is called Xuan Pin (玄牝). The door to reach this Xuan Pin is the root of heaven and earth. It is very soft and continuous as though it existed. When used, it will not be exhausted."[34]

*What is Xuan? It is Yang and is the heaven. What is Pin? It is Yin and is the earth. However, Xuan and Pin two Qi's, all have profound implications. Without meeting those holy men to give instruction in the oral secrets, it cannot be understood easily. The Inner Classic of the Yellow Emperor said, "Original Shen resides in the Heavenly Valley. Protect it, then cultivation can be real." There is a Heavenly Valley called Ni Wan at the top of the body which is the residence of concealed Shen. A corresponding valley named Jiang Gong (heart) in the middle of the body is the residence of concealed Qi. Another divine valley called Guan Yuan (Key Origin) at the bottom of the body is the residence of concealed Jing.*

玄者，陽也，天也；牝者，陰也，地也。然則玄牝二氣，
各有深旨，非遇聖人，授以口訣，不可得而知也。《黃
帝內經》云：'天谷元神，守之自真。'言人身中上有
天谷泥丸，藏神之府也；中有應谷絳宮，藏氣之府也；
下有靈谷關元，藏精之府也。

Xuan Pin (玄牝) here means the interaction of Yin and Yang, to initiate life. Xuan Pin is the mother of life (creation and variations). It is difficult to understand and cultivate Yin and Yang Qi, and make them interact with each other. Usually, you need an experienced teacher to personally direct you on the right path.

This document mentions three valleys in the body to cultivate. The Spiritual

Valley (神谷, Upper Dan Tian) where the Valley Spirit resides is in the head. In the chest is the Jiang Gong (絳宮, Middle Dan Tian) which collects Post-Birth Qi converted from food and air. The third valley is Guan Yuan (關元, Lower Dan Tian) where Pre-Birth Original Qi is converted from Original Essence (Yuan Jing, 元精). These valleys conceal the essence of life.

*The Heavenly Valley is a mysterious palace, the residence of Original Shen, the home of human natural spiritual disposition, and the vital way of spiritual cultivation. Holy men follow the rules of heaven and earth and know the origin of variations. They protect the Shen and keep it at this mysterious palace, and store Qi abundantly at the residence of Pin. Shen and Qi mutually interact, enabling you to accomplish the cultivation of the real Dao naturally, unified with the Dao, and to enter the domain of being without death and without life. Therefore, it is said that when the Spiritual Valley does not die, it is called Xuan Pin. Those holy men know how to apply their cultivation in Xuan Pin, know how to create and vary in a trice. When the Qi of Xuan Pin enters this root (Real Lower Dan Tian), if you hold the breath too much, it becomes urgent. If you allow breathing to act freely, then it is out of control. So keep it very soft and continuous without any gap or interruption.*

天谷，玄宮也，乃元神之室，靈性之所存，是神之要也。
聖人則天地之要，知變化之源，神守于玄宮，氣騰于牝
府，神氣交感，自然成真，與道為一，而入于不死不生，
故曰谷神不死，是謂玄牝也。聖人運用于玄牝之內，造
化于恍惚之中，當其玄牝之氣，入乎其根，閉極則失于
急，任之則失于蕩，欲其綿綿續續，勿令間斷耳。

Spiritual Valley (Shen Gu, 神谷) is also called Mud Pill Palace (Ni Wan Gong, 泥丸宮). The Original Shen (Yuan Shen, 元神) residing in this palace is powerful and marvelous and the origin of creation and variations. It directs your mind and thinking and is the Taiji (太極, Grand Ultimate) of the human universe.

Those who obtain the Dao follow both human and natural Taiji and can thus know the Way of Nature. They unify and resonate their Shen with the natural Shen at its residence, and nourish it continuously with Qi. This is the way to achieve immortality of the Shen, called Xuan Pin (玄牝), the mother of creation and variations.

Keep Shen there through correct breathing, soft as a baby. Have a baby's heart (pure mind) without external attraction, which allows you to feel internally. Only then can you have soft breathing as if it were there and as if it were not there, being regulated without being regulated. Lao Zi said, "When concentrating the Qi to reach its softness, can it be as soft as a baby?"

*What is the meaning of "as if it were existing?" It means retaining it by following nature. After retaining Shen (at its residence) for a long time, it will be tranquil naturally. After practicing breathing for a long time, it will be stabilized naturally. When the temperament has become natural, then it can be used marvelously. Then no need to try hard or force it urgently, and "When used, it cannot be exhausted." Xuan and Pin are the two origins at the top and bottom, and are the correct paths for the Qi mother to ascend and descend. Those worldly seculars do not know these roots or study their origin and say the nose and mouth are Xuan and Pin. If the nose and mouth are Xuan and Pin, how can they be called the doorways of Xuan Pin? This is all because these people cannot comprehend the marvelousness of training. How can they understand if they are not great holy men?*

若存者，順其自然而存之，神久自寧，息久自定，性入
自然，無為妙用，未嘗至于勤勞迫切，故曰用之不勤。
即此而觀，則玄牝為上下二源，氣母升降之正道明矣。
世人不窮其根，不究其源，便以鼻為玄，以口為牝。若
以鼻口為玄牝，則玄牝之門又將何以名之？此皆不能造
其妙，非大聖人安能究是理哉！

This last paragraph talks about Lao Zi's concept in spiritual cultivation. In *Dao De Jing* ( 道德經 ), Chapter 6, it said "The Valley Spirit (Gu Shen, 谷神) does not die, then it is called Xuan Pin. The key to reaching this Xuan Pin ( 玄牝 ) is the root of heaven and earth (nature). It is very soft and continuous as if it were existing. When used, it will not be exhausted."[34]

The meaning of "as if it were existing" (Ruo Cun, 若存) is to practice keeping the Shen at its residence and maintaining and conserving Qi at the Real Lower Dan Tian until it becomes natural, namely regulating without regulating (Bu Tiao Er Tiao, 不調而調).

Xuan Pin ( 玄牝 ) is the interaction between Shen at the Upper Dan Tian and Qi at the Real Lower Dan Tian, namely unification and harmony of Shen and Qi. This is the mother of creation and variations, and the way to achieve immortality. Many seculars falsely believe Xuan Pin to be the nose and the mouth (breathing).

## Five Trainings of Shen

There are five trainings to regulate Shen: 1. Raising up the Shen (Yang Shen, 養神), 2. Protecting the Shen (Shou Shen, 守神), 3. Firming the Shen (Gu Shen, 固神), 4. Stabilizing the Shen (Ding Shen, 定神), and 5. Focusing the Shen (Ning Shen, 凝神). These are called Lian Shen ( 練神 ). Lian ( 練 ) means to refine, train, or discipline. There are also two training keys and two purposes of training Shen.

**Raising the Shen (Yang Shen, 養神).** Yang ( 養 ) means to nourish, raise, or nurse. Yang Shen is the main training task for Scholars and Buddhists. Shen needs to be nourished with Qi. Fire Qi from food and air can raise up Shen easily, but also increases emotional disturbance, leading Shen away from its residence. Using Yi nourished by Water Qi to raise up your Shen is harder, but this Shen is stronger and more concentrated than that from Fire Qi. Adjust Xin (Yang) and Yi (Yin) to raise up your Shen properly so it is raised but not excited and stays at its residence.

Raising the Shen correctly is like raising a child. You need great patience and perseverance. One way is to restrain his attention from the seven emotions and six desires. The other is to let him keep this contact with his human nature, yet educate his wisdom to make clear judgments, which is a long process, demanding understanding and patience. Raising Shen is not about increasing emotional excitement. This scatters the Yi, and Shen becomes confused and loses its center. Yang Shen builds a strong spiritual center and helps it control your life.

**Protecting the Shen (Shou Shen, 守神).** After raising your Shen, keep it at its residence and train it. A child needs to keep his mind with his family instead of straying outside and running wild. Then you can educate him.

Shou (守) means to keep and protect. The training involves keeping Shen at its residence, which is much harder than raising it up. Shou Shen training uses the regulated mind to direct, nurse, watch, and keep the Shen there. It is like keeping your child at home instead of letting him leave home and run wild. Be patient and control your temper, regulating your Xin and Yi. If you lose your temper, you only make the child want to leave home again. Once you have regulated your Xin and Yi will you be able to keep your Shen effectively.

**Firming the Shen (Gu Shen, 固神).** Gu (固) means to coalesce and to firm. After keeping Shen at its residence, you firm and coalesce it (Gu Shen). Gu Shen means training Shen to stay at its residence willingly. After you control your child in the house, make him want from his heart to stay. Only then will his mind be steady and calm. To reach this, you need more love and patience until he understands the importance of staying home and growing up normally. This third step of Shen training is to make the Shen willing to stay at its residence in peace, by regulating thoughts and emotions.

**Stabilizing the Shen (Ding Shen, 定神).** Ding Shen (定神) means to stabilize and calm the Shen. When your child is at peace, he will not be attracted to external distractions. Regulate your Shen to calm it down, so it is energized but not excited, with the mind peaceful and steady.

**Condensing the Shen (Ning Shen, 凝神).** Ning (凝) means to condense, concentrate, refine, focus, and strengthen. The first four processes which raise up, keep, firm and stabilize, are the foundations of Shen cultivation. After this, you condense and focus your Shen into a tiny spot. This is where you train the Shen to a higher spiritual state. When focused in a tiny point, it is like a sunbeam focused through a lens. The smaller the point, the stronger the beam. Here is translation and commentary of an ancient article on condensing the Shen.

# Anthology of Daoist Village
## 《道鄉集》

*What does it mean to condense? It means to gather. What is Shen? It is the right-eous thought in the Xin. What is Xi (profound breathing)? It is to induce Pre-Heaven Real Qi (Original Qi). It has no shape or appearance. Pre-Heaven Qi is generated at the point of extreme nihility and sincere calmness. Xue cavity (Real Lower Dan Tian) is the original root of producing Pre-Heaven Qi. Why condense Shen at this Qi cavity? It is to place and condense righteous thought there and not allow Shen to be distracted and move away. When Shen is condensed, fire (Qi) can be gathered. When fire is gathered and led downward, water rises automatically. This is mutual coordination of fire and water, to condense Shen at the Qi cavity. What is Xi? It is breathing. What is Xi-Xi (Continuous Breathing)? Breathing very soft and unbroken. What is Gui (Returning)? Reversing the path of life and returning to its origin. What is Gen (Root)? Root and foundation of life. Every breath is soft and continuous and returns it to this root. Breathing is not separate from the basic foundation of producing Qi. It is as though existing yet forgotten and seems to be there yet not there. This is how Embryonic Breathing was practiced since ancient times, following the natural way. If Shen condenses at the Qi cavity, breathing is also stabilized at this original root.*

夫凝者聚也，神者心中之正念也。息者，先天之真氣也。
無形無象，生于虛極靜篤之時，穴即生先天氣之本根。
所以凝神氣穴者，即將我心中之正念，凝聚于氣穴，不
令神往外馳。神凝則火聚，火聚于下，水自上升，此水
火調濟之要訣。亦凝神氣穴之妙諦也。息者，呼吸也。
息息者，綿綿不斷之義也。歸者，返回也。根者，基本
也。息息歸根，即呼吸不離生氣根本。若存若忘，似有
似無，昔所謂胎息者是也。須知此息，本乎自然，神既
凝于氣穴，息也定于本根。

This describes mutual unification, coordination, and harmonization of Shen with Pre-Heaven Qi (Xian Tian Qi, 先天氣, Original Qi), which is conceived at the Real Lower Dan Tian. Shen is fire (Yang, son) while Pre-Heaven Qi (mother) is water (Yin). Lead Shen down to unite with Pre-Heaven Qi, so mind and body can be calm and peaceful. Then Qi stays at its residence and is stored there.

Reach this goal through soft, slender, and continuous breathing, focusing your Shen at the Real Lower Dan Tian. This is crucial in Embryonic Breathing, the root of life, so the Spiritual Embryo can be conceived. Regulate Shen through training Embryonic Breathing, the crux of Internal Elixir Qigong (Nei Dan, 內丹). Refer to the previous book, *Qigong Meditation—Embryonic Breathing* for more detail.

## Two Training Keys

Remember, there are two keys in regulating Shen: 1. Mutual dependence of Shen and breathing (Shen Xi Xiang Yi, 神息相依), and 2. Mutual harmony of Shen and Qi (Shen Qi Xiang He, 神氣相合).

**Mutual Dependence of Shen and Breathing (Shen Xi Xiang Yi, 神息相依).** After Shen has been trained to a high degree, put it to work. The first assignment is coordinating with your breathing. In Qigong training, breathing is considered as the strategy. When this is directed by your Shen, it obtains optimum results. This strategy is called Shen Xi Xiang Yi (神息相依), which means Shen and breathing are mutually dependent. Shen Xi (神息) means Shen breathing. Your Shen and breathing become one, and Qi is led efficiently. This daunting task requires you to have regulated your body, breathing, and mind.

### Anthology of Daoist Village[8]
### 《道鄉集》

*"Be calm, then focus on the Real Lower Dan Tian. Where your eyes focus, Xin should follow. When Xin and eyes have reached the place and ceased, then Xin and breathing should accord with each other and gradually enter the Great Steadiness (Da Ding)." "Shen is stabilized in coordination with breathing. Breathing is peaceful in coordination with Shen. When they accord with each other, the Great Steadiness can be reached."*

〝能靜時觀照下田，目之所在，心亦隨之，心目得其所止，而后心與息依，漸入大定。〞又〝神依息而定，息依神而安，互相依附，始歸大定。〞

Eyes focus means the Yi (意). Ancient documents often say, "The eyes observe (Guan, 觀) the nose (breathing), and the nose observes the Xin."[21] Restrain your eyes, and focus on breathing, through which Xin can be observed and regulated.

Qigong society often says, Xin-ape and Yi-horse (Xin Yuan Yi Ma, 心猿意馬). Xin means heart, related to emotional disturbance. Use the Yi-horse to govern the Xin-monkey, using breathing as the strategy. With Xin under control, stabilize Shen at its residence. Shen and breathing mutually harmonize and accord with each other. This is called the Great Steadiness (Da Ding, 大定).

In Buddhist society Da Ding means, "When Xin for Buddhism is clear and bright, it is called Da Ding."[28] The mind is at peace and the body extremely relaxed. Shen and body harmonize and coordinate with each other.

**Mutual Harmony of Shen and Qi (Shen Qi Xiang He, 神氣相合).** The second Shen training key uses Shen to direct the circulation and distribution of Qi, called Shen Qi Xiang He (神氣相合, Shen and Qi combine). In battle, the fighting spirit of the soldiers determines their ability to fight and to execute strategy. Shen is the Son (Zi, 子), while Qi is the Mother (Mu, 母). When mother and son unite in harmony with each other, it is called Mu Zi Xiang He (母子相合, mutual harmony of mother and son). Some ancient documents describe the practice:

### Secrets of spiritual applications of all veracious Holy Embryo
### (Methods of Transporting Qi)
### 《諸真聖胎神用訣》
### （御氣之法）

*Go to the top to Ni Wan (Mud Pill Palace) and to the bottom to Mingmen (Real Lower Dan Tian). Two sceneries follow each other mutually, to save the remaining days and increase longevity. If Shen does not control exhaling, then breathing is not complete. If Shen does not govern inhaling, the breathing is not complete either. Coordinate and harmonize Shen and Qi mutually, in every breath, then the embryo can be conceived from concealed Qi, and Qi can be produced through Embryonic Breathing. Embryonic Qi coalesces internally and never dies.*

上至泥丸，下至命門，兩景相隨，可救殘老矣。若呼不
得神宰，一息不全，吸不得神宰，亦一息不全。若能息
息之中，使神氣相合，則胎從伏氣中結，氣從有胎中息，
胎氣內結，永不死矣。

Ni Wan (泥丸) implies the Upper Dan Tian. The Spiritual Valley (Shen Gu, 神谷) between the two hemispheres of the brain is called Ni Wan Gong (泥丸宮, Mud Pill Palace), referring to the pineal and pituitary glands. When these two glands produce abundant hormones, they promote smooth metabolism. Vital force is strong and Shen high. Mingmen (命門, Life Door) here means the Real Lower Dan Tian instead of the Mingmen cavity of acupuncture. The Real Lower Dan Tian stores Qi, the life force.

Circulate Qi, controlled by Shen, through the Upper Dan Tian and the Real Lower Dan Tian. Shen and Qi mutually coordinate and harmonize with each other, through Embryonic Breathing, so the Spiritual Embryo can be conceived. Two polarities become one. This is the Wuji state, the initiation of life.

## Ten Books of Cultivating Truth: short cut of miscellaneous writing
### 《修真十書 · 雜著捷徑》

*Qi is nourished by Qi, and Qi then meets Shen. When Shen and Qi are not sep-arated, then it is true cultivation. The son does not leave the mother, nor the mother the son. When son and mother stay together, then live long without dying.*

氣養于氣，氣會于神，神氣不散，是為修真。子不離母，
母不放子，子母共守，長生不死。

To accumulate abundant Qi, you must find the extra Qi and store it at the Real Lower Dan Tian (Zhen Xia Dan Tian, 真下丹田) by keeping your Shen there. When Shen and Qi unite in harmony, the Spiritual Embryo (Sheng Tai, 聖胎) can be conceived. Shen and Qi, like son and mother, will not part from each other. This is the way to reach longevity.

## Marvelous applications of maintaining the shape and cultivating internal truth by Great Teacher Da Mo
### 《達摩大師住世留形內真妙用訣》

*Without keeping the son and mother (Shen and Qi) together, even though Qi is stored internally through breathing, nevertheless Shen is constantly labored exter-nally, becoming dirty and confused. Once Shen is dirty, the original harmonious Qi gradually disperses and cannot stay. Daoists often make this mistake, not knowing that shape and Shen are the core of practice. If one does not keep Qi and Shen internally but keeps them externally, their residences will be dangerous and gradually rotten. Non-Daoists labor their Shen and fatigue their thinking. There is not even a respiration leading Qi and Shen to the Qihai (Real Lower Dan Tian). If they expect longevity, isn't it too far to be reached?*

若不知子母相守，氣雖呼吸于內，神常勞役于外，遂使
神常穢濁而神不清。神既不清，即元和之氣漸散而不能
相守也。道人常用之，而不知根本以形神為主。若人不
知守于內而守于外，自然令宅舍虛危，漸見衰壞矣。況
非道之人，勞神役思，無一息神氣注于氣海之中，而欲
望其長生，豈不遠乎！

Shen and the Qi must combine and not separate from each other. First stop the mind from all outside distractions and emotional disturbances, lest your Shen become dirty. Through correct Embryonic Breathing, keeping Shen and Qi at the Real Lower Dan Tian, you attain longevity.

## Chapter of Clear Understanding
## (Mao, Ri-Xin; Song Dynasty)
### 《宋·毛日新；了明篇》

*Qi follows Shen and Shen follows Qi. Shen and Qi mutually follow each other and penetrate into Ni Wan. Keep Jin Guan locked and sealed constantly. Once having caught Jin Pin, then internal joy. Practice this Gongfu diligently and establish strong will, throughout the day (twelve timings). When Yin ends and Yang has completed, Shen can leave the body. When this Gongfu has been accomplished, your name will be on the list of immortality.*

氣隨神，神隨氣，神氣相隨，透入泥丸裡。長把金關牢
鎖閉，捉得金晶，暗地添歡喜。下辛勤，須發志，十二
時中，莫把功夫棄。陰盡陽全神出體，功行成時，名列
神仙位。

This poem describes the mutual dependency of Shen and Qi. Once Shen and Qi enter Ni Wan Gong (泥丸宮, Upper Dan Tian), keep it there firmly. Jin Guan (金關, Golden Gate) means Upper Dan Tian. Jin Pin (金品, Golden Material) implies the Spiritual Embryo. Shi Er Shi (十二時, twelve timings) are the traditional Chinese divisions of the day.

## Secrets of applying Qi with Concentrated Shen[29]
### 《用氣集神訣》
### （延陵先生集新舊服氣經·唐·延陵先生集）

*Shen is gathered from insubstantial and made peaceful with substantial. Shen is wisdom of the Xin. When Xin is peaceful without desire, Shen can be like a king with harmony and righteous Qi. Having reached this stage, let Shen be free without restraint, the longer the better. Practice ceaselessly, so Qi in the body reaches extreme peace. This is delightful for heaven, so you live long. When outside the body (material world) is substantially empty, then it is also (delightful) for heaven. When inside the body is empty and comprehensive (without emotional bondage or desire), then it is also (delightful) for heaven. Practice for a long, long time, then enlightenment can be attained. All these secrets are understood internally. After practicing for a long time, understanding is deep and refined, matching the enlightenment of heaven. Then Qi can develop from Jing internally. Dao can be reached, and this Dao will correspond with De (the virtue of nature). The completeness of the De is that, when it is used, it manifests Ren (benevolence). When divided (expanded), it demonstrates Yi (righteousness).*

神集于虛，而安于實。神，心中知者也。安而無欲，則
神王而氣和正。如此之時，則一任所之，唯久彌善。行
之不已，體氣至安，謂之樂天，樂天則壽。身外虛空亦
天也，身內虛通亦天也，習之久久，乃明生焉。密自內
知之，久習彌廣而精，上合于明，明則內發于精，如是
乃至于道，道應于德。德之成矣，用而為仁，分而為義。

Shen is insubstantial and cannot be seen. However, it can be felt and condensed to a high spiritual level. Though insubstantial, it must be in accord with the material world of secular society. Shen is related to the wisdom mind (Yi, 意) and the emotional mind (Xin, 心). The emotional mind brings confusion and excitement, while the wisdom mind directs you to focused thinking and decisions. Shen can be raised and condensed, so the emotional mind under control becomes peaceful and calm. This results in harmonization of Shen and Qi's circulation, the stage of unification of Shen and Qi (Shen Qi Xiang He, 神氣相合). Practice often to achieve regulating without regulating, bringing health and longevity. Your mind becomes neutral and bright, clear and wise, reaching far and wide. Internally wise, externally you apply the Dao (道) of nature in action, which is called "De" (德). When Dao and De are applied in human society, it is benevolence (Ren, 仁) and righteousness (義).

*Jing Qi leaves from the head in daytime and resides at the abdomen (Real Lower Dan Tian) at night. Therefore, respect the head and the abdomen. Settle the colors (materials) externally, while respecting righteousness within. Whenever there is an opportunity (for taking advantage), there is no slightest thought (of taking it). All in the mind is goodness. Thus, Shen and Qi engage the quality and harmonize into a single body. This is called Great Smoothness (Da Shun). Heaven will protect (you) and (make you) auspicious without any disadvantage. This is because all the marvelous (manifestations of nature) have their roots. The Shen's insubstantial nothingness, inside Xin, connects with its system. The Qi firmly concealed in the intestines should be nourished warmly and patiently. In daily life, close your eyes and observe the internal origin of the Qi. Whenever an event causes disturbance of the Ling (spiritual mind), close your eyes gladly and observe the Xin internally. Reject it as though saying, "My Shen and Qi are concealed and developed from my body, making me able to reach the Dao." Then heaven will bestow auspiciousness, because heaven is the Ling of the insubstantial Qi. Use it to reach the ultimate of the Dao.*

精氣畫出于首，夜栖于腹，當自尊其首，重其腹。色庄
于外，敬直于中，應機無想，唯善是與，此神氣事質，
合吾一體，謂之大順，天保祐之，吉無不利。凡妙本有
所，神在心中之虛，上通其系，氣蘊腸中之實，恆宜溫
養之。平居常宜閉目內視氣源，每行一事利于生靈，則
欣然閉目，內視其心，謝之若曰：‘吾身之神氣，明發
于吾形，使吾達道也。’ 如是則天降之吉。故天者，虛
氣之靈，吾能用之，道極于斯矣。

In daytime, brain function leads Qi upward, and at night, during sleep, Qi returns to the Real Lower Dan Tian for recharging. When you cultivate immortality, you must cultivate both Shen at the top (quality) and Qi at the bottom (quantity).

Many distractions cause emotional disturbance and increase desire. Whatever your thoughts and actions, let them be in the goodness of the Dao (道) and De (德). You feel righteous and enlightened internally, your spirit in harmony and at peace. This follows the way of nature, and nature will protect you.

## Two Purposes of Regulating the Shen

There are two main purposes of regulating the Shen in Qigong practice. For secular society, it is to improve health and extend life, but for Buddhists and Daoists, the goal is to reach Buddhahood or enlightenment.

**Health and Longevity.** Yi is related to Shen. When Yi is strong and concentrated, Shen can be raised high. The most popular and essential purpose of Qigong practice is to attain health, using Yi to lead the Qi (Yi Yi Yin Qi, 以意引氣). If concentrated Yi raises Shen, Qi circulates smoothly, and the body is healthy. Small Circulation meditation increases the Qi circulating in the Conception and Governing Vessels, and in the Twelve Primary Qi Channels.

Qigong also enhances longevity. It raises the spirit up to a high level, then uses it to govern the Qi (Yi Shen Yu Qi, 以神馭氣) and to enhance Qi circulation in the bone marrow and brain. Qi is compared to soldiers in battle, while Shen is their fighting spirit. When the general's spirit is high, the morale of his soldiers is also high, and his orders are carried out effectively. In the same way, Qi nourishes the bone marrow and brain. Healthy marrow enhances production of blood cells, promoting metabolism and leading to longevity.

The following ancient document describes this process.

## Historical Record: Autobiography of Tai Shi Gong
### 《史記・太史公自序》

*How can one be alive? It is because of the existence of the Shen. How can this Shen be relied on to exist? It is because of the shape. When the Shen is greatly used, then exhausted. When the shape is greatly labored, then worn out. When shape and Shen are separated, they die. The dead cannot be revived, and those who are separated cannot be reunited. Therefore, holy men take spiritual cultivation very seriously. Shen is the root of the life while the shape is its vehicle.*

凡人所生者，神也；所托者，形也。神大用則竭，形大勞則敝，形神離則死，死者不可復生，離者不可復反，故聖人重之。由是觀之，神者，生之本也，形者，生之具也。

Buddhists regard the spirit as the root of human life, while the physical body is only the vehicle for its cultivation. To reach Buddhahood, they cultivate the spirit more than the body. But Daoists regard the cultivation of the spirit and the body are being equally important. It takes many years to cultivate the Shen to reach enlightenment. If the physical body is weak and unhealthy, your life will be too short for spiritual cultivation.

To Buddhists, the material world does not exist, so there is nothing to be cultivated or considered. The Buddhist document, *Altar Classic of the Sixth Ancestor* (六祖壇經) said, "Bodhi does not have a tree originally, nor is there a shining mirror in front. There are no objects there originally, so how can they be contaminated by dust or mud (objects or emotions)?"[41] Bodhi means an enlightened mind. Buddha was enlightened under the Bodhi tree. Shining mirror means a pure and clean Shen. When you cultivate Shen, the material world disappears, so there is no tree or mirror stand. With no material concept in your mind, how can it be cleaned of secular emotions and desires?

A Daoist document, *The Thesis of Nourishing Life* (養生論), contrasts this, "Utter and receive Qi (Tu Na, 吐納) through breathing, absorb food to nourish the body, thus allow the shape (physical body) and Shen to be harmonized. This means the mutual coordination of external and internal."[42] Tu Na (吐納) means uttering and receiving, an ancient term for cultivating Qi through breathing.

**Enlightenment.** To spiritual cultivators, the final goal of regulating Shen is reaching enlightenment. That means comprehending the meaning of nature and human life, then unifying the human spirit with nature to become as one. This is the final goal of the unification of Heaven and Man (Tian Ren He Yi, 天人合一).

To reach this, one must open the third eye for communication. First build up abundant Qi at the Real Lower Dan Tian. This is led up through the Thrusting

Vessel to activate the brain, and enhance the resonance of the Spiritual Valley. When spiritual energy reaches a certain level, the third eye reopens.

To reach this high level of cultivation, first regulate your mind. If it is trapped in emotional bondage, how can you build up your spirit and keep it neutral? Buddhists and Daoists define four steps in spiritual cultivation.

## Four Steps to Cultivate Spiritual Enlightenment

**Self-recognition (Zi Shi, 自識).** First set your spirit free from emotional bondage, otherwise the spirit stays in the emotional mud of secular society. Once the spirit is free from this bondage, it can reach the neutral state and finally unify with the natural spirit. Self-recognition (Zi Shi, 自識) means observing the heart (Guan Xin, 觀心), that is, observing the initiation of thoughts and emotions to discover your true identity.

*Important Script of Similar Contents* (同指要抄) said, "All religious styles, throughout generations, all considered observing the Xin (Guan Xin, 觀心) as the most important in cultivation."[43]

*The Complete Book of Principal Contents of Human Life and Temperament* (性命圭旨全書) said, "When learning the Dao, first comprehend your own Xin. The deep hidden place of your own Xin is the hardest place to find. Once you have found it and no other place can be found, you realize that a secular's Xin can be just like a Buddha's."[44] This describes the difficulty of discovering your true self hiding behind the mask. Once you have discovered this hidden Xin, you recognize it and cultivate it. This cultivated Xin can reach the same level as Buddha.

**Self-awareness (Zi Jue, 自覺).** Having recognized your true identity, ponder deeply, and clearly discriminate truth from illusion. From discriminating between truth and falsehood, awareness arises. Your mind establishes contact with events and phenomena in your life. The feeling of self-awareness can be profound.

To Buddhist society, this is the stage where observation is stopped. It is the beginning of regulating the temperament and spirit towards goodness. *Anthology of Daoist Village* (道鄉集) said, "The real meaning of Buddhahood which has been handed down is: observation is stopped. What is observation? It means to place my vision warmly on the ultimate goodness. What is stop? It means to focus my real intention on the ultimate goodness."[45] Buddhist society has three observations (San Guan, 三觀): 1. Observing Emptiness, is observing the emptiness of all natural laws and events, 2. Observing Falseness, is observing the falseness of all natural laws, 3. Observing Between, is observing the non-emptiness and non-falseness of natural laws, keeping the neutral viewpoint. It also means double observation.[18] Zhi Guan (止觀, Stop Observation) is the way to reach Guan Zhi (觀止, Observation is Stopped). Observe and analyze events and occurrences. Once you see through the events in your mind, nothing troubles you. This is the stage of Guan Zhi, reached by cultivating your mind to the stage of ultimate goodness. Pay attention to all goodness, then nothing bothers you. You are kind, righteous and gentle, with no inner conflict. You are free from the affinity of emotions and desires.

Extreme calmness and peace within are the key to this self-awareness, reached through practicing Embryonic Breathing (Tai Xi, 胎息), as described in the book, *Qigong Meditation—Embryonic Breathing.*

**Self-awakening (Zi Xing, 自醒)(Zi Wu, 自悟).** Through Embryonic Breathing, you reach self-awakening. Your mind is clear and allows you to comprehend accurately the truth of your life and nature. This stage is called entering the observation (Ru Guan, 入觀). Entering means to comprehend the observation and the temperament (Wu Xing, 悟性).[46] This is the stage of enlightenment and Buddhahood (Fo, 佛), called understanding the heart and seeing through the temperament (Ming Xin Jian Xing, 明心見性). Comprehension is no longer necessary (Liao Wu, 了悟).

How is Buddhahood defined? It means to achieve awareness and wisdom, to awaken through understanding and observation, to awaken through knowing the reasons behind natural laws, and to discriminate them clearly. It is like being awakened from sleep and is called 'awakening through realization'. Comprehend vexations through observation so they are not harmful. It is like observing and sensing 'thieves' (contaminated thoughts) in secular society, so it is called awakening through observation.[47] *Thesis of Buddha Ground* (佛地論) said, "All laws and all manifestations of nature can bloom and be awakened by themselves. We can also bloom and be awakened from emotional bondage, like being awakened from sleep and like the blooming of the lotus flower. This is called Buddha."[48]

To Buddhists, we are born and grow in emotional mud (Chen Tu, 塵土, human matrix). We create dignity, glory, pride, happiness, sadness, jealousy, and desire. We lie and cover our faces with masks, and we all experience significant spiritual pain living in this human matrix. The mud makes us blind and deaf, and nothing is clear in our minds. The conscious mind is active, while the sub-conscious Shen is asleep. We are dreaming in the human matrix and not awakening.

Nevertheless, each of us has a lotus seed, our Original Shen. Through meditation, it buds and grows from deep in the mud. The subconscious mind grows, and after long practice, the lotus flower emerges from the matrix, and you see everything clearly. To awaken your Shen, bring all thoughts to your Shen center and keep the Shen there. This Upper Dan Tian or Spiritual Mountain (Ling Shan, 靈山), in which there is the Spiritual Valley (Shen Gu, 神谷), is where the Valley Spirit (Gu Shen, 谷神) lives.

Remember the song which says, "Do not search far for Buddha since he is in the Spiritual Mountain. Where is the Spiritual Mountain? In your mind."[39]

In a state of extreme calmness and emptiness, your mind is clear to comprehend the truth of nature. *The Righteous Rules of Heavenly Immortality: Straight Discussion of Two Qi's Pre-Heaven and Post-Heaven* (天仙正理・先天后天二氣直論) said, "Those who apply Qi, how do they know it is true pre-heaven practice? When calmness

(Jing, 靜) and emptiness (Xu, 虛) have reached their extremities, there is no single slight thought involved in consciousness. This is the true pre-heaven practice."[49] Pre-Heaven truth (Xian Tian Zhi Zhen, 先天之真) means the truthful state before birth, where the mind is simple and pure, extremely calm and sincere. However, how do you know you have reached this state in practice? When there is not even the smallest thought existing or initiating in your mind. Your subconscious mind (Pre-Heaven truthful mind) awakens to activity.

Qigong society classifies the conscious mind as Yang, generated by the brain since birth. The subconscious mind is Yin and is born with you. The conscious mind and memory are generated from conditioning by the environment and are not truthful. A thick facade covers the falseness of this conscious mind. However, the subconscious mind is truthful, connected with spiritual memory, which is active only when your body is calm and activities of your conscious mind have ceased.

To return to the Pre-Birth stage, cease physical and mental activity. Then the subconscious mind acts, and directs you to the true path of spiritual cultivation.

**Freedom from Self-bondage** (Zi Tuo, 自脫). The last stage of spiritual cultivation is to free yourself from physical, mental, and spiritual bondage. Once you have awakened spiritually, you see clearly who you are and how you want to be. Free yourself from the bondage of the human matrix. In Buddhist terms, the third eye opens. The lotus grows, and the flower emerges from the mud. Your spirit is reunited with the spirit of nature.

**Freedom from Material Bondage.** Set yourself free from the bondage of your physical body and all material attractions around you. Your body is only recycled material, and beauty is only temporary. Material concerns trigger mental bondage. Take care of this recycled material, protect it and nourish it, but free yourself from attaching to it.

What you need from the material world is enough energy supply for your physical strength, without sinking into the mud of materialism and losing the feeling of your life. Most material things you own will last longer than you, and you own them only as long as you live. If you pursue material enjoyment, your mind stays focused on materialistic concerns. To set yourself free from material bondage, the first step is to gain enough for comfortable living. Any extra beyond that entangles you deeper in the mud. To reach profound spiritual cultivation, Buddhists believe you must cultivate a neutral state separate from the four emptinesses of earth, water, fire, and wind (Si Da Jie Kong, 四大皆空, material world). They believe this is crucial to reaching Buddhahood.

**Freedom from Mental Bondage.** Mental bondage means the thoughts generated from the emotional matrix, and desires for both the mental and material worlds. Again, human suffering is caused by the seven passions and six desires (Qi Qing Liu Yu, 七情六慾). The seven passions are happiness (Xi, 喜), anger (Nu, 怒), sorrow (Ai, 哀), joy (Le, 樂), love (Ai, 愛), hate (Hen, 恨) and desire (Yu, 慾). The six desires are the sensory pleasures derived from the eyes, ears, nose, tongue, body, and mind.

We humans, in order to survive in the harsh reality of this world, lie and trick each other. Truth within is hidden behind the mask we wear, decorated with glory, dignity and honor, which are tools to enslave the souls and bodies of others. Lust for wealth and power has become the common core education for the next generation. A human emotional matrix has been created and all of us suffer within it.

To escape from this matrix, first awaken deep in your heart. With a neutral and open mind, see through the matrix we have created. The truth should always be in your mind, else the search for the Dao will be in vain. Ponder the words of Michael Faraday (1791-1867): "*The philosopher should be a man willing to listen to every suggestion, but determined to judge for himself. He should not be biased by appearances, have no favorite hypothesis, be of no school, and in doctrine have no master. He should not be a respecter of persons, but of things. Truth should be his primary object. If to these qualities be added industry, he may indeed hope to walk within the veil of the temple of Nature.*" Once you have this truth in your mind, you have achieved a peaceful mind, and your spirit can awaken and be cultivated.

**Freedom from Spiritual Bondage.** You need to be free from mental bondage before setting out to escape from spiritual bondage. The spirit is overshadowed and blinded by traditional religious doctrines, based on the emotions of the past.

The various religions bind us in their spiritual religious matrix, created by those considered holy men in the past. The concepts of God, heaven, and hell were created in the human mind and worship was initiated. As time passed, we have been led deeper and deeper away from the truth, and trapped in humanly-created spiritual bondage. *Lao Zi*, Chapter 1, said, "Dao, if it can be spoken (described), then it is not the true everlasting Dao. Name, if it can be named, then it is not the true everlasting name."[50] We humans, before really knowing the Dao, have already talked about Dao. Even if we know the true path to search for it, we still cling stubbornly to the old path and dare not change it.

To achieve this true Dao, we must continue to search for it, talking and exchanging opinions. Always keep in mind that the Dao we are talking about may not yet be true. Having seen the truth, *we should not be afraid to face it, challenging our old thoughts and beliefs, and daring to accept mistakes and to dream about the future.* Science should search for the true Dao, helping us to escape from the traditional religious matrix.

Escape from the traditional matrix and free yourself from spiritual bondage and doctrines. Awaken your subconscious spiritual mind, by bringing your mind and spiritual feeling to the day you were conceived. From this Daoist principle were derived the theory and techniques of Embryonic Breathing.

To return to the embryonic state, first get rid of the human emotional matrix. Focus the mind on the pineal and pituitary glands at the Mud Pill Palace (Ni Wan Gong, 泥丸宮). Where there are brain cells, that is where conscious thought and the human matrix can be created. However, the lower center of the Spiritual Valley has no brain cells, so no matrix can be generated. Through this center, where the subconscious mind resides, we can resonate or communicate with the natural spirit. By calming the activity of the brain through absence of thought, we bring our spiritual awareness to a high level.

For strong resonance between your spirit and the natural spirit, you need strong spiritual energy at this Mud Pill Palace. Store abundant Qi at your Real Lower Dan Tian (Zhen Xia Dan Tian, 真下丹田), and lead it up to nourish the Mud Pill Palace, raising spiritual energy up to a high level. Spiritual cultivation is discussed in more detail in my previous book, *Qigong Meditation—Embryonic Breathing*.

Once you bring your spiritual energy to a very high level, you reopen your third eye, called Tian Yan (heaven eye, 天眼) by Daoist society and Yintang (M-NH-3, sealed hall, 印堂) by Chinese medicine. Having reopened the third eye, your spirit can unite with the natural spirit without obstacle. This is the final stage of spiritual cultivation, the Unification of Heaven and Man (Tian Ren He Yi, 天人合一).

## References

1. 真調為無調而自調。

2. 形不正，則氣不順。氣不順，則意不寧。意不寧，則氣散亂。

3. 解剖生理學 (*A Study of Anatomic Physiology*)，李文森編著。華杏出版股份有限公司。 Taipei, 1986.

4. 《莊子·大宗師》：〝古之真人，···其息深深。真人之息以踵，眾人之息以喉。〞

5. 《性命圭旨全書·火候》：〝神息者，火候也。〞指文火安神定息，任其自如，謂之神息。即〝不得勤，不得息者，是皆神息之自然火候之微旨也。〞

6. 《性命圭旨全書·蟄藏氣穴，眾妙歸根》：〝調息要調真息息，煉神須煉不神神。〞

7. 《天仙正理·伏氣直論》：〝古人托名調息者，隨順往來之理而不執滯往來之形，欲合乎似無之呼吸也。〞

8. *Chinese Qigong Dictionary* (中國氣功辭典), by Lu, Guang-Rong (呂光榮), 人民衛生出版社, Beijing, China, 1988.

9. Teens' Troubles Tied to Brain, Michael Lasalandra, *Boston Herald*, June 12, 1998.

10. Inside the Teen Brain, by Shannon Brownlee, pp. 44-54, *U.S. News*, August 9, 1999.

11. 《備急千金要方・卷二十七・養性》：〝多思則神殆，多念則志散，多欲則志昏，多事則形勞，多語則氣乏，多笑則臟傷，多愁則心懾，多樂則意溢，多喜則忘錯昏亂，多怒則百脈不定，多好則專迷不理，多惡則憔悴無歡。此十二多不除，則榮衛失度，血氣妄行，喪生之本也。〞

12. 《性命圭旨全書・亨集》：〝身不動而心自安，心不動而神自守

13. 《性命圭旨全書・蟄藏氣穴，眾妙歸根》：〝合真人深深之息，則心息相依，息調心靜。〞

14. 《聽心齋客問》：〝心依著事物已久，一旦離境，不能自立。所以用調息功夫，拴系此心，便心息相依。調字亦不是用意，只是一呼一吸系念耳。至心離境，則無人無我，更無息可調，只綿綿若存，久之，自然純熟。〞

15. 《道藏・坐忘論》：〝夫心者一身之主，百神之帥，靜則生慧，動則生昏，欣迷動靜之中。〞

16. 《至游子・集要篇》：〝不畏念起，惟畏覺遲。〞

17. 《道藏・重陽立教十五論》：〝欲界、色界、無色界，此乃三界也。心忘慮念，即超欲界；心忘諸境，即超色界；不著空見，即超無色界。〞

18. 〔三觀〕：一・空觀：觀諸法之空諦。二・假觀：觀諸法之假。三・中觀：一觀諸法亦非空，亦非假，即中也。二觀諸法亦空亦假，即是中，謂為雙照之觀。

19. 《性命圭旨全書・亨集》：〝一念動時皆是火，萬緣寂處即生春。〞

20. 《維摩經》：〝系心于緣謂之止，分別深達謂之觀。〞〝念念歸一為止，了了分明為觀。〞

21. 眼觀鼻，鼻觀心

22. 《莊子・人間世》：〝若一志，無聽之以耳而聽之以心；無聽之以心而聽之以氣。聽止于耳，心止于符。氣也者，虛而待物者也。唯道集虛，虛者心齋也。〞

23. 《道鄉集》：〝余今傳汝止念之法。譬如我心看水，此念即在水上；我心看月，此念即在月上；設想此眼光專看氣穴，我心即在氣穴矣。〞

24. 《中和集》：〝諦觀三教聖人書，息之一字最簡直。若于息上做功夫，為佛為仙不勞力。息緣達本禪之機，息心明理儒之極，息氣凝神道之玄，三息相須無不克。〞

25. 《慧苑音義・上》：〝禪那，此云靜心思慮也。〞

26. 孔子曰：〝知止而后有定，定而后能靜，靜而后能安，安而后能慮，慮而後能得。〞

27. 《智度論》：〝正心行處，見慮凝心，心定于一處而不動，故曰定；正受所觀之法，故曰受；調心之暴，直心之曲，定心之散，故曰調直定；正心之行動，使合于法之依處，故曰正心行處；息止緣慮，凝結心念，故曰息慮凝心。〞

28. 《管子・內業》：〝佛心澄明，謂之大定。〞指腦神安靜，形體放鬆，神形相對協調與穩定。

29. *The Great Completion of Chinese Qigong* (中國氣功大成), by Fang, Chun-Yang (方春陽), 吉林科學技術出版社, Jilin, China, 1989.

30. *The Complete Book of Nourishing the Life in Chinese Daoist Qigong* (中國道教氣功養生大全), by Li, Yuan-Guo (李遠國), 四川辭書出版社, Chengdu, Sichuan China, 1991.

31. 《道德經・十六章》：〝致虛極，守靜篤。〞

32. 意不在氣，在氣則滯。

33. 行氣如九曲珠，無微不到。

34. 《道德經・六章》：〝谷神不死，是謂玄牝。玄牝之門，是謂天地根，綿綿若存，用之不勤。〞

35. 〝指造化生育萬物之根本，亦即天地萬物之母，即道之別稱也。〞

36. 《武當修真圖》：〝明堂下，兩眉連線中點上方。有神光出，而曰天目。〞

37. 《云笈七籤》：〝兩眉間為泥丸之玉門。〞

38. 〝人人身中有一神，一神中有一靈光，靈光獨耀超千谷，道化無窮徹萬方。〞

39.〝佛在靈山莫遠求，靈山只在汝心頭。人人有個靈山塔，好向靈山塔下修。〞

40.《本草綱目》：〝腦為元神之府。〞

41.《六祖壇經》：〝菩提本無樹，明鏡亦非台，本來無一物，何處惹塵埃。〞

42.《養生論》：〝呼吸吐納，服食養身，使形神相親，表裡既濟也。〞

43.《同指要抄》：〝一代教門，皆以觀心為要。〞

44.《性命圭旨全書・涵養本源，救護命寶》：〝學道先須學自心，自心深處最難尋。若還尋到無尋處，方悟凡心即佛心。〞指覺悟之心。

45.《道鄉集》：〝佛之真傳，在于觀止。〞〝觀者何？將我目光，溫煦于至善地之義也。〞〝止者何？將我真意止于至善地之義也。〞

46.入觀：觀為觀想之義。入為悟性，即悟真理。

47.即覺或智之意。如覺悟、覺察、覺知諸法之事理，而了了分明。如睡夢之寤，謂之覺悟。覺察煩惱，使不為害，如世人之覺之為賊者，故云覺察。

48.《佛地論》：〝于一切法，一切種相，能自開覺，亦開覺一切有情，如睡夢覺醒，如蓮花開，故名佛。〞

49.《天仙正理・先天后天二氣直論》：〝夫用此氣者，由何以知先天之真也。當靜虛至極時。亦未涉一念覺知，此正真先天之真境界也。〞

50.老子・第一章：〝道、可道，非、常道；名、可名，非、常名。〞

## CHAPTER 5

# Theoretical Root of Small Circulation Meditation
# 小周天靜坐之理論根基

## 5-1. INTRODUCTION 介紹

There are six general purposes of Small Circulation Meditation:

1. Search for a peaceful mind.

2. Improve physical and mental health.

3. Find the center of self-being.

4. Comprehend the meaning of life.

5. Search for spiritual freedom.

6. Comprehend the meaning of the universe.

Through Small Circulation Meditation we rebuild the body from weak to strong and train the mind to be calm and focused. The Qi in the Eight Vessels and Twelve Primary Qi Channels becomes abundant, strengthening the immune system. Small Circulation is the first step in Internal Elixir practice, the foundation of Muscle/Tendon Changing and Marrow/Brain Washing Qigong.

There are various styles of Small Circulation, each with a different name. In Buddhist society it is called Turning the Wheel of Natural Law (Zhuan Fa Lun, 轉法輪). Every style has its own theory and method. Study and compare them, and take the best from each.

There is a Chinese story about six blind men who touch an elephant to know what it looks like. The first one touches the elephant's ear and says, "An elephant is like a large fan." The second one touches the side of its body and says, "No, it is like a wall." The third one describes the leg, "No, the elephant is like a pillar." The fourth one touches the nose and shouts, "The elephant is like a large moving branch of a tree." The fifth one touches the ivory, and says, "It is a large horn sticking out of a huge mouth." The sixth one who touches the tail says loudly, "An elephant is a large swinging broom sticking out of the wall." If they were to put all of the information together, they would have a reasonable description of the elephant. This story shows we should not stubbornly insist there is only one viewpoint, as we often see only part of the story.

When you practice, don't waste time in just theoretical research. Practice and theory should go together. From practice, you gain experience, and from theory, you have a clear guideline for practice. Some people hesitate due to the danger involved, accomplishing nothing and simply wasting time. Be cautious but determined, and learn from the experience of others, and you will find the right path.

A priest staying in a church is told the dam wall has broken, and the church will be flooded. He refuses to leave, and says God will save him. As water enters the church and rises quickly, he climbs up on the roof and prays for mercy and a miracle to save him. A boat comes to rescue him, but he refuses, waiting for God's miracle to save him. The boat leaves as the waters keep rising. Another boat comes to rescue him, but is again rejected. A third rescue boat receives the same answer. The waters engulf the church, and the priest drowns.

He blames God for not working a miracle to save him, but God says, "I sent three boats to save you but you rejected them all." Will you wait for the perfect theory, or grasp the opportunity while you can?

When Buddha traveled the countryside, he came to a river. An old Qigong master lived there, who asked him, "You are the Buddha? If so, can you do the same thing I can? I cross the river by walking on top of the water." Buddha said, "That is very impressive. But how long have you practiced it?" The old man replied, "It took me nearly forty years to achieve it." The Buddha looked at him and said, "It took you forty years! It takes me only a few coins to cross it on the ferryboat."

Often we spend too much time on unimportant things. Treat your time preciously and use it efficiently. Get rid of your dignity. If you take your dignity too seriously, you will not find a sincere teacher willing to teach from the heart.

A young Samurai swordsman entered the house of a famous Zen master. He looked at the master, bowed and said, "Master! I have reached a deep level of Zen, both in theory and practice. I have heard you are great so I come here to bow to you and hope you can teach me something."

The Zen master looked at this proud young man. Without a word, he went into the back room and brought out a teapot and a teacup. He placed the cup in front of the young man and started to pour the tea into the cup. The tea filled the cup quickly and soon began to overflow. The young man looked at the old man with a confused expression. He said, "Stop, master! The teacup is overflowing."

The old Zen master put the teapot down and smiled at him. He said, "This is you. You are too full already. I cannot teach you. If you wish to learn, you must first empty your cup." Can you be as humble as an empty cup?

When you find a good qualified teacher or source of learning, treat it preciously, so you don't miss the opportunity of learning. This chance may not come again. Traditionally, it was very difficult to find a qualified teacher. Even if you found one, you would not necessarily be accepted.

Today, it is easier to collect information since there are so many books, videotapes, and DVDs available. But the guidance of an experienced teacher is generally crucial to reach the final goal. Subtle advice can save you a great deal of time and effort. When you are lost in a big city, even though you have read the map, guidance from a passerby could save a lot of effort.

A young man had already spent more than seven years searching for a good master. He came to where a great teacher lived deep in the remote mountains with a few students. He was received kindly and expressed his intention of learning from the master. The master looked at him for a while, then brought out a teapot and a teacup. He poured tea into the cup, stopping when the tea reached the brim. He put the tea pot down with a smile, hinting to the young man that the place was already full. He could not accept another student.

The young man looked at the cup and realized what it meant. He lowered his head in sadness. Noticing a rice straw on the floor, he picked it up and carefully stuck it into the tea. The tea did not overflow. He looked at the master's face with hope, showing him, "Look, there is still space for me. The tea did not overflow."

Through this silent communication, the old master realized that the young man was one of those rare intelligent ones who could comprehend the profound feeling of the art. He accepted him with delight. It is very difficult to find an intelligent student able to comprehend the art deeply and to develop it. When a teacher finds this kind of student, it will be like a precious pearl in his hands.

In the next section, I review the history of Small Circulation practice. Then I summarize those acupuncture cavities related to the practice in section 5-3. We discuss the theory of Small Circulation in section 5-4. In section 5-5, crucial obstacles to Small Circulation, The Three Gates, are explained. We discuss different Small Circulation paths in section 5-6. Finally, an illustration of Internal Elixir meditation passed down from the Chinese Tang Dynasty (618-907 A.D., 唐代) is introduced and interpreted.

## 5-2. SMALL CIRCULATION—PAST AND PRESENT 小周天之過去與現在

After more than 1500 years of study and development, the practice of Small Circulation Qigong meditation has gradually evolved, from initial limited knowledge to a stage which allows practitioners to have a clear understanding of the practice.

## Small Circulation Practice in the Past

The practice of Small Circulation (Small Cyclic Heaven, Xiao Zhou Tian, 小周天) probably started in China around 500 A.D., when Da Mo's *Muscle/Tendon Changing and Marrow/Brain Washing Classic* (Yi Jin Jing, Xi Sui Jing; 易筋經 · 洗髓經) became available. There are a few reasons for this conclusion:

1. There are almost no Chinese documents available about the subject from before 500 A.D.

2. Small Circulation is a necessary prerequisite to reach advanced accomplishment in Muscle/Tendon Changing.

3. Da Mo (483-536 A.D., 達磨) was originally from India. When he arrived in China during the Liang Dynasty (502-557 A.D., 梁朝), Indian Yoga had already existed for 800 years. Small Circulation practice was an advanced level of practice in Indian Yoga, called Microcosmic Orbit Meditation.

4. Daoist practice of Small Circulation was originally from Buddhist society, called Turning the Wheel of Natural Law (Zhuan Fa Lun, 轉法輪). Even though Buddhism was imported into China during the reign of the Ming Emperor of the East Han Dynasty (58-76 A.D., 東漢明帝), documents on Qigong spiritual enlightenment practice were very scarce. It was not until Da Mo arrived, that actual Qigong practices were passed down.

Later, theory and practice of Small Circulation and Grand Circulation meditation were studied, researched, and developed in China. They blended with traditional Chinese Daoist theory based on the *Dao De Jing* (道德經), written by Lao Zi (老子, 604-531 B.C.), and a new understanding and practice developed. The most important influence from *Dao De Jing* was the theory of Embryonic Breathing (Tai Xi, 胎息). Without it, reaching the final goal of spiritual enlightenment would be very difficult.

With the addition of Chinese medical knowledge of Qi meridians and vessels, the theory and practice of Small Circulation were revised continuously and reached a profound level during the Qing Dynasty (1644-1912 A.D., 清朝). Many documents were written about Small Circulation during this period. I present some of them here with commentary.

# A Small Cyclic Heaven of Yin-Yang Circulation
## Antithetic writing of regulating the path
### (Wu, Shi-Ji, Qing Dynasty)

陰陽循環一小周天
（理瀹駢文・清・吳師機著）

*It (Small Circulation) is actually called 'Small Cyclic Heaven of Yin-Yang Circulation.' Close the eyes and sit quietly. The nose inhales clean air. Expand the abdomen to enable internal Qi to descend to the Lower Dan Tian under the navel. Transport Qi past Huiyin and up the Governing Vessel. Pass the Tailbone (Weilu), Squeezing Spine (Jiaji, between the shoulder blades) and Jade Pillow (Yuzhen), Three Gates. Reach Baihui (Gv-20) cavity on top of the head, follow the face to the tongue and connect with the Conception Vessel, descend down along the front of the chest, finally reach the Dan Tian and again circulate through the original path. Where there is a problem (Qi stagnation or pain), inhale and think of the place, and exhale to lead the Qi back to the Dan Tian. This strengthens the body and repels sickness. It is also named San Mei Yin.*

全稱為陰陽循環一小周天。閉目靜坐，鼻吸清氣，鼓腹
使內氣下降臍下丹田，運氣過肛門，沿督脈尾閭、夾脊、
玉枕三關，到頭頂百會穴，順面部至舌與任脈接，沿前
胸而下，至丹田復順原徑路循行。患在何處，收氣即存
想其處，放氣則歸於丹田。可強身卻病。又名三昧印。

This document, which was written by Wu, Ji-Shi (吳師機) in 1864, discusses a few key points. First, to meditate, close your eyes to cut off the connection between your eyes and your surroundings. Second, to circulate the Qi smoothly, sit quietly with your body calm and relaxed. This is the pre-condition for Qi circulation. Third, breathe correctly. Breathing is the strategy of Qigong practice. When breathing correctly, Qi can be guided efficiently. Fourth, generate and accumulate Qi at the Lower Dan Tian. Without abundant Qi stored there, the path of Qi circulating in the Conception and Governing Vessels cannot be widened, so regulating the Qi in the Twelve Primary Qi Channels will not be effective. Fifth, the path of Qi circulation is from the Lower Dan Tian, via the Huiyin, past the tailbone (Weilu, 尾閭, Changqiang, 長強), Jiaji (夾脊, Lingtai, 靈臺) and Yuzhen (玉枕, Naohu, 腦戶), the Three Gates (San Guan, 三關), then over the head, and down the front center line back to the Lower Dan Tian. Small Circulation practice is the foundation of Muscle/Tendon Changing, which can change your body from weak to strong. It is also called San Mei Yin (三昧印) in Buddhist society, or San Mo Di (三摩地, Samadhi) a special Buddhist term which means steadiness of the mind and body (Ding, 定).

# Small Cyclic Heaven
## (Original truth of using no herbs)
## (Wang Yang, Qing Dynasty)

小周天
（勿藥元詮・清・汪昂輯）

*First, stop the Nian (the thoughts lingering in the mind), calm the body and the heart, face east, and sit with crossed legs (Jia Zuo). The breathing is peaceful and harmonious. Use San Mei Yin and maintain it under the navel. Knock the teeth sixty-six times and gather your spirit in the whole body. The tongue circles the mouth sixty-six times both internally and externally, while you also circle both eyes following the circles of the tongue. The tongue touches the palate, count the breathing calmly until it reaches three hundred and sixty times. Wait until the spiritual water (saliva) is full, rinse (the mouth) several times. Use Four Secret Words (Si Zi Jue), lead Qi from the Conception Vessel, past the grain path (Huiyin), and reach the tailbone (Changqiang). Use Yi to transport, slowly lead Qi up to the central gate, Jiaji (Lingtai cavity). Gradually speed up. Close your eyes and look up, inhale but do not exhale through the nose, thrust through Yuzhen (Naohu cavity). Use the eye to lead it forward and pass Kunlun (Baihui), down to Que Qiao (magpie bridge, tongue), then divide the saliva and send it down the Chong Lou (throat), enter Li palace (heart, Middle Dan Tian), and finally reach the Qihai (Lower Dan Tian). Pause for a moment, use the same method and repeat it three times. Divide the saliva in the mouth into three gulps and send it down. This is what is called "reversed flow of heavenly river water."*

先要止念，身心澄清，面東跏坐，呼吸平和，用三昧印，
按于臍下；叩齒三十六通，以集身神；赤龍攪海，內外
三十六遍；雙目隨轉運，舌抵上齶，靜心數息，三百六
十周天畢，待神水滿，漱津數遍；用〝四字訣〞，從任
脈撮過穀道到尾閭，以意運送，徐徐上夾脊中關，漸漸
速些；閉目上視，鼻吸莫呼，衝過玉枕，將目往前一忍，
直轉崑崙，倒下鵲橋，分津送下重樓，入離宮，而至氣
海；略定一定，復用前法，連行三次，口中之津，分三
次咽下，所謂天河水逆流也。

This document was written by Wang, Ang (汪昂) in 1682 A.D. during the Qing Dynasty (1644-1912 A.D., 清朝). The Qi path is the same as in the previous document, but it also describes the preparation for Small Circulation.

Nian (念) is the thought lingering your mind and hard to get rid of. Jia Zuo (跏坐) is a special Buddhist meditation term which means to sit with crossed legs. San Mei Yin comes from Indian Samadhi and means great steadiness of the mind and body. Si Zi Jue (四字訣) means Four Secret Words, namely Cuo (撮), Di (抵), Bi (閉), and Xi (吸). Cuo means to condense, to focus, to concentrate. It implies the concentration of the mind and Qi. Di means to press up, namely the tongue is pressing up against the palate of the mouth. Bi means to close, as in close or hold up the Huiyin (perinium). Xi means to suck in, as in "leading the Qi up the spine in coordination with inhalation."

Que Qiao (鵲橋) means magpie bridge, or tongue, which bridges the Conception and Governing Vessels. Chong Lou (重樓) means layers of stories, namely the throat area. Li Gong (離宮) means Li palace, or heart. In the Eight Trigrams (Bagua, 八卦), Li represents fire, and the heart belongs to fire in the Five Elements (Wuxing, 五行). Qihai (氣海) is the Lower Dan Tian (Xia Dan Tian, 下丹田), which belongs to water, and is called Kan palace (Kan Gong, 坎宮) in the Eight Trigrams.

To lead the Qi from Huiyin (Co-1, 會陰, perineum, sea bottom) up the back to the crown is called reversed flow of the heavenly river water (Tian He Shui Ni Liu, 天河水逆流).

> *Sit quietly for a while. Let the left and right hand each rub the Lower Dan Tian one hundred and eight times, including the navel. Then cover the navel with clothes to keep the wind off. Rub the back of the thumbs until they are warm, and wipe the eyes with them fourteen times to get rid of (excess Yang) heart fire. Rub the nose thirty-six times to moisten the lungs. Rub the ears fourteen times to nourish the kidneys. Rub the face fourteen times to strengthen the spleen. Cover the ears with the hands and beat the heavenly drum (Ming Tian Gu). Raise the hands up gradually as if worshipping heaven, and repeat three times. Slowly exhale dirty air and inhale clean air. Hold the shoulders, move and shift the tendons and bones a few times. Rub Yuzhen gate twenty-four times, rub kidney eyes one hundred and eight times, and also the center of each foot one hundred and eight times.*

靜坐片時，將手左右擦丹田各一百八下，連臍抱住，放手時將衣被圍住臍輪，勿令風入；次將大指背擦熱，拭目十四遍，去心火；擦鼻三十六遍，潤肺；擦耳十四遍，補腎；擦面十四遍，健脾。雙手掩耳鳴天鼓，徐徐將手往上，即朝天椊，如此者三，徐徐呵出濁氣四、五口，收清氣；雙手抱肩，移筋換骨數遍；擦玉枕關二十四下；擦腰眼各一百八下，擦足心各一百八下。

This document describes the recovery Qigong exercises right after Small Circulation meditation. Ming Tian Gu (鳴天鼓) means to 'beat the heavenly drum.' Cover the ears with the palms, using the fingers to tap the base of the skull and the two major neck muscles. Refer to the YMAA book, *Eight Simple Qigong Exercises* (*The Eight Pieces of Brocade, Ba Duan Jin, 八段錦*).

These documents briefly describe the practice of Small Circulation, but without giving detail of how to build up Qi and the attendant dangers. The basic theory remains the same, though with different approaches to the final goal.

Small Circulation meditation is commonly practiced in Chinese martial arts society, as the foundation of Muscle/Tendon Changing, which strengthens martial power significantly. The common procedures as learned from a master are:

1. **Build up abundant Qi.** A master would teach how to build the Qi to a very high level at the Lower Dan Tian through abdominal breathing. The student would spend up to ten years building this Qi and conditioning the Lower Dan Tian.

2. **Circulate Qi in the Small Circulation path.** Since Qi is already abundant, it can be dangerous without correct technique. The crucial keys were often kept secret by the master, namely to control the Huiyin cavity in coordination with breathing and to touch the tongue to the palate of the mouth. Only when the student had earned his trust were these secrets revealed. There are three places, called Three Gates (San Guan, 三關), which are dangerous in practice. The student would obey the master's order step by step to get through these three gates. The danger of being unable to control this abundant Qi, is that it can enter the wrong path, called 'entering the fire' (Zou Huo, 走火). We discuss these three gates and their dangers in detail in section 5-5.

An important point is that Embryonic Breathing (Tai Xi, 胎息) is the Yin side of Internal Elixir (Nei Dan, 內丹) practice. It is the crucial key in practicing Marrow/Brain Washing and is unknown in secular society. Even in Buddhist and Daoist monasteries, only a few monks reach a profound level to understand it. Whenever stored Qi is built up to an abundant level at the False Lower Dan Tian, the excess is immediately distributed through the Conception and Governing Vessels and the Twelve Primary Qi Channels. The body, including the twelve internal organs, grows stronger. This is the fundamental concept of Muscle/Tendon Changing.

With Small Circulation training accomplished, the body and the manifestation of martial power are significantly enhanced. But too much Muscle/Tendon Changing training can also cause a serious problem called energy dispersion (San Gong, 散功). When the physical body has been over-energized, it can lead to high blood pressure and stroke. To balance this, practice the Yin side of training, Marrow/Brain Washing Qigong. The first step is Embryonic Breathing (Tai Xi, 胎息), described in detail in the previous book in this series, *Qigong Meditation—Embryonic Breathing*.

## Modified Practice in Present Day

Though Small Circulation has been known in Indian Yoga, Chinese Buddhist Chan (禪, Japanese Zen, 忍), and Chinese Daoist societies, still only a few Qigong practitioners dare to practice it, due to the following reasons:

1. **Lack of understanding of theory and practice.** There is very little information available to read and study.

2. **Dangers during practice.** The Three Gates (San Guan, 三關) are dangerous.

3. **Lack of an experienced teacher.** Often experience is essential for guidance, especially when there is a problem.

The following practice methods have developed from my personal practice, teaching, and study over more than 25 years. I believe this new approach has reduced the danger to the minimum.

1. **Teach theory first.** Theory is like a map of a city. Without it, the student can easily get lost, especially in today's environment where he does not live and practice together with the master. Most practitioners in the past did not know the theory, but this has now been understood and revealed. For any beginner, understanding the theory has become crucial for successful practice.

2. **Teach Embryonic Breathing first.** To prevent too much Yang developing and the problem of energy dispersion, a student should first learn the Yin side of training, namely the theory and methods of Embryonic Breathing. With this tool, he can manipulate the situation and balance the body's Yin and Yang easily and effectively.

3. **Build up Qi only as much as necessary.** Traditionally a student would build up Qi to a highly abundant level, encountering the attendant dangers. Before he has accumulated too much Qi, he should learn to circulate it. In this way, there is not enough Qi to cause the problem of 'entering the fire' (Zou Huo, 走火).

4. **Use the mind to circulate before the Qi storage reaches a harmful level.** Traditionally one accumulated abundant Qi, then learned to circulate it. If we reverse this procedure, before a student's Qi has reached a harmful level, he can already lead it smoothly. That is like teaching a beginner driver with a small car. Only when he is a skilled driver, is a bigger and more powerful car provided. The disadvantage of this is that weaker Qi takes longer to overcome blockages and widen its path. It is like opening a blocked water pipe.

5. **First practice Small Small Circulation** (Xiao Xiao Zhou Tian, 小小周天) **to avoid danger**, especially at the tailbone area, and circulate Qi in coordination with the breathing, abdomen, and perineum.

6. **Carefully select the Qi turning points to avoid the problem of Qi stagnation.** Before completing the whole small circulation, first train the correct turning points where Qi can be returned to the Lower Dan Tian. If the turning points are wrong, Qi stagnation can occur, and also 'entering the fire'. These turning points were kept secret in the past. I have modified them, and believe these are safer than the traditional points used in the past. Once you understand the theory, you can modify the training path without causing any problem.

## 5-3. SMALL CIRCULATION AND QI NETWORK 小周天與經絡學

### Qi Network

1. **Diaphragm** (Heng Ge Mo, 橫膈膜, Junction of Upper and Lower Level Qi)

   A. The diaphragm is a good electric conductor sandwiched between fasciae, which are poor conductors. This area acts as a battery to store fire Qi (Huo Qi, 火氣), and is called the Middle Dan Tian (Zhong Dan Tian, 中丹田).

   B. It divides the body into upper and lower bodies, in terms of Qi. The chest area above it is where the External Qi (Wai Qi, 外氣, oxygen and carbon dioxide) is exchanged. The diaphragm pumps the air in and out. The stomach and abdomen below the diaphragm constitute the biobattery where Internal Qi (Nei Qi, 內氣, bioelectricity) is stored. This Lower Dan Tian (Xia Dan Tian, 下丹田) produces Qi and stores it. The abdomen is the Qi pump, while the Huiyin (Co-1, 會陰, perineum) is the controlling gate which regulates its flow.

   C. External Qi (air) and internal Qi (bioelectricity) are closely related to one other. Oxygen (air) and bioelectricity are proportional to each other. When oxygen supply is more abundant, more glucose will be converted into Qi to manifest as physical action, heat, and light.

   D. When too much Qi accumulates at the Middle Dan Tian, the heartbeat will be faster and breathing heavier, disturbing the emotional mind.

## 2. Jing ( 經 , Primary Qi channels)

A. There are twelve primary Qi channels, six Yin and six Yang. They act as rivers which follow the limbs and distribute Qi throughout the body. Three Yang (large intestines, Triple Burner, and small intestines) and three Yin (lungs, pericardium and heart) channels connect six internal organs with the upper extremities. Another three Yang (stomach, bladder, and gall bladder) and three Yin (spleen, kidneys, and liver) channels connect the other six internal organs with the lower extremities. When Qi circulation stagnates in these rivers, sickness is initiated.

B. The heart, lungs, and pericardium coexist and are isolated from the other organs by the diaphragm. These three Yin organs are closely related and harmonize with each other. For example, when the heart beats faster, the breathing is faster. When the breathing is slower, the heartbeat slows. The pericardium acts as a cooler for the heart which, like a car engine, needs a radiator to maintain its function. These three Yin organs are connected to the thumb (lungs), middle finger (pericardium), and pinky (heart) and to three Yang organs, namely large intestine (index finger), triple burner (middle finger), and small intestine (pinky).

## 3. Luo ( 絡 , Secondary Qi channels)

A. There are millions of secondary channels, called Luo, branching out like streams from the primary channels and distributing Qi throughout the body. They are like capillaries in the blood system. They branch out from the primary channels, circulating Qi laterally.

B. Luo connect the primary channels to the skin surface and bone marrow, and to the organs. When more Qi is led out through the Luo from the primary Qi channels (Jing), the Guardian Qi (Wei Qi, 衛氣 ) is strengthened, Qi manifests more externally, so the body becomes warmer. When more Qi is led in through Luo from the primary Qi channels, the Marrow Qi (Sui Qi, 髓氣 ) is enhanced. More Qi is stored internally and physical manifestation is weakened, so you feel chilly.

C. When exhalation is longer than inhalation, more Qi is led out and manifested. When inhalation is longer than exhalation, more Qi is led in and stored. With the sound of Ha ( 哈 ) and Hen ( 哼 ), manifestation and storage are more effective.

### 4. Mai （脈, Vessels）

Vessels (Mai, 脈) are like reservoirs which regulate Qi in the Twelve Primary Channels. One of the oldest Chinese medical books, Nan Jing (難經), said, "Mai includes strange meridians eight vessels, which do not belong to the Twelve Meridians."[1] Li, Shi-Zhen (李時珍) also explains in his book, *The Study of Strange Meridians and Eight Vessels* (奇經八脈考), "Strange meridians include eight vessels which are not restrained like twelve meridians. There is no matching and coordination on the surface or internally, so they are called strange."[2]

Chinese medicine recognizes the importance of the Conception and Governing Vessels (任脈・督脈) used in acupuncture practice. Due to limited understanding of the other six vessels, acupuncture usually does not manipulate them. That is why, together with the Twelve Primary Qi Channels (Shi Er Jing, 十二經), they are commonly called Fourteen Channels (Shi Si Jing, 十四經) in Chinese acupuncture. In the book, *The Study of Practical Chinese Medical Qigong* (實用中醫氣功學), it says, "Governing Vessel originates from Huiyin, Qi moves up the back of the body, and is the total governor of the Yang vessels. Therefore, it is called the ocean of the Yang vessel. Conception Vessel begins from Huiyin, (Qi) circulates along the abdomen up the front of the body and is responsible for all Yin vessels. Therefore, it is called ocean of the Yin vessels. If one circulates Qi smoothly in these two, then hundreds of vessels all transport. Qi circulates through the body without hindrance or stagnation. The Dao of longevity depends on this."[3,4]

How do these two vessels control the Qi status of the whole body? Let us conclude this from available documents.

### Conception Vessel—Ocean of Yin Vessels (Ren Mai, 任脈) (陰脈之海) (Figure 5-1)[4,5]

1. It circulates at the right center of the chest and abdomen to meet three Yin primary Qi channels of the feet (liver, spleen, and kidneys) at Zhongji (Co-3, 中極) and Guanyuan (Co-4, 關元) cavities. It joins Yang Linking Vessel (Yangwei Mai, 陽維脈) at Tiantu (Co-22, 天突) and Lianquan (Co-23, 廉泉) cavities, and connects with Thrusting Vessel (Chong Mai, 衝脈) at Yinjiao (Co-7, 陰交).

2. The three Yin primary Qi channels of the feet join the three Yin primary Qi channels of the hands (heart, lungs, and pericardium). Through this network, the Conception Vessel regulates all six Yin channels.

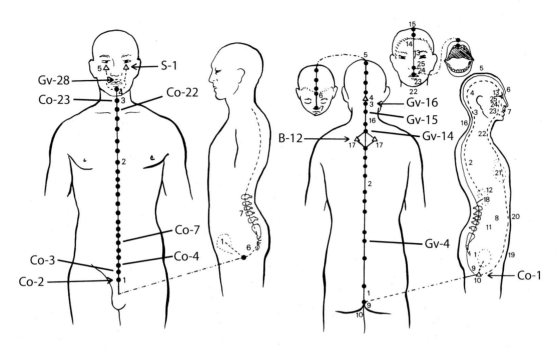

Figure 5-1. Conception Vessel (Ren Mai)-
Ocean of Yin Vessels

Figure 5-2. Governing Vessel (Du Mai)—
Ocean of Yang Vessels

## Governing Vessel—Oean of Yang Vessels (Du Mai, 督脈 ) ( 陽脈之海 ) (Figure 5-2)[4,6]

1. This vessel circulates at the right center of the back. It meets several times with the six Yang primary Qi channels of the hands and feet. The most central place is Dazhui (Gv-14, 大椎 ) cavity. All three Yang channels of the hands and feet meet here.

2. The Girdle Vessel (Dai Mai, 帶脈 ) begins below the hypochondrium at the level of the 2nd lumbar vertebra connecting Mingmen (Gv-4, 命門 ) and encircles the waist like a girdle. Yang Linking Vessel (Yangwei Mai, 陽維脈 ) also connects the Governing Vessel (Du Mai, 督脈 ) at Fengfu (Gv-16, 風府 ) and Yamen (Gv-15, 啞門 ). In this way, the Governing Vessel governs the function of the Yang vessels.

## Mai and Internal Elixir Meditation

How important are the vessels to Internal Elixir (Nei Dan, 內丹 ) practice? Li, Shi-Zhen ( 李時珍 , 1518-1593 A.D.) explains this in his book, *The Study of Strange Meridians and Eight Vessels* ( 奇經八脈考 ), "The Eight Vessels introduced in all existing books are too brief and not understood in detail. So for those doctors who do not know them, it is harder to explore the origin of sickness. For those immortal family (Qigong practitioners for enlightenment) who do not know them, it is hard to install the furnace and tripod (position spirit and Qi). Shi-Zhen is not wise, so refers to all available discussions and gathers information here, so those immortal family and doctors can use it. If those doctors know these Eight Vessels, then the major contents of Twelve Primary Qi Channels and fifteen secondary Qi channels can be understood. If those immortal researchers know these Eight Vessels, then the marvelousness of ascending and descending, tiger and dragon, and the hidden profound detail of Xuan Pin can be obtained."[7] Xuan Pin (玄牝) is what is called Taiji (太極, Grand Ultimate) in *Yi Jing* (*The Book of Change*). This Taiji is the Dao (道) of lives in the great nature. Therefore, Xuan Pin can be called the root of creation, variation, bearing, and raising of millions of lives. It is the mother of millions of objects of heaven and earth, another name for Dao.

Finally, I summarize the key points of the Eight Vessels.

**1. Conception Vessel** (Ren Mai, 任脈)

    a. A Yin vessel which balances the Qi status of the Yang Governing Vessel.

    b. Responsible for regulating Qi in the six Yin primary channels. When Qi is abundant, it circulates smoothly in the six Yin primary Qi channels.

    c. With the Yang Governing Vessel, it completes the Small Circulation. When Qi circulates smoothly in Small Circulation, the physical body can be conditioned and health improved. Small Circulation is the fire path (Huo Lu, 火路) of Internal Elixir (Nei Dan, 內丹) practice. Qi circulates strongly in the fire path during the daytime.

**2. Governing Vessel** (Du Mai, 督脈)

    a. A Yang vessel which balances the Qi of the Yin Conception Vessel.

    b. Governs and regulates the Qi in the six primary Yang Qi channels. When Qi is abundant in this vessel, it circulates smoothly in the six primary Yang Qi channels.

    c. With the Yin Conception Vessel, it completes the Small Circulation.

**3. Thrusting Vessel** (Chong Mai, 衝脈)

    a. The main section of the Thrusting Vessel is the spinal cord, which connects the brain (Upper Dan Tian) with the second brain (Real Lower Dan Tian), constituting the central Qi system. Upper and lower brains are the two poles of this system.

b. Qi circulates strongly at night, and the brain obtains its energetic nourishment at this time. Due to abundant Qi supply at night, hormone production is enhanced and the pituitary and pineal glands, adrenals, testicles, and ovaries function fully.

c. This path is responsible for spiritual growth, while the Small Circulation accounts for physical life. So circulating Qi in the Thrusting Vessel (water path) is for spiritual cultivation (marrow/brain washing), while circulating it in the Small Circulation (fire path) is for physical conditioning (muscle/tendon changing).

d. Among the Eight Vessels, this vessel is classified as extreme Yin and balances the Girdle Vessel which is classified as extreme Yang. When Qi accumulates here, the body is calm, and the marrow and brain obtain nourishment (marrow washing).

e. This central energy line gives a feeling of being centered.

## 4. Girdle Vessel (Dai Mai, 帶脈)

a. Its Qi circulates strongly whenever you are standing up. This gives a feeling of physical and mental balance, from which you find your center. This vessel is classified as extreme Yang and balances the Thrusting Vessel. One provides balance, while the other provides centered feeling. That means though there are two vessels, they function as one.

b. The Qi circulating in this vessel is responsible for the body's Guardian Qi (Wei Qi, 衛氣). When this Qi expands abundantly, you are more balanced and the immune system functions well.

c. How much the Guardian Qi can expand depends on the abundance of Qi stored in the Real Lower Dan Tian. The more Qi stored in the Real Lower Dan Tian, the more healthy, balanced, and centered you are.

## 5. Yin Heel Vessel (Yinqiao Mai, 陰蹻脈) and Yin Linking Vessel (Yinwei Mai, 陰維脈)

a. These two vessels connect at the Huiyin (Co-1) (會陰) with the Conception and Thrusting Vessels. At the bottom, they connect to the concave area of the feet. When sexual energy is strong, the Qi stored in these two vessels is strong, manifesting as the strength of the legs. When sexual energy is depleted, the legs are weak.

b. These two vessels balance the Qi status of the Yang Heel and Yang Linking Vessels. While the Yin vessels store the Qi, the Yang vessels manifest it.

**6. Yang Heel Vessel** (Yangqiao Mai, 陽蹻脈) and **Yang Linking Vessel** (Yangwei Mai, 陽維脈)

a. These two vessels balance the Qi status of the Yin Heel and Yin Linking Vessels. While the Yin vessels store Qi, the Yang vessels manifest it. When the Qi is strong, the lower part of the body will be strong.

b. These two Yang vessels balance the above two Yin vessels. Though physically they are two, in function they are one.

## Zi and Wu Major Qi Flow (Zi Wu Liu Zhu, 子午流注)

To understand the Qi network, recognize that the body is alive and the Qi circulation in it is affected by nature. This relationship with the cycles of nature is called Zi Wu Liu Zhu (子午流注), which you need to follow to circulate Qi efficiently.

Zi (子) is the period between 11 P.M. and 1 A.M., and Wu (午) between 11 A.M. and 1 P.M. Liu (流) means flow, and Zhu (注) means tendency. So Zi Wu Liu Zhu (子午流注) means 'the major Qi flow tendency which follows the time changes'.

The *Inner Classic* (內經) calls this the correspondence of heaven and man.[8] The major Qi flows of the Twelve Primary Qi Channels differ from each other. Qi flowing in the Conception and Governing Vessels (fire path) is also affected by the natural cycle. As it circulates, the Qi level in one part of the path is always higher than elsewhere. This area of stronger Qi moves around the path regularly every twenty-four hours. It is this area of higher Qi potential which keeps the Qi flowing. Just as water only flows from a higher to a lower level, Qi only moves from a place of higher potential to one of lower potential.

*Great Collection of Golden Elixir* (金丹大成集) said, "Zi and Wu are the middle points of heaven and earth. In heaven, they are the sun and the moon; in humans, they are the heart and kidneys; in time, they are Zi (子, midnight) and Wu (午, noon); in the Eight Trigrams, they are Kan (坎, Water) and Li (離, Fire); in orientation, they are the south and the north."[9] Also, Dr. Yang, Ji-Zhou (楊繼洲, 1522-1620 A.D.) explained in his book, *The Complete Book of Acupuncture and Moxibustion* (針灸大成), "Conception and Governing Vessels of a human body, back and front are analogous to nature's Zi-Wu (子午, midnight-noon). If analogous to south and north, they can be divided and combined. When divided, Yin and Yang are not disordered, and when combined, they coordinate seamlessly with each other. One is two and two is one."[10] In the Small Circulation fire path, Qi circulates more strongly in the Conception Vessel (Ren Mai, 任脈) than in the Governing Vessel (Du Mai, 督脈) during daytime, while it circulates more strongly in the Governing Vessel at night. It seems they are two vessels, but in function they are one, since they belong to the same circuit.

Li, Shi-Zhen (李時珍, 1518-1593 A.D.) discussed this in *The Study of Strange Meridians and Eight Vessels* (奇經八脈考), "Conception and Governing Vessels are the body's Zi-Wu (子午). It is the Dao of ascending and descending of Yang-Huo (陽火) and Yin-Fu (陰符), used by the Elixir Family (Dan Jia, 丹家, Qigong society). It is the key place of Kan and Li."[11] Yang-Huo (陽火, Yang fire) means the way to increase the body's fire to make it more Yang. Yin-Fu (陰符, Yin magic water) is the way to enhance the body's water, making its Yang more Yin. Fu (符) is the magic water (Fu Shui, 符水) for curing disease.

In the Fire Path, the major Qi flow at noon is at the Middle Dan Tian (Zhong Dan Tian, 中丹田). It moves down to the Lower Dan Tian between 2 and 4 P.M. It goes down to Huiyin (Co-1, 會陰) at sunset and moves to the back in the evening, reaching the top of the Baihui (Gv-20, 百會) at midnight. At sunrise, the Qi is in

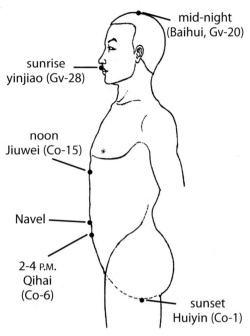

Figure 5-3. Natural Qi Circulation in the Fire Path

the face, and by noon, it has reached the Middle Dan Tian to complete the cycle. This cycle is used by martial artists for vital cavity strikes (Dian Xue, 點穴) (Figure 5-3).

## Cavities Related to Meditation 靜坐有關之穴道

Let us summarize the important cavities used in Small Circulation practice, so it will be easier to follow the discussion in the rest of the book.

1. **Shang Dan Tian** (上丹田, Upper Elixir Field)
   The whole brain is regarded as the Upper Dan Tian. Brain cells are highly conductive and can store and consume a lot of electricity. The space between the two hemispheres of the brain is called the Spiritual Valley (Shen Gu, 神谷) where the Valley Spirit (Gu Shen, 谷神) resides. At the bottom center of the valley, where the pituitary and pineal glands are situated, is the Mud Pill Palace (Ni Wan Gong, 泥丸宮). The brain is responsible for conscious thought, while this space without any brain cells is related to your subconscious mind. It is where you connect with nature since birth. While your conscious mind is in the false human matrix, your subconscious mind is free and truthful.
   Baihui (Gv-20, 百會) at the crown and Yintang (M-NH-3, 印堂, third eye) are the two gates where your spirit communicates with the natural

energy and spirit. Though Baihui is open, Yintang has been sealed in humans for a long time.

2. **Zhong Dan Tian** (中丹田, Middle Elixir Field)

There are different opinions about the location of the Middle Dan Tian. Some documents believe Shanzhong (Co-17, 膻中) is the Middle Dan Tian since behind it is the thymus gland, related to your heart (emotional mind). Others claim the heart itself is the Middle Dan Tian since it relates to your emotional mind and stores Post-birth fire Qi. Others again believe that Jiuwei (Co-15, 鳩尾, Wide Pigeon's Tail, lower sternum) is where it is located (Figure 5-4).

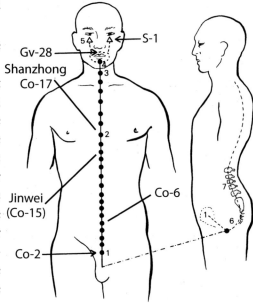

Figure 5-4. Shanzhong (Co-17) and Jiuwei (Co-15)

Looking at the body's structure, we see the diaphragm, a good electric conductor, sandwiched between fasciae (poor conductors) on both sides. This is like a battery, able to store charge to an abundant level. It is between the lungs where air is exchanged and the stomach where food is converted, so Post-birth Qi can be stored to a high level. Qi stored in this area also affects the emotional mind.

3. **Jia Xia Dan Tian** (假下丹田, False Lower Elixir Field)

The False Lower Dan Tian is located about two inches below the navel in the abdominal area. This is Qihai (Co-6, 氣海, Ocean of Qi) in Chinese medicine (Figure 5-5). Daoists call it Dan Lu (丹爐, Elixir Furnace). These names indicate that this area can produce Qi (grow elixir) as abundantly as the ocean.

When you move your abdomen up and down through abdominal breathing, you produce Qi. This movement is called Qi Huo (起火) and means to start the fire. Two ways of breathing build up the fire and store Qi. One is Normal Abdominal Breathing (Zheng Fu Hu Xi, 正腹呼吸), the other Reverse Abdominal Breathing (Fan, Ni Fu Hu Xi, 反·逆腹呼吸). The abdominal breathing is also called Returning to Childhood Breathing (Fan Tong Hu Xi, 返童呼吸) or Post-Heaven Breathing (Xian Tian Hu Xi, 先天呼吸). A fetus uses this pumping movement to suck in nutrition and oxygen from its mother through the umbilical cord. Most small children retain this habit of abdominal movement. These two ways of breathing have been discussed in section 4-3 and will be scientifically analyzed in the next section.

4. **Zhen Xia Dan Tian** (真下丹田, Real Lower Elixir Field)

Daoists regard the regular Lower Dan Tian at the abdomen as the false one. The real one is inside the body under the stomach, in front of the kidneys (Nei Shen, 內腎) and above the External Kidneys (Wai Shen, 外腎, testicles). The Real Lower Dan Tian is the Large and Small Intestines where the second brain or biobattery is located, as understood by scientists today (Figure 5-5). Daoist regard the regular Lower Dan Tian as false because when Qi accumulates there, it automatically enters the Conception Vessel and disperses into the Twelve Primary Qi Channels. So, though it generates Qi and stores it to some level, it

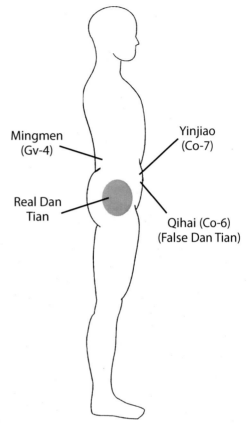

Figure 5-5. Real and False Lower Dan Tian

cannot reach an abundant level. Though Qi stored at the False Lower Dan Tian is beneficial for health, it is not enough for spiritual enlightenment. The Real Lower Dan Tian is the lower pole of the central energy line, connected with the brain (Upper Dan Tian) through the spinal cord (Thrusting Vessel). To have enough Qi to nourish the brain for spiritual enlightenment, first condition your biobattery, and store Qi there to an abundant level.

The document, *Observing Vessels* (脈望) says, "(Real) Dan Tian is the root of life. This is why Daoists who meditate for spiritual cultivation and Buddhists who meditate for Buddhahood all gather real Qi (Original Qi) under the navel. There is a Spiritual Turtle (Shen Gui, 神龜) in the Dan Tian which inhales and exhales this Real Qi (Zhen Qi). This respiration is not breathing through the mouth and nose, which are only the doors for respiration. Dan Tian is the origin of Qi and the place for those holy men to begin their cultivation. This is the place where they keep and store the Real Oneness (Zhen Yi), so it is called Embryonic Breathing."[12]

Zhen Yi (真一) means Real One or True Singularity, namely the central Qi system constituted by the Two Poles. The Yang pole at the Real Lower Dan Tian provides the quantity of Qi, and the Yin pole at the Upper Dan Tian controls the quality of its manifestation as life (spirit). Physically, there are Two Polarities but in function there is only one, since they are the Yin and Yang of the same thing. If you keep your mind in this Real One or True Singularity, you raise up your Spirit of Vitality (Jing Shen, 精神) and establish abundant Qi storage.

### 5. Huang Ting (黃庭, Yellow Yard)

Huang Ting (黃庭) can imply various places in the body. Liang, Qiu-Zi (梁丘子) interpreted Huang Ting, in *Classic of Huang Ting's Internal Scene* (黃庭內景經), "Yellow (Huang), is the middle (color) of colors. Yard (Ting) is the center of a square. Externally, it means the center of heaven (Tian Zhong, 天中), the center of a man (Ren Zhong, 人中), and the center of the earth (Di Zhong, 地中). Internally, it means the center of the brain (Nao Zhong, 腦中), the center of the heart (Xin Zhong, 心中), and the center of the spleen (Pi Zhong, 脾中)."[13] So Huang Ting can imply the center of many things.

Shi, He-Yang (石和陽) interpreted Huang Ting in *Classic of Huang Ting's External Scene* (黃庭外景經), "Above Mingmen, there are two esoteric marvelous apertures, left is Xuan (玄) and right is Pin (牝, two internal kidneys). There is an empty place between named Huang Ting."[14]

The document, *Secret Recording of Nourishing Life* (養生秘錄·金丹問答) said, "Where exactly is Huang Ting? Above the bladder, under the spleen, in front of the kidneys, left of the liver, and right of the lungs."[15] So Huang Ting is the center of where the internal organs are located (i.e., center of gravity).

Huang Ting is also called Yu Huan Xue (玉環穴, Jade Ring Cavity), the name first used in the *Illustration of Brass Acupuncture and Moxibustion* (銅人俞穴針灸圖), by Dr. Wang, Wei-Yi (王唯一). The Daoist book *Wang Lu Shi Yu* (王錄識餘) said, "In the *Illustration of Brass Acupuncture and Moxibustion* it was recorded that within the body's cavities of viscera and bowels, there is a Jade Ring (Yu Huan), but I do not know what the Jade Ring is." Later, Zhang, Zi-Yang (張紫陽) described the place the immortals use to form the elixir, "The heart is on top, the kidneys are underneath, the spleen is to the left, and the liver is to the right. The life door (Sheng Men, 生門, navel) is in front, the closed door is to the rear, they are connected like a ring, white like cotton, an inch in diameter. It encompasses the Essence and the refinement of the whole body. It is opposite the navel and is the root of life. This is the Jade Ring."[16] The life door in the front means the Qi door is open in front, and closed to the rear. This concept was also confirmed in the document, *Muscle/Tendon Changing Classic; Appendix* (易筋經・附錄).[17]

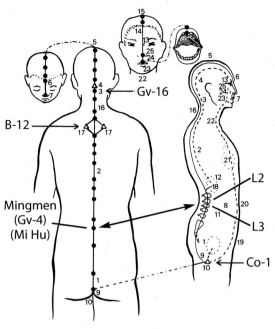

Figure 5-6. Mi Hu (Mingmen, Gv-4)

Mi Hu (密戶) means Concealed Door (Mingmen, Gv-4, 命門) located between L2 and L3 vertebrae (Figure 5-6). So Huang Ting is actually the second brain, the Real Lower Dan Tian (Zhen Xia Dan Tian, 真下丹田) or biobattery of the body. This place is the center of gravity which stores abundant Qi or bioelectricity. Other documents claim Huang Ting to be between the kidneys, while others place it under the heart. I believe Huang Ting means the place above the Real Lower Dan Tian, behind the navel, and in front of the kidneys. In Daoist spiritual enlightenment practice, this is where Kan and Li interact. Water Qi is stored at the Real Lower Dan Tian while Fire Qi is accumulated at the Middle Dan Tian. Water and fire Qi interact at Huang Ting, to conceive the Spiritual Embryo.

6. **Baihui** (Gv-20, 百會, Hundred Meetings)

Baihui is located on top of the head and is where the whole body's Qi gathers (hundred meetings). This is the most Yang part of the body, just as Huiyin (Co-1, 會陰, perineum) is the most Yin part of the body. Through the Thrusting Vessel, these two cavities relate to each other (Figure 5-7). When Qi manifests at Baihui, the spirit (Shen, 神) can be raised high and the body's Qi governed efficiently by the mind.

Baihui is the gate where the spirit exits and enters. Through it, the spirit leaves the body and enters to return to its residence, the Mud Pill Palace (Ni Wan Gong, 泥丸宮).

7. Yintang (M-NH-3, 印堂, Sealed Hall)

Yintang (M-NH-3, 印堂) cavity in Chinese medicine, is called Tian Yan or Tian Mu (天眼・天目, heaven eye) in Daoist society and the third eye in the West (Figure 5-8). It is called heaven eye because when it is open, you can communicate with the Qi and spirit of heaven. You can communicate telepathically with other living beings. You are enlightened, knowing many natural secrets and seeing true reality.

This is a paired cavity with Qiangjian (Gv-18, 強間). These two cavities are located at the end of the Spiritual Valley (Shen Gu, 神谷).

8. **Yinjiao** (Gv-28, 齦交, Gum's Junction) (Figure 5-8)

This is the last cavity in the Governing Vessel (Du Mai, 督脈) and connects with the Conception Vessel (Ren Mai, 任脈). Yinjiao cavity is the junction or connecting bridge between the Yin Conception and Yang Governing vessels.

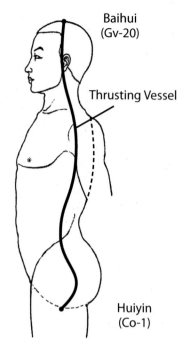

Figure 5-7. Baihui (Gv-20) and Huiyin (Co-1) connected by Thrusting Vessel

9. **Renzhong** (Gv-26, 人中, Philtrum) or **Shuigou** (水溝, Water Ditch) (Figure 5-8)

This cavity under the nose is also called Shuigou (水溝, water ditch). It is a matching cavity with Naohu (Gv-17, 腦戶, Brain's Household) at the top of the neck. It connects with the conscious mind, and when one is unconscious, pressing this cavity can awaken you.

10. **Tiantu** (Co-22, 天突, Heaven's Prominence) (Figure 5-8)

Tiantu is at the bottom of the throat. When attacked, breathing capability can be affected. Its Qi corresponds with that of Dazhui (Gv-14, 大椎) on the back.

11. **Jiuwei** (Co-15, 鳩尾, Wide Pigeon's Tail) or **Xinkan** (心坎, Heart Pit) (Figure 5-9)

Jiuwei is at the bottom of the sternum. It is connected with the heart and with Lingtai (Gv-10, 靈臺), its paired cavity on the back. When these two cavities are struck at noon time, heart attack can occur. Jiuwei is called Xinkan (心坎) in Chinese martial arts society.

12. **Zhongwan** (Co-12, 中脘, Middle Cavity, Solar Plexus) (Figure 5-9)

Zhongwan is at the solar plexus and called 'center' in Qigong society. Behind it is the Huang Ting (黃庭) cavity. Through Yin and Yang interaction of fire and water Qi at Huang Ting, the Spiritual Embryo is conceived.

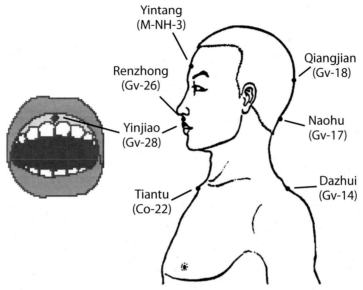

Figure 5-8. Yintang (M-NH-3), Qiangjian (Gv-18), Yinjiao (Gv-28), Renzhong (Gv-26), Naohu (Gv-17), Tiantu (Co-22), and Dazhui (Gv-14)

This cavity is one of the vital cavities in martial arts society. When struck upward with force, heart attack can occur. When struck straight forward, nausea can occur. When struck downward, the lungs can be sealed and breathing prevented.

13. **Abdomen Yinjiao** (Co-7, 陰交, Yin Junction) (Figure 5-9)
This should not be confused with Yinjiao (Gv-28) at the mouth. This cavity is the junction of the Yin Conception Vessel and Yin Thrusting Vessel. It connects to the Real Lower Dan Tian and allows Qi to enter and exit from the human biobattery. It is a paired cavity with Mingmen (Gv-4, 命門, Life's Door) located between L2 and L3 vertebrae.

14. **Qihai** (Co-6, 氣海, Sea of Qi) (Figure 5-9)
Qihai is about two inches below the navel and regarded as the False Lower Dan Tian in Daoist society. It is also called Elixir Furnace (Dan Lu, 丹爐), since it produces Qi. When moved up and down, fat (food essence) is converted into Qi.

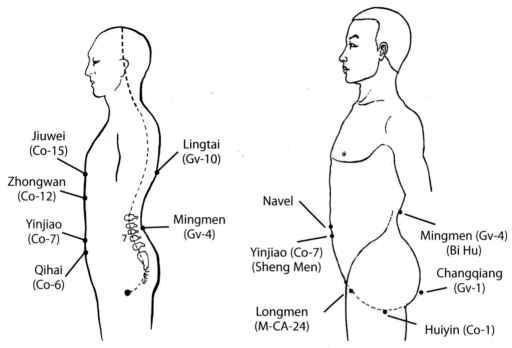

Figure 5-9. Jiuwei (Co-15), Lingtai (Gv-10), Zhongwan (Co-12), Abdomen Yinjiao (Co-7), Mingmen (Gv-4), and Qihai (Co-6)

Figure 5-10. Longmen (M-CA-24), Changqiang (Gv-1), Huiyin (Co-1)

15. **Longmen** (M-CA-24, 龍門, Dragon's Gate) or **Xiayin** (下陰, Low Yin) (Figure 5-10)

The groin area is called Longmen. It is also called Xiayin (下陰, Low Yin) since the Qi here is Yin. It and Changqiang (Gv-1, 長強, Long Strength, Weilu, 尾閭, Coccyx) are considered as a pair of corresponding Qi cavities.

16. **Huiyin** (Co-1, 會陰, perineum) (Figure 5-10)

Huiyin means to meet Yin, since it connects the four main Yin vessels, Conception, Thrusting, Yin-Heel, and Yin-Linking Vessels. It is regarded as a secret gate (Qiao Men, 竅門) in Internal Elixir Qigong. When opened (pushed out), Qi stored in the body can be released, and when closed (held up), Qi can be retained and stored. This gate is the pump of the body's inner Qi, which controls Qi storage and manifestation. This cavity and Baihui (Gv-20, 百會, Hundred Meetings) are corresponding paired gates in the body's central Qi system.

17. **Changqiang** (Gv-1, 長強, Long Strength) or **Weilu** (尾閭, Coccyx) (Figure 5-10)

Changqiang is the first gate obstructing the path of Small Circulation meditation. The Qi passage is narrow here due to the structure of the area. Since there is little conductive muscle or tendon here, the passage of this area becomes narrower as one gets older. To widen this gate is the first task of Small Circulation. This is the first dangerous gate. When one does not know the correct way to lead Qi past it, the Qi can flow into the legs instead, damaging the nerves.

18. **Mingmen** (Gv-4, 命門, Life's Door) (Figure 5-11)

Mingmen means life door, connected to the Real Lower Dan

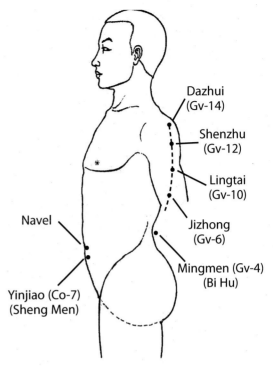

Figure 5-11. Mingmen (Gv-4), Yinjiao (Co-7), Jizhong (Gv-6), Lingtai (Gv-10), Shenzhu (Gv-12), and Dazhui (Gv-14)

Tian. It should not be confused with Gv-10 (靈臺) behind the back, called Lingtai in medical society but Mingmen by martial arts society.

Mingmen is a corresponding cavity with Yinjiao (Co-7, 陰交) at the abdominal area. Qi stored at the Real Lower Dan Tian can be led either from Yinjiao or from Mingmen to enter the Small Circulation orbit.

19. **Jizhong** (Gv-6, 脊中, Mid-spine) (Figure 5-11)

Jizhong is located at the middle of the spine. It is a Qi turning point for beginners in Small Circulation practice.

20. **Lingtai** (Gv-10, 靈臺, Spiritual Platform) or **Jiaji** (夾脊, Squeeze the spine) or **Mingmen** (命門, Life Door) (Figure 5-11)

Lingtai is a Chinese medical name. Due to its location between the shoulder blades, it is called Jiaji (Squeeze the spine) in Daoist society. It is often called Mingmen (life door) in martial arts society, because when it is struck at the right time, the heart can be shocked.

Lingtai is the second dangerous gate or obstacle in Small Circulation meditation. There is no anatomic structure to cause Qi stagnation, but it is connected to the heart. When excess Qi is led there, it can go to the heart and

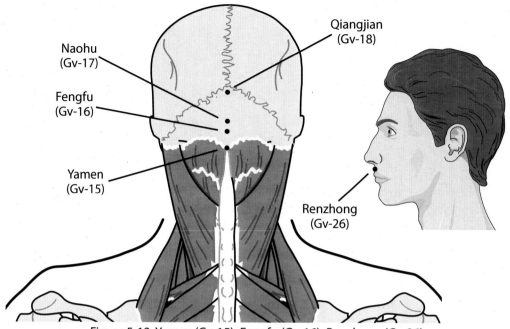

Figure 5-12. Yamen (Gv-15), Fengfu (Gv-16), Renzhong (Gv-26), Naohu (Gv-17), and Qiangjian (Gv-18)

make it too Yang, causing faster heartbeat. This may induce one to pay attention to the heart and thus lead more Qi there, precipitating a heart attack. So it is a dangerous cavity. When you practice, beware of it. If the heartbeat increases, simply ignore it and continue leading Qi up the spine.

21. **Shenzhu** (Gv-12, 身柱, Body Pillar) and **Dazhui** (Gv-14, 大椎, Big Vertebra) (Figure 5-11)
Both Shenzhu and Dazhui cavities can be used as turning points, because they join the path of the spine with that of the arms. Any Qi stagnation can be removed easily.

22. **Yamen** (Gv-15, 啞門, Door of Muteness) (Figure 5-12)
Yamen is at the rear center of the neck. Neck movement easily removes stagnant Qi in this area, so it can also be used as a Qi turning point.

23. **Fengfu** (Gv-16, 風府, Wind's Dwelling) (Figure 5-12)
Fengfu is a pairing cavity of Renzhong (Gv-26, 人中) and located exactly opposite it. It is a major cavity for treatment of stiff neck, numbness of the limbs, common cold, headache, stroke, and mental illness.

24. **Naohu** (Gv-17, 腦戶, Brain's Household) or **Yuzhen** (玉枕, Jade Pillow) (Figure 5-12)
Naohu is about one inch above Fengfu, also called Jade Pillow (Yuzhen, 玉枕) by Daoist society. It is the Third Gate of Small Circulation practice. When abundant Qi reaches this cavity, excess Qi may enter and cause brain damage, so one needs caution here. We discuss the Three Gates (San Guan, 三關) in more detail later.

25. **Qiangjian** (Gv-18, 強間, Between Strength) (Figure 5-12)
Qiangjian is opposite the heaven eye (Tian Yan, 天眼, third eye). These two are corresponding cavities, although Naohu (Gv-17, 腦戶) is also often considered a paired cavity of the Third Eye.

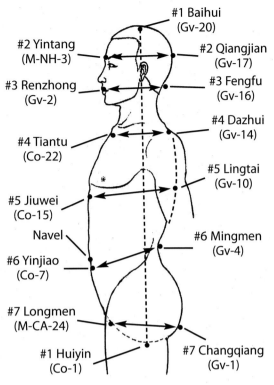

Figure 5-13. Seven Pairs of Corresponding Qi Gates

**Seven Pairs of Corresponding Qi Gates**
The human body has seven major pairs of corresponding Qi gates from which its Qi structure is constituted: 1. Huiyin (Co-1, 會陰) and Baihui (Gv-20, 百會); 2. Yintang (M-HN-3, 印堂) and Qiangjian (Gv-17, 強間) [or Naohu (Gv-18, 腦戶)]; 3. Renzhong (Gv-26, 人中) and Fengfu (Gv-16, 風府); 4. Tiantu (Co-22, 天突) and Dazhui (Gv-14, 大椎); 5. Jiuwei (Co-15, 鳩尾) and Lingtai (Gv-10, 靈臺); 6. Yinjiao (Co-7, 陰交) and Mingmen (Gv-4, 命門); and 7. Longmen (M-CA-24, 龍門) [or Xiayin (下陰)] and Changqiang (Gv-1, 長強) [or Weilu (尾閭)]. Among these seven, two pairs are the most important: Huiyin (Yin) and Baihui (Yang), and Yinjiao (Yin) and Mingmen (Yang). Huiyin is connected to Baihui through the Thrusting Vessel ,which establishes the central balance of Qi distribution in the body. Yinjiao is also connected to Mingmen through the Thrusting Vessel and joins the Conception Vessel in front and the Governing Vessel behind, providing front and rear Qi balance to the body. These four are the main Qi gates (Figure 5-13).

Tiantu controls vocal vibrations and generates the sounds of Hen (哼, Yin) and Ha (哈, Yang) for manifestation of Qi. It is a gate of expression, and its energy is balanced with Yintang, where the spirit resides. When spirit is high in Yintang, the energy manifested is strong, and alertness and awareness are high. Jiuwei and Lingtai connect to the heart (emotional mind) and offer strong driving force to raise up the spirit. These four minor gates control manifestation of Qi in the body. So the Eight Gates are defined.

## 5-4. THEORY OF SMALL CIRCULATION MEDITATION 小周天之理論

In this section, I propose a theory of Small Circulation practice from both Eastern and Western understanding. If any ancient practice has survived thousands of years with its function and effectiveness verified, it must be correct. Then we should be able to interpret it in terms of modern scientific logic. Ancient theory and practice should be consistent with modern scientific interpretation, else either theory or practice need to be modified. I propose to demonstrate this connection and offer a new theoretical concept of this practice.

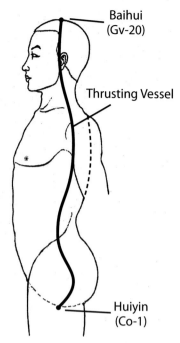

Figure 5-14. Qi Circulates in Thrusting Vessel and Bone Marrow at Night

## General Concepts

1. From Chinese medicine and Qigong, we understand that the major Qi flow during daytime is in the Conception and Governing Vessels, while at night time it is in the Thrusting Vessel. The Conception Vessel regulates Qi circulation in the six primary Yin channels, while the Governing Vessel regulates the six primary Yang channels. These Twelve Primary Qi Channels (Shi Er Jing, 十二經) distribute Qi throughout the body via millions of secondary Qi channels (Luo, 絡). During the day, when there is physical activity, Qi circulates strongly in these two vessels. Exhalation is longer than inhalation and Guardian Qi (Wei Qi, 衛氣) expands.

At night, your body relaxes and rests. Inhalation is longer than exhalation, leading Qi into the Thrusting Vessel and bone marrow (Figure 5-14). The brain and glands are nourished with Qi, while hormone production increases.

We conclude that Qi in the Small Circulation path nourishes the body (muscle/tendon changing), while that in the Thrusting Vessel promotes longevity and spiritual cultivation (marrow/brain washing).

2. Qi is stronger in the Conception Vessel during the day and in the Governing Vessel at night. During daytime, nature is Yang around you and Yin Qi in the Conception Vessel balances external Yang. At night, the external environment is Yin, and Qi in the Yang Governing Vessel balances natural Yin (Figure 5-15).

3. There are three major obstacles to Qi circulation in the Small Circulation orbit, all located in the Governing Vessel. There is no obstacle in the Conception Vessel.

4. Conception and Governing Vessels are constructed from many different layers of tendon and fascia (Figure 5-16). Since the conductivity of tendons is higher than that of the surrounding muscles, we can assume that Qi circulation at this

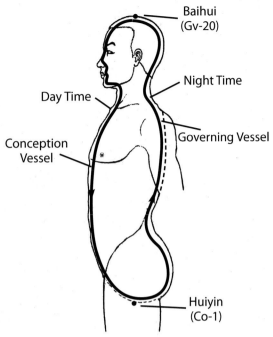

Figure 5-15. Qi is Stronger in the Conception Vessel during the Day and in the Governing Vessel at Night

center line is more abundant than in the surrounding areas. Many layers of tendon and fascia (poor conductors) are sandwiched at these two vessels like a battery, able to store Qi to an abundant level.

We assume electrical conductivity of tendons is higher than that of muscles, for the following reasons:

a. The cross section area of a tendon connected to a muscle is much smaller than that of the muscle itself. Since both are insulated with fasciae which is a poor conductor, and the same current passes through both areas, the current must flow faster through the tendon than through the muscle. So the electric conductivity of tendons is higher than that of muscles (Figure 5-17).

b. Tendon is stronger than muscle, so its Qi must circulate stronger than in muscle.

c. After physical exercise, tendons are colder than muscles. More Qi is trapped in the muscle and manifested as heat, which means the muscle has more resistance.

These conclusions are derived from logical analysis, but require verification with modern scientific equipment.

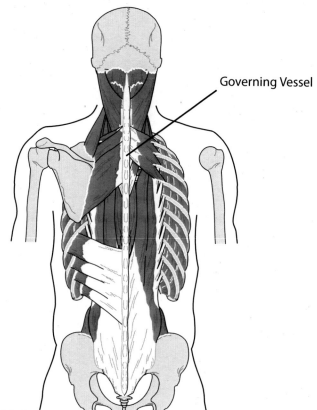

Figure 5-16. Conception and Governing Vessels are Constructed
from Many Different Layers of Tendon and Fascia

### Producing Qi (Sheng Qi, 生氣)

Let us summarize the methods of producing and increasing Qi in the body.

**1. From metabolism of food and air.** The biochemical reaction is:

$$\text{glucose} + 6O_2 \longrightarrow 6CO_2 + 6H_2O$$

$$\Delta G^{o\prime} = -686 \text{ Kcal (energy content)}$$

From digestion of food and inhalation of oxygen, energy is generated.
Different foods produce different quantity and quality of Qi, and herbs
especially are used to manipulate the Qi status of the body. This is called
Fire Qi (Huo Qi, 火氣) or Post-Heaven Qi (Hou Tian Qi, 後天氣).

**2. From abdominal exercise.** The Lower Elixir Field (Xia Dan Tian, 下丹田), called Qi Ocean (Qihai, Co-6, 氣海) by Chinese medicine, is at the front of the abdomen a few inches below the navel. Qi is generated here as abundantly as the ocean. This center is also called Furnace Tripod (Ding Lu, 鼎爐) or Elixir Furnace (Dan Lu, 丹爐), but is said to be a False Dan Tian (Jia Dan Tian, 假丹田) by Daoists. Even though it produces Qi, it cannot store it to an abundant level.

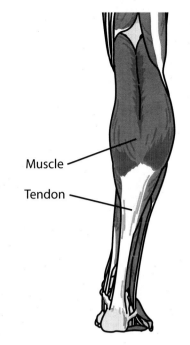

Muscle

Tendon

Figure 5-17. Electric Conductivity of Tendons is Higher Than That of Muscles

The up-and-down movements of 'back to childhood breathing' facilitate the biochemical reaction that converts stored fat into Qi. This is called Water Qi (Shui Qi, 水氣), Pre-Heaven Qi (Xian Tian Qi, 先天氣), or Original Qi (Yuan Qi, 元氣). It is pure and clean like water to calm you physically and mentally. Fat is the essence of food, which is processed, purified, and stored in the body. Fat has a high calorific content and can be converted into energy efficiently.

It is also called Pre-Heaven Qi or Original Qi because your Qi is converted from your Original Essence (Yuan Jing, 元精, hormone). In my view, however, since hormones act as catalysts in the body's biochemical reactions, they cannot be converted into Qi. All they do is facilitate the process of converting fat into Qi.

How is Qi generated at the Lower Dan Tian? The abdomen has six layers of muscle and fascia. A lot of fat is stored in the layers of fascia. When you move your abdomen up and down, your mind controls contraction and relaxation of the muscles. This causes food essence to be converted into Qi through biochemical reaction. When those places where fat is stored are exercised, the fat gradually disappears and turns into energy, so it is reasonable to assume the same happens when we move the abdomen.

Since muscles are good conductors, while fasciae are poor conductors, this area can act like a battery to store the Qi. All animals store fat (food essence) to survive in nature. In this way, extra food is stored for when there is none available. The largest storage place is the abdomen. Qi is converted and stored more abundantly here than any other place in the body and distributed efficiently to the body through the Conception and Governing Vessels.

Abdominal movement is coordinated with breathing in Qigong practice. This is called 'Starting the Fire' (Qi Huo, 起火), and there are two ways of doing so. One is Normal Abdominal Breathing (Zheng Fu Hu Xi, 正腹呼吸) and the other Reversed Abdominal Breathing (Fan, Ni Fu Hu Xi, 反、逆腹呼吸).

According to the intensity of Qi production, the practice is classified as Martial Fire (Wu Huo, 武火), or Scholar Fire (Wen Huo, 文火). Rapid breathing quickly generates Martial Fire Qi to an abundant level, which is used to energize the body for battle, or for Wai Dan Qigong practice. It is hard to store this Qi in the Real Lower Dan Tian. If you intend to store Qi internally, breathe softly and slenderly, then lead it to the Real Lower Dan Tian and store it there. This is called Scholar Fire (Wen Huo, 文火) breathing.

3. **From massaging the abdominal area.** In muscle/tendon changing, massage combined with herbs converts the fat into Qi, as described in *Qigong—The Secret of Youth*.

## Storing Qi to an Abundant Level (Xu Qi, 蓄氣)

Having produced extra Qi at the False Lower Dan Tian, lead it inward, and store it at the Real Lower Dan Tian. When it is left at the False Lower Dan Tian on the Conception Vessel, it is distributed through the Small Circulation path to the Twelve Primary Qi Channels. This improves strength and health, but it is then not available to nourish the brain for enlightenment. Remember, each brain cell requires up to twelve times more Qi than other cells. To achieve enlightenment, along with mental conditioning, you need to lead considerable Qi to the brain from storage at the Real Lower Dan Tian. My book, *Qigong Meditation—Embryonic Breathing* discusses this in detail. Here, I summarize key theories and training methods.

1. **Condition the battery at the Lower Dan Tian to store abundant Qi, far stronger than that of other people.** Conditioning is achieved through massage and physical stimulation (pounding and beating) of the stomach and abdominal area (Huang Ting, 黃庭). This converts fat into Qi and reduces fat between the layers of muscle, allowing more charge to be stored. The most important factor is conditioning the nervous system in this area to raise its pain threshold. Qi cannot generally be stored abundantly because it causes pain and tension when storage reaches its thresh-

old of tolerance, leading the Qi to disperse. Conditioning increases the tolerance of the nerves, allowing Qi storage to increase.

2. **Increase the efficiency of conversion of fat into Qi, which depends on the hormones (Original Essence) to regulate metabolism.** Hormones act as catalysts for the biochemical reaction that converts food into Qi. When they are adequate, the reaction proceeds smoothly.

   There are three major glands surrounding the abdominal area (Huang Ting), namely adrenals at the back, pancreas in front, and testicles or ovaries at the bottom. To increase their production of hormones, supply them with extra Qi through massage.

   There are two ways to massage the adrenals located on top of the kidneys. One is through alternating pressure on the lower back. The other is to massage the kidneys directly. When you reach a high level of practice, you can lead Qi directly to the kidneys using the mind.

   Massage the pancreas through abdominal exercise and massage. In the past, Qigong practitioners seldom used the mind to lead Qi to the pancreas, because they did not recognize its capability of producing Original Essence.

   Testicles and ovaries are massaged directly, or the focused mind leads Qi there with the assistance of correct breathing. Qi is also led there by tensing and relaxing the Huiyin (Co-1, 會陰, perineum).

3. **Store Qi to an abundant level at the Real Lower Dan Tian to reach spiritual enlightenment.** Embryonic Breathing (Tai Xi, 胎息) is the way to achieve this. Locate the two polarities of the body, Mud Pill Palace and Real Lower Dan Tian, and focus your mind there. Focus at the Mud Pill Palace so your mind is calm, centered and focused, and the spirit raised. Focus at the Real Lower Dan Tian to conserve Qi and lead it back to its residence.

   Once you synchronize these two centers, the strength of the central Qi system is firmly established. Next, bring your mind to the Huang Ting, where spirit and Qi are united, returning your being to the beginning of life. This is called Unification of Mother (Qi) and Son (Spirit), namely Mu Zi Xiang Shou (母子相守), or Wuji Breathing (Wuji Hu Xi, 無極呼吸).

## Circulating Qi (Xing Qi, 行氣)

There are two main reasons to practice Small Circulation. One is to accumulate abundant Qi in the Conception and Governing Vessels, and the other is to circulate it smoothly in these vessels to regulate Qi in the Twelve Primary Qi Channels. Qi already circulates naturally in these two vessels, otherwise you would have encountered some physical problem. But this circulation becomes stagnant as we age, and the path of circulation becomes narrow. Small Circulation widens this path so Qi can circulate smoothly and abundantly again. There are three places, called Three Gates (San Guan, 三關), where the path is especially narrow, causing Qi circulation to stagnate. The aim of practice is to open and widen these three gates, a process called 'Through Three Gates' (Tong San Guan, 通三關).

We now describe natural small circulation, the theory of opening the gates, and the traditional and modified methods of Small Circulation practice. Since the Three Gates are so important, we discuss them separately in the next section.

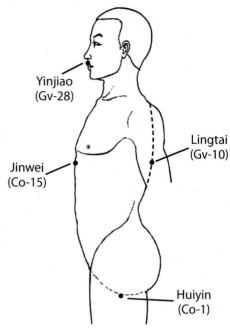

Figure 5-18. Huiyin (Co-1), Yinjiao (Gv-28), Jiuwei (Co-15), and Lingtai (Gv-10)

1. **Natural Qi Circulation in the Small Circulation Orbit.** "Internal Qi circulation in the Governing Vessel is from the bottom to the top. It connects at Yinjiao (Gv-28, 齦交, Gum's Junction) with the Conception Vessel and circulates down the Conception Vessel, becoming cyclic circulation. The junctions of the Governing and Conception Vessels, at the top and bottom, are called upper magpie bridge (Shang Que Qiao, 上鵲橋) and lower magpie bridge (Xia Que Qiao, 下鵲橋)."[18,19] Qi circulates from top to bottom in front of the body, and from bottom to top at the back. The two vessels are joined at the magpie bridges. They are Huiyin (Co-1, 會陰) and Yinjiao (Gv-28, 齦交), which control Qi in Small Circulation practice (Figure 5-18).

The major Qi flow in these two vessels is determined by the time of day and thus controlled by the sun. At midnight (11 P.M. to 1 A.M.) Qi accumulates at Baihui, connected with its corresponding gate, Huiyin, so Huiyin can also be classified as midnight. At dawn, depending on the season, the major Qi flow is at the mouth (Yinjiao). Since external Qi is changing from Yin (night) to Yang (day), internal Qi circulation also changes from Yang (Governing Vessel) to Yin (Conception Vessel). At noon, the major Qi flow is at Jiuwei (Co-15, 鳩尾) and its corresponding gate Lingtai (Gv-10, 靈台) at the back. If these cavities are attacked at noon, a heart attack can be triggered. At dusk, the major Qi flow is at

Huiyin, where Qi circulation is changing from Yin to Yang, while external Qi is changing from Yang to Yin. That Qi flow corresponds to the time of the day was considered top secret in Chinese martial arts society, since serious injury can follow an attack on these cavities.

2. **Theory of Opening the Gates.** As you age, the Qi channels gradually block, choking the flow of Qi. Age spots, wrinkles, pain, numbness, and organ malfunctions develop, made worse by lack of exercise. As the channels get narrower, the Qi circulation slows, narrowing them still further.

    In Qigong we widen the path of Qi circulation in the Conception and Governing Vessels. Qi stagnation is more serious at cavities like Changqiang and Naohu. The path is widened through abundant Qi circulation, just as when a river is blocked with garbage, abundant water flushes it away and restores the flow.

    Small Circulation practice accumulates abundant Qi and uses the mind to circulate it. The Conception and Governing Vessels control Qi circulation in the Twelve Primary Qi Channels, spreading Qi to the whole body, so once Small Circulation is accomplished, the body becomes strong and healthy.

3. **Traditional Method and Modified Method.** In traditional practice, the master would teach his student to produce extra Qi in the Lower Dan Tian through abdominal breathing. After a long time, about ten years of practice, this area would be conditioned and plenty of Qi stored. Only then would the master teach his trusted student to lead the Qi. The main goal, besides increasing the quantity of Qi circulating in the Conception and Governing Vessels, would be to widen the Three Gates, so Qi could circulate smoothly. Qi was stored to an abundant level first, to be able to re-activate Qi flow and widen the path. However, this may cause injury if it enters the wrong path, causing shock to the nervous system and affecting normal function. To avoid the danger of injury, I have modified the ancient training procedures through twenty years of teaching experience, in three major ways. I teach students Embryonic Breathing first, rather than abdominal breathing. This is the root of Internal Elixir practice. In the past, Embryonic Breathing was not practiced for Small Circulation, due to the secrecy surrounding it. It was hidden in Buddhist and Daoist monasteries for spiritual enlightenment practice. Having mastered Embryonic Breathing, you can manipulate Qi even if it is very strong.

    Second, I reverse the order of traditional teaching. When a student has some Qi, I teach him to circulate it immediately. There is no danger since the Qi is not strong enough to cause harm. Having learned to circulate it, he spends the rest of his life accumulating Qi and gradually widening the path. Naturally, this revised method takes longer to achieve.

Third, to prevent danger caused from passing the first gate at Weilu (尾閭, Changqiang, Gv-1, 長強), I teach circulating Qi in a smaller orbit called Small Small Circulation (Xiao Xiao Zhou Tian, 小小周天). The student leads the Qi to Huiyin, passes Weilu and re-enters the Real Lower Dan Tian through Mingmen (Gv-4, 命門) to complete this Small Small Orbit. Only then is he taught regular Small Circulation.

## Practicing Theory and Keys

If you grasp the theory, you can achieve the goal more quickly. You should study the book, *Qigong Meditation—Embryonic Breathing*. The theory and practice of Embryonic Breathing is the essential root of Internal Elixir Qigong.

1. **The Body is the Battlefield** (Tiao Shen, 調身).
   The body is a battlefield and Qi like soldiers engaged in battle against sickness and aging. For religious Qigong, Qi generates crucial power to reopen the Third Eye. Qigong practice aims to increase the quantity of Qi and to improve the quality of its manifestation. So arrange the battlefield in your favor.
   Regulating the body (Tiao Shen, 調身) means keeping the torso upright, neck relaxed, joints opened, and legs crossed comfortably, as you strive for extreme relaxation of the whole body. This reduces to a minimum the resistance to Qi flow, so it circulates smoothly and abundantly. Blood flows smoothly too, carrying oxygen, water, nutrients and Qi throughout the body. The body's metabolism is effective, so damage to the body can be repaired and the aging process slowed.
   Most important of all, your mind becomes peaceful and calm, so it can focus on leading the Qi. This is called harmonious balance of body and mind (Shen Xin Ping Heng, 身心平衡).

2. **Breathing as Strategy** (Tiao Xi, 調息)
   Breathing is the strategy in Qigong practice. When you breathe correctly, Qi circulates smoothly, and when it is awkward, Qi stagnates. The keys to regulating the breath are: A. Calm and silent (Jing, 靜), B. Slender (Xi, 細), C. Deep (Shen, 深), D. Long (Chang, 長), E. Continuous (You, 悠), F. Uniform (Yun, 勻), G. Slow (Huan, 緩), and H. Soft (Mian, 綿).
   Once you reach this stage, oxygen and carbon dioxide exchange smoothly and the metabolism is healthy. Your mind is calm and peaceful and the body relaxed. This is called Mutual Dependence of the Xin and Breathing (Xin Xi Xiang Yi, 神氣相合). Xin is the emotional mind which makes you excited, confused, or distracts you from leading the Qi.

3. **Mind is the General** (Tiao Xin, 內氣)

Mind is the general in charge of the battlefield (body), strategies (breathing), and soldiers (Qi). If the general's mind is calm and clear, he controls the situation effectively. If it is confused and scattered, his control will be weak and shallow.

The mind generates EMF so Qi can be directed. When this mind is confused and weak, the Qi is poorly led. A highly concentrated mind can be achieved in a drowsy, semi-hypnotic state. Your conscious mind is there, yet not there. *Entering the Herbal Mirror* (入藥鏡) describes this state, "The state of trance, remote and profound. Body and mind are naturally comfortable, as though drunk and like an idiot. Muscles and skin are refreshed and transparent. Its beauty is hidden within."[20] Li, Shi-Zhen (李時珍) describes this state in his book, *The Study of Strange Meridians and Eight Vessels* (奇經八脈考), "Dusky (tranced) and silent, like a drunk and like an idiot."[21]

To reach this state, your wisdom mind (Yi) governs your emotional mind (Xin). Once emotion is calm, use Yi to lead your Qi.

4. **Spirit is the Soldiers' Morale** (Tiao Shen, 調神)

The spirit of practice is more important than the mind, Qi, or body. Spirit is invisible but controls the morale of the army. When morale is high, orders are executed effectively. When your spirit is down, your immune system is weak and you easily get sick. Raise up the spirit with a firm mind and strong will. Keep your motivation to practice high at all times, and govern Xin with Yi. Be decisive, with confusion reduced to a minimum. Keeping spirit at a high level, you harmonize Spirit and Qi (Shen Qi Xiang He, 神氣相合), so Qi is led effectively.

5. **Huiyin is the Pump, and the Abdomen is the Bellows.**

The Huiyin cavity is the crucial valve controlling Qi in the four Yin vessels. When it is pushed out, the stored Qi is released, and when it is held up, the valve is closed, holding Qi in and conserving it. So the Huiyin pumps Internal Qi (Nei Qi, 內氣) and governs the manifestation or preservation of the body's Qi. Controlling Huiyin in your practice makes a significant difference. Traditionally this was one tricky place which the master would keep secret until the student was trustworthy.

6. **Tongue is the Bridge of Yin and Yang.**

The tongue is the bridge or switch which connects the Yin Conception and Yang Governing Vessels, necessary so Qi can circulate smoothly between the two vessels. Your tongue should touch your palate whenever you practice Qigong.

## 5-5. THREE GATES 三關

If one does not follow the correct method, practicing Internal Elixir Qigong can be very dangerous. There are two dangers to be faced. One is Zou Huo (走火), which means 'entering the fire'. Qi enters into the wrong path, which may cause physical and mental damage. The other is Ru Mo (入魔), which means 'enter the demon', or being bewitched. The mind enters the state of illusion or imagination during meditation.

Each organ or part of the body has its own Qi threshold. When Qi becomes deficient or exceeds this threshold, damage can occur. For example, if too much Qi enters the heart, it can cause heart attack.

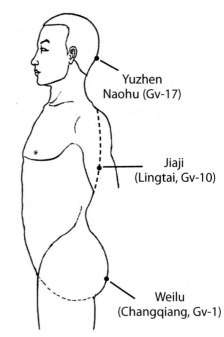

Figure 5-19. Three Gates (San Guan): Yuzhen, Jiaji, and Weilu

When you meditate, you accumulate abundant Qi at your Lower Dan Tian and then circulate it. If your mind directs this Qi and keeps it in the Small Circulation orbit, there will be no problem. But if it strays from this path and enters the wrong one, damage can follow. So your mind plays a key role when you meditate.

In the meditative state, your body is extremely relaxed and your mind calm and clear, so you are vulnerable to disturbing energy around you. These disturbances can cause illusion which can lead your mind astray, as when a cold breeze lets you feel you are in the presence of a ghost.

There are three gates (San Guan, 三關) which can cause one to walk into the fire and enter the demon. They are: Yuzhen (玉枕), Jiaji (夾脊), and Weilu (尾閭). *The Collection of Great Achievements in Golden Elixir* (金丹大成集) said, "Behind the brain is Yuzhen Guan. Jiaji is called Lulu Guan, while the junction of water and fire is called Weilu Guan."(Figure 5-19)[22] Yuzhen means jade pillow. In ancient times, rich people would thread small pieces of jade together to make a pillow. Yuzhen is a Daoist term, known in acupuncture as Naohu. Jiaji means squeeze the spine, the center of the spine between the shoulder blades. Jiaji, or Lulu Guan (轆轤關) means windlass gate, so called since it is at the center where the shoulders turn. Jiaji is called Mingmen (命門, lifedoor) by martial artists since it is connected to the heart and can cause death when struck. In acupuncture it is called Lingtai (Gv-10, 靈臺, spiritual platform). Weilu (tailbone) is the junction where Qi enters the water or fire path. In acupuncture, Weilu is called Changqiang (Gv-1, 長強, long strength), but has always been confused in Qigong society with Huiyin (Co-1, 會陰, perineum).

**First Gate:** Weilu (尾閭), Changqiang (Gv-1, 長強)

The Weilu cavity is also called Xuwei (虛危穴, Endangered Cavity). It has many names, due to its importance in Internal Elixir cultivation. *The Complete Book of Principal Contents of Human Life and Temperament* (性命圭旨全書) lists them:[23]

- Tian Ren He Fa Zhi Ji (天人合發之機): The pivotal place for unification of heaven and man.
- Zi Mu Fen Tai Zhi Lu (子母分胎之路): The path of separation of son (embryo) and mother.
- Ren Du Jie Jiao Zhi Chu (任督接交之處): The junction of Conception and Governing Vessels.
- Yin Yang Bian Hua Zhi Xiang (陰陽變化之鄉): The village (location) of variations of Yin and Yang.
- Jiu Ling Tie Gu (九靈鐵鼓): The iron drum of nine spirits (meaning unknown).
- San Zu Ji Chan (三足金蟾): Golden toad with three legs (meaning unknown).
- Tai Xuan Guan (太玄關): Grand mysterious gate.
- Cang Jin Dou (藏金斗): Hidden golden dipper (meaning unknown).
- Weilu Xue (尾閭穴): Tailbone cavity.
- Sheng Si Xue (生死穴): Cavity of life and death.
- Chao Tian Ling (朝天岭): Approach remote heaven.
- Qihai Men (氣海門): The gate to the Qi ocean.
- Cao Xi Lu (曹溪路): Cao Xi road (meaning unknown).
- San Cha Kou (三岔口): The junction of three paths.
- Ping Yi Xue (平易穴): Peace and easy cavity (meaning unknown).
- Xian Chi (咸池): Pond of wholeness.
- Yin Duan (陰端): Yin extremity.
- Jin Men (禁門): Forbidden gate.
- Huiyin (會陰): Meet Yin.
- Gu Dao (穀道): Grain path.
- Long Hu Xue (龍虎穴): Cavity of dragon and tiger (Yin and Yang).
- San Cha Gu (三岔骨): Junction bone of three paths.
- He Che Lu (河車路): The path of river car (transporting Qi)
- Shang Tian Ti (上天梯): The ladder to heaven (enlightenment)

Much attention has been focused on this cavity in Chinese Qigong history. *The Complete Book of Principal Contents of Human Life and Temperament* (性命圭旨全書) said, "It is because this cavity is where Jing (essence) and Qi are gathered and dispersed, where water and fire begin, where Yin and Yang vary, where the substantial (body) and insubstantial (spirit) enter and leave, where son and mother separate." "This cavity is the center between the Conception and Governing Vessels. Upward, it communicates with Tian Gu (Spiritual Valley), and downward, it reaches Yongquan." "This cavity has the strongest influence (on life), it is the key of one's life and death. So the immortals called it the hole of life and death." The book, *Can Tong Qi* (參同契), said, "This is where to establish and to firm the spiritual cultivation, the place to retain the storage, and the controlling gate of Qi." *Yellow Yard Classic* (黃庭經) said, "This is where to seal and close the life door so the jade (precious life) can be protected. This is also where to seal the path of sperm, so you may live long."[24]

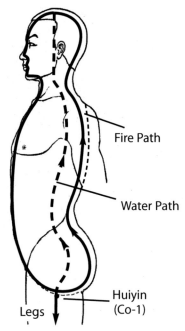

Figure 5-20. Huiyin (Co-1) is the Junction of Fire Path, Wind Path, and Legs

The documents are not clear on where exactly the cavity is, whether it refers to the tailbone (Weilu, 尾閭), or to the Huiyin. The anus is also sometimes considered to be the place and is commonly called Gu Dao (穀道), or grain path.

If we analyze the anatomy and the historical background, the confusion disappears. Almost everyone in those days was illiterate and had difficulty understanding special medical terminology such as Huiyin. Since the muscles of the anus area are connected with the perineum, it was easier to write anus instead of Huiyin. Through contraction and relaxation of the perineum, Qi can be regulated. If the anus is gently held up, the perineum tightens and seals the Qi gate. When it is gently pushed out, the perineum relaxes, and the Qi gate opens.

Also recognize that Huiyin is the key cavity where Qi divides into three paths, Fire Path (Huo Lu, 火路) through the Governing Vessel, Water Path (Shui Lu, 水路) through the Thrusting Vessel, and also down to the bottom of the feet through the Yin Heel Vessels (Yinqiao Mai, 陰蹻脈) and Yin Linking Vessels (Yinwei Mai, 陰維脈) (Figure 5-20). When Qi circulates abundantly in the Fire Path, then the Twelve Primary Qi Channels (Shi Er Jing, 十二經) will also be full.

If Qi is led up strongly through the Water Path, the brain is nourished and energized. This is the key to Marrow/Brain Washing for spiritual enlightenment. Huiyin also regulates Qi flow from the sexual organ to the legs, so when sexual energy is strong, the legs are strong.

Qi enters the Fire or Water paths through the tricky gate at Weilu (tailbone, Changqiang, 長強). Contracting and relaxing the Huiyin muscles pumps Qi through Weilu into the Fire Path or the Water Path. In the beginning, Qi will tend to flow down to the legs instead, because the Qi paths to the legs are wide open.

This is not a problem if the Qi is weak, but abundant Qi can be dangerous if you don't lead it into the correct path. When abundant Qi encounters its first obstacle at the Weilu gate, it may instead

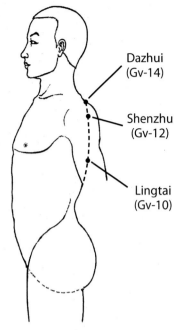

Figure 5-21. Lingtai (Gv-10), Dazhui (Gv-14), and Shenzhu (Gv-12)

rush down to the legs and damage the nervous system there. This is called 'walking into the fire' (Zou Huo, 走火), well known as the first danger of practice, which can paralyze the legs. When you meditate, it is important to sit with crossed legs, to block off the Qi flow to the legs. If too much Qi nevertheless rushes there during meditation, first try to lead it back to the Lower Dan Tian. Then hit the legs to stimulate them, leading Qi from deep inside to dissipate at the skin.

**Second Gate:** Jiaji (夾脊), Lulu (轆轤), Lingtai (Gv-10, 靈臺)

This gate is not narrow and can be passed easily, but is dangerous because abundant Qi there can enter the heart, causing palpitations. A beginner may be distracted by this, focusing on the heart and triggering a heart attack.

In practice, simply ignore this cavity. If you sense Qi flow to the heart, focus on the Dazhui (Gv-14, 大椎) or Shenzhu (Gv-12, 身柱) cavities and lead the Qi there instead (Figure 5-21). With practice you get used to it and find that as long as your mind is calm and clear, there is no problem leading Qi past this cavity.

**Third Gate:** Yuzhen (玉枕, Jade Pillow), Naohu (Gv-17, 腦戶)

This is at the base of the skull and is dangerous due to its physical structure. There is a thin layer of muscle between the skull and the skin. The Qi path suddenly narrows as the neck tendons end. When abundant Qi accumulates here, some of

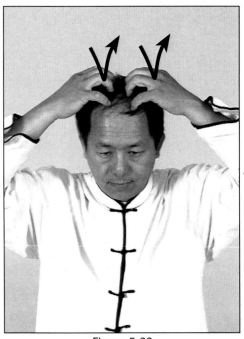

Figure 5-22

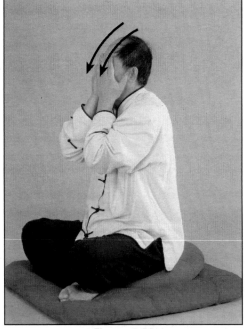

Figure 5-23

it can enter the brain through Naohu, which can excite the nervous system in the brain, damage its function, or even cause mental disorder.

Be careful when you lead Qi past this cavity. Various sensations are generated. Pay attention to Baihui, and Qi will go there. If some Qi enters the brain through Naohu, first lead it back to the Lower Dan Tian. Tap the head with your fingertips to lead Qi to the surface (Figure 5-22), then brush it forward and down the Fire Path with your palms (Figure 5-23).

Having opened and widened these three gates, you complete the Small Circulation path. As you continue your practice, you accumulate more abundant Qi circulating in this Fire Path. The more abundant it is, the better your health and the stronger your foundation for Muscle/Tendon Changing practice.

## 5-6. DIFFERENT PATHS FOR SMALL CIRCULATION 小周天之不同途徑

According to the Qi network and the physical structure, we can conclude a few possible paths for Small Circulation. Due to lack of information and personal experience, I will only discuss those paths I am familiar with.

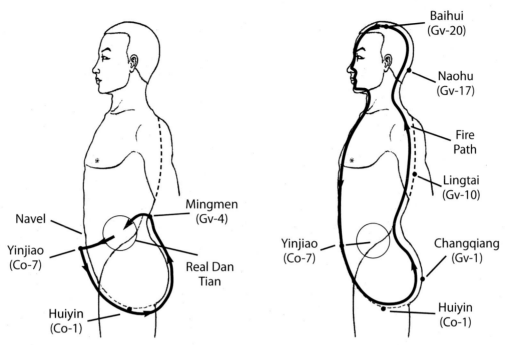

Figure 5-24. Small Small Circulation

Figure 5-25. Fire Path

1. **Small Small Circulation** (Foundation, Xiao Xiao Zhou Tian, 小小周天-根基)

This path is very safe, and much easier for beginners learning to pass the first gate at Weilu. Practice this path first until you can lead the Qi smoothly, before continuing the Fire Path practice.

Lead the Qi down from the Real Lower Dan Tian, through Yinjiao, down to Huiyin, up past Changqiang, and finally enter Mingmen to reach the Qi residence at the Real Lower Dan Tian (Figure 5-24). This is described in detail in Chapter 8.

2. **Fire Path** (Regular Path, Huo Lu, 火路, Shun Xing, 順行)

Fire Path is the regular path that follows natural Qi circulation and is the one most commonly practiced. It is often called Large Returning Elixir (Da Huan Dan, 大還丹). *Returning Elixir Secret* (還丹訣) said, "Keep the body upright and sit correctly, transport Qi from Weilu, with one breath pass through San Guan (Three Gates) up to Ni Wan, harmonize with the spiritual water (saliva) and descend back to Dan Tian. This is Large Returning Elixir (Da Huan Dan). From kidneys to liver, from liver to heart, from heart to spleen, to lungs, and then repeat. Finally end at the Dan Tian. This is called Small Returning Elixir (Xiao Huan Dan,小還丹 )."[25]

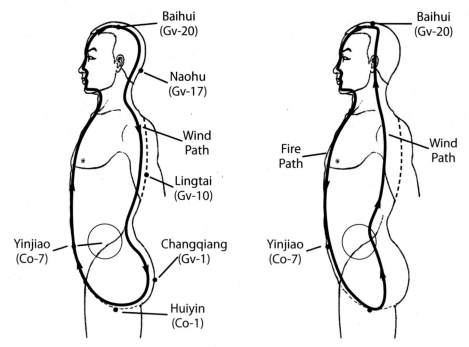

Figure 5-26. Wind Path

Figure 5-27. Combination of Water Path and Front Fire Path.

In this path, you lead Qi from the Real Lower Dan Tian, passing Yinjiao, Huiyin, Changqiang, Lingtai, Naohu, and Baihui, then down through the Conception Vessel back to Yinjiao and the Real Lower Dan Tian (Figure 5-25). This is also described in detail in Chapter 8.

3. **Wind Path** (Reversed Regular Path, Feng Lu, 風路, Ni Xing, 逆行)
Wind Path is the reverse of the natural path, so it generates resistance (wind) (Figure 5-26). Its purpose is to slow down Qi circulation in the fire path.
Lead Qi up the front, down the back, then back to the Real Lower Dan Tian.

4. **Combination of Water Path and Front Fire Path**
Qi is led up the Thrusting Vessel (Water Path) to Baihui, then down the Conception Vessel back to the Real Lower Dan Tian (Figure 5-27). This can be done by those with abundant Qi at the Real Lower Dan Tian and who are able to lead it up to nourish the brain. You may feel Qi moving by itself in the Thrusting Vessel, as all paths are already open to some extent. What you practice is to build abundant Qi, to circulate and to nourish.

## 5. Combination of Back Fire Path and Reverse Water Path

This path brings fire Qi down through the Thrusting Vessel. Qi follows the Fire Path up to Baihui, and then goes down through the Thrusting Vessel back to the Real Lower Dan Tian (Figure 5-28). When the Qi is led up the Thrusting Vessel, the Shen is raised up and Qi activity increases. But when the Qi is led down the Thrusting Vessel, it returns to its residence. Physical and mental activities gradually cease. Once you complete the Fire Path, try this path, which is relatively safe and very efficient in bringing your fire Qi down.

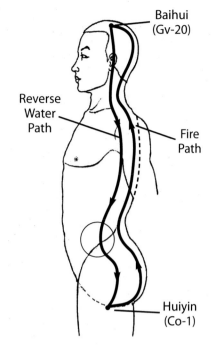

Figure 5-28. Combination of Back Fire Path and Reverse Water Path.

## 6. Back Fire Path—Dazhui— Tiantu —Front Fire Path

This path is little known and seldom practiced. Qi is led up the Fire Path to Dazhui (Gv-14, 大椎), then forward to Tiantu (Co-22, 天突). It then goes down the Conception Vessel to Yinjiao, returning to the Real Lower Dan Tian (Figure 5-29).

## 7. Back Fire Path—Dazhui—Reverse Water Path

To avoid Qi going to the wrong path in the head, some practitioners use this path to cool down the fire, instead of path number 5. Qi is led up the Fire Path to Dazhui, forward to the Thrusting Vessel, then down to the Real Lower Dan Tian (Figure 5-30).

There is no path which enters Jiaji cavity and then goes forward. This would lead extra Qi to the heart, and would be extremely dangerous.

All paths are already open to some extent. Too much stagnation or blockage would have made you sick already. You aim to increase the level of Qi circulating there, to smooth its flow and to widen the path. Follow five basic steps: 1. Train yourself (Lian Ji, 練己), 2. Modulate the herbs (Tiao Yao, 調藥), 3. Produce the herbs (Chan Yao, 產藥), 4. Pick the herbs (Cai Yao, 采藥), and 5. Refine the herbs (Lian Yao, 煉藥). That means to regulate your emotional mind and cultivate your temperament. Be patient and study the method of cultivation. After that, use this calm mind

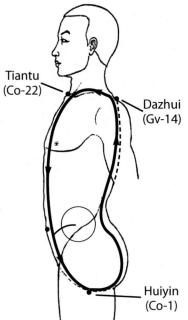

Figure 5-29. Back Fire Path—Dazhui—Tiantu—Front Fire Path.

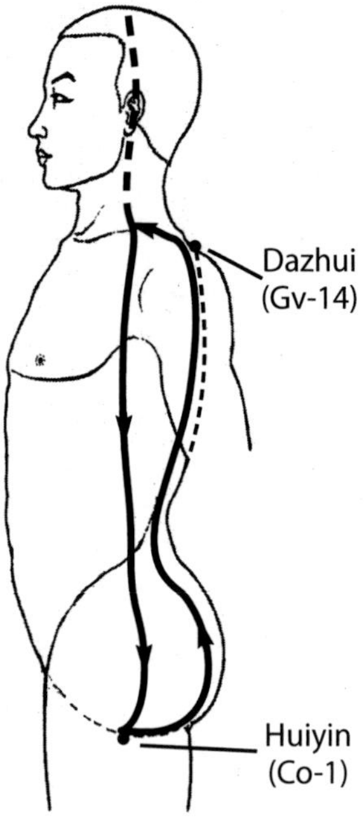

Figure 5-30. Back Fire Path—Dazhui—Reverse Water Path.

to regulate your breathing and Qi flow. You accumulate abundant Qi through abdominal and embryonic breathing, then use it for muscle/tendon changing and marrow/brain washing. Constantly refine your breathing, build up your Qi, and circulate it for the rest of your life.

Once your mind can lead the Qi efficiently, you can lead it any way you like in your body. "Transport Qi as though through a pearl with a nine-curved hole, it will reach even the tiniest place."[26]

## 5-7. TANG DYNASTY INTERNAL ELIXIR MEDITATION ILLUSTRATION
唐代內丹靜坐內景圖

This was painted during the Tang Dynasty (618-907 A.D., 唐代) and revealed to secular society by a Daoist, Su Yun (素雲). Internal Elixir cultivation (Nei Dan, 內丹) is specified very clearly even though it was still in its early stages. Internal Elixir for longevity and enlightenment was brought to China from India by Da Mo during the Liang Dynasty (502-557 A.D., 梁朝). His two classics, *Yi Jin Jing* (易筋經, Muscle/Tendon Changing) and *Xi Sui Jing* (洗髓經, Marrow/Brain Washing) have strongly influenced Chinese Qigong society.

This illustration was revealed more than a thousand years ago. Even though disagreements and discrepancies crept in later, the main structure and contents remain accurate today. Keep a few things in mind:

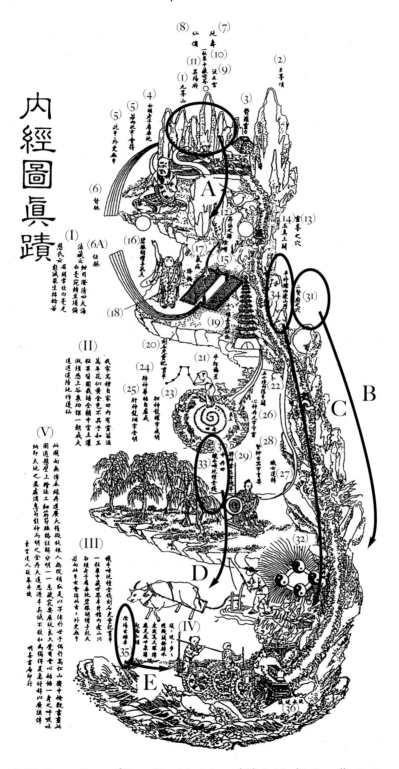

Figure 5-31. Corrections of Tang Dynasty Internal Elixir Meditation Illustration

1. Always question what you see and read. Think and challenge the source. Then you will see much more clearly. If you simply believe, you can easily be led astray.

2. This illustration can be interpreted in various ways, so refer to all of them, and depend on your own thinking, experience, and judgment.

3. At least five functions were deliberately misplaced in the illustration (Figure 5-31): A. The Mud Pill Palace, which refers to the pituitary and pineal glands, is located at the top of the head. It should be at the center of the head behind the eyes. B. The right hand column of characters behind the throat should be at the kidneys behind the spine, where the lady is weaving. C. The left hand column of characters behind the throat refers to the small boiler under the Real Lower Dan Tian, where the four Yin-Yang symbols are located. D. The column of Chinese characters under the heart should be placed above the Iron Bull cultivating the land, which symbolizes cultivating Qi in the Dan Tian. E. The column of Chinese characters below the bull's head should be placed near the water wheels.

4. The following interpretations derive from my current understanding, which may change in the future, and should not be taken at face value (Figure 5-31).

*(I)*

*Fa Zang said:*
*Use the Buddhist heart (mind) and viewpoint to understand the four great oceans (world). Then your spirit will reach the fullness of virtue gradually and softly.*

法藏云：

紺目澄清四大海

白毫宛轉至須彌

Gan (紺) means Buddhist temple, and implies using the Buddhist heart to make judgment. Mu (目) means eyes and implies viewing and observing. Bai Hao (白毫) means many tiny white beams and implies the spiritual light emitted from the head (the third eye). Wan Zhuan (宛轉) means soft, gradual, and gentle. Xu Mi (須彌) is the Daoist term for the spiritual being in the fullness of human virtue.

As long as you have a Buddha heart, you will have a neutral and clear point of view to judge whatever you see. You will be able to cultivate your temperament in the fullness of human virtue.

*Ci Shi said:*
*Once the space between the eyebrows (third eye) can emit tiny white beams frequently, it can help seculars to eradicate the suffering of reincarnation.*

慈氏云：

眉間常放白毫光

能滅眾生轉輪苦

Continuously cultivate your spirit to open the third eye located between the eyebrows to achieve enlightenment. Countless tiny beams of spiritual white light will emit from this place. You reach the first stage of Buddhahood and are able to solve secular emotional suffering, which arises from recurrent reincarnation.

*(II)*

*I am engrossed in cultivating my own land in my family (body). There is a spiritual seed in it which can live ten thousand years (longevity).*

*Its flower is like yellow gold without different color (precious), and its fruits are like jade granules all around.*

*To plant and cultivate, rely on the Earth in the Central Palace, and to irrigate it, depend on the spring in the Upper Valley.*

*When the achievement of reaching the great Dao has been completed through practice, you become an immortal who lives leisurely without worry in this land.*

我家峀種自家田

內有靈苗活萬年

花似黃金色不異

子如玉粒果皆圓

栽培全賴中宮土

灌溉須憑上谷泉

功課一朝成大道

逍遙陸地作蓬仙

The spirit is like a seed, precious as gold. Cultivate it correctly, so it allows you to live long. When cultivated and bearing fruit, it makes your spirit full. To cultivate it, rely on two things. First, build up elixir Qi at the Central Palace (Zhong Gong,

中宮), the Huang Ting (黃庭) or the Real Lower Dan Tian. Also cultivate the spirit residing in the Spiritual Valley (Shen Gu, 神谷). The holy Spiritual Embryo conceived at the Huang Ting establishes the seed of spiritual enlightenment. The quantity of Qi at the Real Lower Dan Tian provides healthy physical life. The spirit at the Upper Dan Tian governs the quality of Qi which manifests as life.

Having cultivated these two, unify them at the Real Lower Dan Tian. This is called the unification and harmonization of Shen and Qi (Shen Qi Xiang He, 神氣相合). This is the goal of Embryonic Breathing. Water Qi at the Real Lower Dan Tian is led up to interact with fire Qi descending from the Middle Dan Tian, to conceive the Spiritual Embryo at the Huang Ting. This is the first step to reaching spiritual enlightenment. Having reached enlightenment, you live as an immortal in this secular world.

*(III)*

*Iron Bull tills the land to plant the golden coins.*

*The stone-carving child threads them (golden coins) together.*

鐵牛耕地種金錢 (33)

刻石兒童把貫串 (20)

The False Lower Dan Tian is where the elixir land is plowed and the precious golden coins (Qi) grown. To build up Qi (start the fire) through Abdominal Breathing (Fu Hu Xi, 腹呼吸), you must be patient and persistent like the stubborn Iron Bull. (The Chinese characters were misplaced, and should be near the bull.)

To store abundant Qi (thread coins together), you need a childlike, innocent heart, free from emotional bondage. The child at the heart area (Middle Dan Tian area) means the innocent and pure mind. Stone carving is hard work demanding patience, as needed to store Qi to an abundant level.

*A single grain of rice can conceal the world,*

*Half liter boiler can heat the mountains and the rivers.*

一粒米中藏世界 (10)

半升鐺內煮山川 (34)

A single grain of rice is very small. It refers to the Mud Pill Palace (Ni Wan Gong, 泥丸宮) where the Shen resides. Keep your spirit there without being distracted by secular Xin, then you can use this Shen to govern your life. The physical body is heaven and earth (Tian Di, 天地), country (Guo, 國), world (Shi Jie, 世界), or mountains and rivers (Shan Chuan, 山川). Qi is called the people, and spirit is called the king.

The tiny boiler at the Lower Dan Tian produces enough Qi to supply the mountains and rivers (physical body). Abundant Qi at the Lower Dan Tian will supply the whole body's needs. Maintain your Shen at its residence to govern the quality of Qi manifestation, which means the quality of life. (The Chinese characters behind the throat were misplaced and should be under the four Yin-Yang symbols.)

*The eyebrows of the white-headed old man reach to the ground.*

*The northern foreign monk with the blue eyes holds up heaven with his hands.*

白頭老子眉垂地 (4)

碧眼胡僧手托天 (16)

The long eyebrows and white hair imply very old age and mean immortality can be reached through cultivation. Hands holding up heaven means the tongue is touching the palate of the mouth. This technique originated from Da Mo (達磨), also known as Bodhidharma, who had been a prince in southern India. From the Mahayana school of Buddhism, he was considered to have been a bodhisattva, an enlightened being who renounced nirvana to save others. From fragmentary historical records, it is believed he was born about 483 A.D. He arrived in Canton in 527 A.D. during the reign of the Wei Xiao Ming emperor (魏孝明帝, 516-528 A.D.) or the Liang Wu emperor (梁武帝, 502-557 A.D.).

*If one comprehends the knack of this mystery,*

*then beyond it, there is no more mystery.*

若向此鄉玄會得 (5)

此玄玄外更無鄉 (5)

These are the secrets of spiritual cultivation. Grasp them, then there is nothing more to be understood.

*(IV)*

*Repeatedly and continuously, step by step repeat the cycle.*
*The pump turns the water and makes it flow to the East.*
*When the bottom of a deep lake of ten thousand fathoms can be seen,*
*then the sweet spring will emerge from the end of the southern mountains.*

復復連連步步週
機關撥轉水東流
萬丈深潭應見底
甘泉湧起南山頭

Huiyin is the secret cavity which controls manifestation of the body's Yin and Yang. From this area, you lead Qi in the Fire Path. Your body is strong and healthy, manifesting Qi into physical form.

However, if you lead the Qi up through the Thrusting Vessel, you enter the water path, which calms the body and raises the spirit.

The boy and girl represent Yin and Yang, manifesting through continuously pumping the water wheel (Huiyin). Yin manifests the water path, while Yang manifests the fire path.

There was said to be an island called Peng Lai Xian Dao (蓬萊仙島), in the eastern ocean, where the immortals lived. Through cultivation, you can attain immortality.

Your mind must be clear and calm like a very deep lake through which the bottom can be seen clearly. This means you are not in emotional bondage, and your spirit is free and pure.

Once your mind is calm and peaceful and the spirit clear and focused, then saliva (sweet spring) is generated in the mouth, to the south of the head.

## 九峰山 (1)

Nine-peaked mountain. The top of the head is commonly referred to as the peak of a mountain or of heaven. Nine-peaked mountains means the brain in the top half of the head. Brain is also called Jiu Gong (九宮) which means nine palaces.

## 巨峰頂 (2)

Top of giant peak. The brain at the back of the head right behind Baihui.

## 鬱羅靈臺 (3)

Obscure spiritual platform. Baihui is where spirit leaves and enters its residence.

## 督脈 (6)

Governing Vessel. One of four Yang vessels regulating the Qi status of the six primary Yang channels.

## 任脈 (6A)

**Conception Vessel.** One of four Yin vessels regulating the Qi status of the six primary Yin channels.

## 延壽 (7)

**Extending life.** Embryonic Breathing (Tai Xi, 胎息) condenses the spirit at the Mud Pill Palace (Ni Wan Gong, 泥丸宮), where growth hormone and melatonin are produced in the pituitary and pineal glands. This is the key to longevity and immortality. (Mud Pill Palace is misplaced and should be at the center of the head.)

## 仙儡 (8)

**Immortal realm.** The same as 7 above.

## 泥丸宮 (9)

**Mud Pill Palace.** Center of the head where pituitary and pineal glands are situated. Considered the Yin center (Yin He, 陰核) of the Yang Shen's (陽神) manifestation, and the residence of Original Shen (Yuan Shen, 元神). Condensing the spirit here through Embryonic Breathing produces hormones, the secret of longevity. When this center is firmed and under control, manifestation of Yang can be elevated to a magnificent level without inducing chaos. (These Chinese characters were misplaced, and should be at the center of the head.)

## 昇陽府 (11)

**Uprising Yang residence.** Same as Mud Pill Palace above.

## 昇法之源 (12)

**The origin of natural rule in spiritual raising.** Same as Mud Pill Palace above.

## 靈峰之穴 (13)

**Cavity of spiritual peak.** Called Jade Pillow (Yu Zhen, 玉枕) by Daoists or Naohu (Gv-17, 腦戶) by Chinese medicine. The Qi at this cavity balances that at the Tian Yan (天眼, third eye), called Yintang (M-NH-3, 印堂) by Chinese medicine. Through the Qi balance of this gate, the third eye can be opened. This is the third gate needing to be opened in Small Circulation meditation. It is very precious in training, like jade. Because it helps open the third eye to reach the truth, it is a true gate.

## 玉真上關 (14)

**Jade true upper gate.** Another name for Jade Pillow, see 13 above.

## 飡咽 (15)

**Food swallowing.** The entrance of food into the body. When saliva is correctly swallowed with a sound En (嗯), health is maintained and significant progress made in meditation.

## 氣疾 (17)

**Qi urgency.** This Qi is Kong Qi (空氣, air). In meditation you regulate your breathing to be slender, soft, smooth, and natural. Without first calming body and mind, the mouth will be dry and breathing urgent. Calm the body and mind through correct breathing, then saliva will be generated.

## 降橋 (18)

**Descending bridge.** Under this bridge, saliva (heavenly water, Tian Chi Shui, 天池水) is generated. If swallowed correctly, Qi descends and strengthens the Yin, assisting physical and mental calm during meditation.

## 十二樓臺藏秘訣 (19)

**In the twelve-storied pagoda, secrets are hidden.** Twelve-storied pagoda is the throat. Sounds express emotions, controlling the body's Qi. For example, Ha (哈) sound on exhalation raises the spirit and leads Qi outward, strengthening Guardian Qi (Wei Qi, 衛氣). Hen (哼) sound on inhalation calms the spirit, leading Qi inward and nourishing Marrow Qi (Sui Qi, 髓氣).

This sentence can also be interpreted that through asking, you will learn all hidden secrets of practice.

## 牛郎橋星 (21)

**Cowherd bridge stars.** The bridge joins Cowherd (Niu Lang, 牛郎) and Weaving Lady (Zhi Nu, 織女), so the baby embryo can be conceived. This bridge is the Xin (heart). The mind brings Yin and Yang together so they can interact.

## 五十境內隱鄉關 (22)

**In the fifty realms, the mysterious gateways are concealed.** Fifty realms are the vertebrae within which the spinal cord (Thrusting Vessel) is concealed. Mysterious gateways refers to the Water Path (Shui Lu, 水路), circulating in the Thrusting Vessel. Water path meditation is crucial to brain washing (Xi Sui, 洗髓) for spiritual enlightenment. Its secrets have been concealed in Buddhist and Daoist monasteries for more than fifteen centuries.

### 膽神龍曜字威明 (23)

**Gall bladder spirit, Long Yao, means majestic and bright.** The spirit of the gall bladder is called Long Yao (龍曜). It is also associated with the liver. When it manifests, the eyes are bright and majestic. The gall bladder (Yang organ) is the paired organ of the liver (Yin organ).

### 肺神華皓自虛成 (24)

**Lung spirit, Hua Hao, is completed from emptiness.** The spirit of the lungs is called Hua Hao (華皓). It is associated with the nose, which takes in air (emptiness) and fills the lungs with life.

### 肝神龍煙字含明 (25)

**Liver spirit, Long Yan, contains brightness.** The spirit of the liver, called Long Yan (龍煙), is associated with the eyes. When the liver is healthy, the eyes are bright and sharp.

### 心神丹元字守靈 (26)

**Heart spirit, Dan Yuan, contains and maintains the Ling.** The spirit of the heart is called Dan Yuan (丹元). It contains the Ling (靈) and maintains its activities.

### 織女運轉 (27)

**Weaving lady circulates and turns the wheel.** This is the Huang Ting (黃庭) cavity where the Spiritual Embryo is conceived. The lady is preparing for the baby's birth.

### 腎神玄冥字育嬰 (28)

**Kidney spirit, Xuan Ming, (玄冥) contains nourishment for the baby.** It nourishes the production of sperm. The kidneys are called Internal Kidneys (Nei Shen, 內腎), while the testicles are called External Kidneys (Wai Shen, 外腎). They are related to each other in function, responsible for reproduction and nourishment of new life.

脾神常在宇魂亭 (29)

**Spleen spirit, Chang Zai, is concealed in the soul pavilion.** The spleen spirit, Chang Zai (常在), is related to the soul.

中丹田 (30)

**Middle Dan Tian.** The diaphragm, under the heart.

二腎府之穴 (31)

**Cavities of two kidney residences.** These two cavities are also called Shenshu (B-23, 腎俞, Kidney's Hollow). Through them, the kidney Qi enters and leaves at the back. (The descriptive characters should be behind the kidneys, not the throat.)

正丹田 (32)

**Real Lower Dan Tian.** Second brain or biobattery where abundant Qi is accumulated in Qigong practice. This maintains physical strength and health. From here, Qi is led up through the Thrusting Vessel (Chong Mai, 衝脈) to nourish the brain, open the third eye and attain spiritual enlightenment.

陰陽玄踏車 (35)

**Stepping car (water pump) of Yin-Yang mystery.** Water pump or water wheel, which implies the Huiyin. Through control of the Huiyin cavity, you can lead Qi to the Fire Path (Huo Lu, 火路, Yang) or the Water Path (Shui Lu, 水路, Yin). This method of controlling the body's Yin and Yang was kept secret in the past. (Chinese characters should be placed closer to the water pump.)

坎水逆流 (36)

**Kan water flows in the reverse direction. Kan** (坎) represents water in the Eight **Trigrams.** Kan water (Kan Shui, 坎水) refers to the Qi circulating in the body. Through the pumping action of the Huiyin, Kan water is led up to nourish the brain.

*"This illustration has never before been passed down to others, because this Elixir Dao (丹道, Dao of refining elixir) is so wide and refined. Those not wise enough will not be able to gain (the key), so it is rarely seen in this world. By accident, I found this illustration and writing in Gao Song Mountain (高松山, high pine mountain). It was hanging on the wall. The skills of this drawing are very refined, and the tendons, joints, vessels, and Qi channels are clearly indicated and interpreted. Every one conceals the important key in detail. I looked and pondered it for a long time, and feel I have comprehended some meaning within. Consequently, I started to realize deeply that the uttering and taking (Tu Na, 吐納) of the whole body is just like the substantial and insubstantial of heaven and earth. If one can enlighten it and comprehend it clearly, then more than half of the achievement of reaching Great Dao of Golden Elixir (Jin Dan Da Dao, 金丹大道) will have been achieved already. I dare not keep this secret to myself and thus publish it enthusiastically so it can be spread to the public."*

— Copied and discerned by Su Yun Daoist

此圖向無傳本，緣丹道廣大精微，鈍根人無從領取，是以罕傳於世。予偶於高松山齋中檢觀書畫。此圖適懸壁上，繪法工細，筋、節、脈、絡註解分明。一一悉藏竅要，展玩良久，覺有會心。始悟一身之呼吸吐納，即天地之盈虛消息。茍能神而明之，金丹大道，思過半矣！誠不敢私為獨得，爰急付梓，以廣流傳。

素雲道人敬摹并識

## References

1. 《難經・二十七難》：〝脈有奇經八脈者，不拘于十二經。〞

2. 李時珍《奇經八脈考》：〝奇經凡八脈，不拘制于十二正經，無表里配合，故謂之奇。〞

3. 《實用氣功學》：〝督脈起於會陰，循背而行于身之后，為陽脈之總督，故曰陽脈之海。任脈起於會陰，循腹而行于身之前，為陰脈之承任，故曰陰脈之海。〞〝人能通此兩脈，則百脈皆通，自然周身流轉，無有停壅之患，而長生久視之道斷在此矣。〞

4. *The Study of Practical Chinese Medical Qigong* (實用中醫氣功學), by Ma, Ji-Ren (馬濟人), 上海科學技術出版社, Shanghai, China, 1992.

5. 任脈：一・它循行于胸腹之正中，并在中極、關元穴與足三陰經交會，在天突、廉泉穴與陰維脈交會，在陰交穴與衝脈交會。二・足三陰經上接手三陰經。這樣任脈就可以溝通手、足三陰經的全部六條陰經了。

6. 督脈（總督諸陽）：一・它循行于背部之正中，其脈氣多次與十二正經的手、足的全部六條陽經相交會。最集中的地點是大椎穴，手足三陽經都在這裡左右相會。二・帶脈出于第二腰椎繞腰一轉，陽維脈與督脈也交會在風府、啞門，這樣督脈就起著統率的作用了。

7. 李時珍《奇經八脈考》：〝八脈散在群書者，略而不悉。醫不知此，罔探病機；仙家不知此，難安爐鼎。時珍不敏，參考諸說，萃集于左，所以備學仙、醫者筌蹄之用云。〞 〝是故醫而知乎八脈，則十二經、十五絡之大旨得矣；仙而知乎八脈，則虎龍升降、玄牝幽微之竅妙得矣。〞

8. 《內經》：〝天人相應。

9. 《金丹大成集》：〝子午乃天地之中也，在天為日、月，在人為心、腎，在時為子、午，在卦為坎、離，在位為南、北。〞

10. 楊繼洲在《針灸大成》：〝人身之任督，以背腹言，天地之子午；以南北言，可以分，可以合者也。分之以見陰陽不雜，合之以見渾淪之無間，一而二，二而一也。〞

11. 李時珍在《奇經八脈考》：〝任督兩脈，乃身之子午也，乃丹家陽火陰符升降之道，坎水離火交媾之鄉。〞

12. 《脈望》：〝丹田，性命之本。道士思神，比丘坐禪，皆聚真氣于臍下，良由此也。丹田內有神龜，呼吸真氣，非口鼻之呼吸也。口鼻只是呼吸之門戶，丹田為氣之本源，聖人下手之處，收藏真一所居，故曰胎息。〞

13. 《黃庭內景經・梁丘子注》：〝黃者，中之色也；庭者，四方之中也。外指事即天中，人中，地中；內指事即腦中，心中，脾中。〞

14. 《黃庭外景經・石和陽注》：〝命門之上，有玄關二竅，左玄右牝，中虛一處，名曰黃庭。〞

15. 《養生秘錄・金丹問答》：〝黃庭正在何處？答曰：在膀胱之上，脾之下，腎之前，肝之左，肺之右也。〞

16. 王錄識餘云：〝銅人針灸圖，載臟腑一身俞穴有玉環，余不知玉環是何物。〞張紫陽玉清金華祕文，論神仙結丹處曰：〝心上腎下，脾左肝右，生門在前，密戶居後，其連如環，其白如棉，方圓徑寸，密裹一身之精粹，此即玉環。〞

17. 《易筋經・附錄》：〝神仙結丹處。曰：心下腎上脾左肝右，生門在前，密戶居后，其連如環，其白如綿，方圓徑寸，包裹一身之精粹。・・・其處與臍相對。人之命脈根蒂也。〞

18. 〝督脈的內氣循行上向是自下而上，但至上唇齦交穴與任脈交接后，內氣則沿任脈上而下。成循環周流的情況。督脈與任脈上下交接處，分別稱為上鵲橋與下鵲橋。〞

19. *The Study of Practical Chinese Medical Qigong* (實用中醫氣功學), by Ma, Ji-Ren (馬濟人), 上海科學技術出版社, Shanghai, China, p. 682, 1992.

20. 《入藥鏡》：〝恍恍惚惚，杳杳冥冥，自然身心如暢，如醉如痴，肌膚爽透，美在其中。〞

21. 《奇經八脈考》：〝昏昏默默，如醉如痴。〞

22. 《金丹大成集》：〝腦後曰玉枕關，夾脊曰轆轤關，水火之際曰尾閭關。〞

23. 據《性命圭旨全書・采藥歸壺圖》所列：天人合發之機；子母分胎之路；任督接交之處；陰陽變化之鄉；九靈鐵鼓；三足金蟾；太玄關；藏金斗；尾閭穴；生死穴；朝天嶺；氣海門；曹溪路；三岔口；平易穴；咸池；陰端；禁門；會陰；穀道；龍虎穴；三岔骨；河車路；上天梯等。

24. 《性命圭旨全書・天人合發采藥歸壺》：〝蓋精氣聚散常在此處，水火發端也在此處，陰陽變化也在此處，有無出入也在此處，子母分胎也在此處。〞〝其穴言于任督二脈中間，上通天谷，下達湧泉。〞又〝此穴干涉最大，系人生死岸頭。故仙家名為生死窟。《參同契》云：筑固靈株者此也。拘畜禁門者此也。《黃庭經》云：閉塞命門保玉都者此也。閉子精路可長活者，此也。〞

25. 《還丹訣》：〝端身正坐，運氣自尾閭起，一撞三關至泥丸。合而神水下降，復還丹田。曰大還丹。自腎轉肝，自肝傳心，自心傳脾，傳肺，周而復始，再至丹田，曰小還丹。〞

26. 行氣如九曲珠，無微不到。

CHAPTER 6

# Embryonic Breathing
# 胎息

## 6-1. Introduction 介紹

More than a hundred ancient documents which discuss Embryonic Breathing (Tai Xi, 胎息), were written by experienced Qigong masters in different historical periods. Embryonic Breathing is one of the very few subjects discussed seriously and in depth. Why has this subject been regarded as so important to Nei Dan (內丹, Internal Elixir) Qigong practitioners?

In the previous chapter, we discussed the body's circulatory network of bioelectricity, or Qi. For this Qi to circulate smoothly, we must first concern ourselves with the biobattery, the energy supply source of this network. For longevity we need a strong and healthy body, and an efficient Qi system. When this Qi system performs efficiently, we cannot only maintain physical health, but also lead extra Qi up the spinal cord (Chong Mai, 衝脈) to nourish the brain, which enhances the spirit of vitality. The method of using Qi to strengthen the body is called Muscle/Tendon Changing Qigong (Yi Jin Gong, 易筋功), while using it to nourish the marrow and brain for enlightenment is called Marrow/Brain Washing Qigong (Xi Sui Gong, 洗髓功).

In realizing these benefits, we need to condition the biobattery, the Real Lower Dan Tian, to produce the Qi and store it abundantly. Embryonic Breathing is the method developed through thousands of years of experience.

Embryonic Breathing is also called Cavity Breathing (Xue Wei Hu Xi, 穴位呼吸) or Dan Tian Breathing (Dan Tian Hu Xi, 丹田呼吸). I call it No Extremity Breathing (Wuji Hu Xi, 無極呼吸) or Second Brain Breathing. It is also called Wuji breathing because its final goal is the Wuji state, where you focus only at the center of your Real Lower Dan Tian (Zhen Xia Dan Tian, 真下丹田).

The purposes of Embryonic Breathing are:

1. **To calm the body and mind.** The first goal is to establish the mind in a state of extreme calm, in the Real Lower Dan Tian. Then Qi is not led away from the center and consumed. The brain is not agitated nor the body excited,

and Qi can be accumulated in abundance. *Dao De Jing*, Chapter 16 (道德經 · 十六章) said, "Approach the nothingness (emptiness) to its extremity, and maintain calmness with sincerity..."[1] This implies extreme calm of the body and mind. Your conscious mind gradually disappears, and the subconscious mind connected to the spirit awakens.

2. **To condition the Real Lower Dan Tian (biobattery) and improve the storage capacity of Qi.** To increase Qi storage capacity higher than ordinary people, the Real Lower Dan Tian must be conditioned. Refer to *Qigong—The Secret of Youth*.

3. **To accumulate abundant Qi in the Real Lower Dan Tian.** This process charges the biobattery to an abundant level and facilitates the Qigong practice of muscle/tendon changing and marrow/brain washing.

4. **To stimulate production of hormones (Original Essence) in the adrenals, testicles or ovaries, and pancreas.** Hormones catalyze the body's biochemical reactions. Abundant healthy hormones keep the body's metabolism and Qi production smooth and healthy. Establishing healthy hormone levels is the key to longevity.

5. **To make the body strong and healthy through muscle/tendon changing.** When abundant Qi accumulates in the Real Lower Dan Tian, that in the Eight Vessels (Ba Mai, 八脈) and Twelve Primary Qi Channels (Shi Er Jing, 十二經) will also flow strongly. This is crucial to maintaining physical health.

6. **For longevity and enlightenment, through marrow/brain washing.** When abundant Qi is led into the bone marrow, the production of blood cells proceeds smoothly. This is vital in slowing down the aging process, because blood cells are the main carriers of oxygen and nutrition. Also, when abundant Qi is led up through the spinal cord to nourish the brain, the spirit of vitality is raised and the third eye can open. This is the achievement of Buddhahood or enlightenment.

## 6-2. THEORY OF EMBRYONIC BREATHING 胎息理論之簡介

Since so many documents are available, we cannot include them all in this book. Here we briefly discuss the concepts and methods of Embryonic Breathing, as they relate to spiritual cultivation. Again, for a more detailed discussion, refer to the book, *Qigong Meditation—Embryonic Breathing*.

**Definition of Embryonic Breathing** 胎息之定義. According to the ancient documents, there are two definitions of Embryonic Breathing. One is to locate the spiritual center and the Qi center, then unite Shen and Qi at the Real Lower Dan Tian.

These two centers are the two poles of the energy body. Bring the Shen down to unite with the Qi at the Real Lower Dan Tian, which is the Qi center (Figure 6-1). Thus you return to the Wuji state, the origin of life. You are returning to the Real Lower Dan Tian where you were conceived as a fetus. In this Wuji state, you return your being to nature.

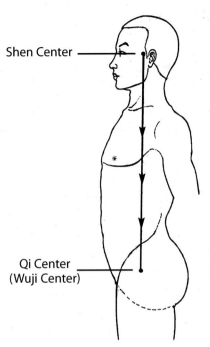

Figure 6-1. Unification of Shen and Qi at the Wuji Center

The earliest document in which this concept of Embryonic Breathing was propounded is Lao Zi's *Dao De Jing*. Chapter 16 says, "Approach the nothingness (emptiness) to its extremity, and maintain calmness with sincerity. Millions of objects (lives) in action allow me to observe their cyclic repetition. Though there are so many objects, each individual must repeatedly return to its root (origin). When it returns to the root, it means calmness. When it is calmed, it means repetition of a life. When the life repeats, it means constant natural cycle."[2] From this document we see the purpose of Embryonic Breathing in tracing back the root of our lives, and understanding the cyclic repetition of nature. That means returning our spiritual being to the Wuji state (無極, No Extremity, neutral state) of human life and thus reaching the origin of our spiritual nature.

Regulate Shen through cultivating the mind to an empty, neutral state. Shen finds its center and stays at its residence. Without this, we remain locked in the human emotional matrix. The mind cannot see the origin of the spirit, nor can we lead Qi to its residence (Real Lower Dan Tian) and keep it there. The very beginning of Embryonic Breathing is searching for the spiritual origin in the center of the brain (Upper Dan Tian) and the origin of Qi at the center of physical gravity, the Real Lower Dan Tian.

To regulate Shen, Chapter 6 of *Dao De Jing* said, "The Valley Spirit (Gu Shen, 谷神) does not die, then it is called Xuan Pin (玄牝). The door (key) to reach this Xuan Pin is the root of heaven and earth (nature). It is very soft and continuous as though it existed. When used, it will not be exhausted."[3] Shen is called Valley Spirit (Gu Shen, 谷神) because it resides in the Spiritual Valley (Shen Gu, 神谷), the space between the two hemispheres of the brain. Xuan Pin (玄牝) means the marvelous and mysterious Dao, the mother of creation of millions of objects. The goal of regulating the Shen is to keep it at the Spiritual Valley, its residence.

Breathe softly, slenderly, and deeply like a newborn baby. Chapter 10 of *Dao De Jing* said, "When bearing and managing the Po (魄, Vital Spirit) and embracing the state of oneness (Bao Yi, 抱一), can it be not separate? When concentrating Qi to reach softness, can it be soft as a baby? When cleansing the thought to reach purity, can it be without flaw?"[4] *Ling Jian Zi's Dao Yin Zi-Wu Recording* (靈劍子導引子午記注) said, "What is Embryonic Breathing? It is a method of Embracing Oneness (Bao Yi, 抱一) and keeping it in the neutral state."[5]

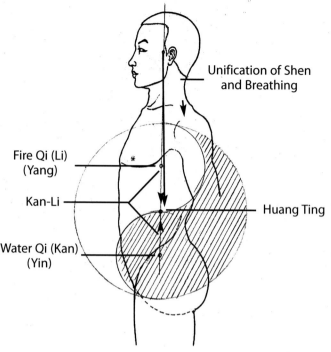

Figure 6-2. Conceiving the Spiritual Embryo

Embryonic Breathing means to regulate the mind and Shen to their most calm and concentrated state, and to accumulate abundant Qi at the Real Lower Dan Tian, then unite the Shen and Qi to return the being to its origin. Embryonic Breathing has always been very important in Chinese Qigong practice, being the method of storing Qi in the Real Lower Dan Tian. Through Embryonic Breathing you charge your biobattery to a high level. Then your vital energy is raised, the immune system is strengthened and the body reconditioned.

In Buddhist and Daoist tradition, Embryonic Breathing is defined as conceiving a Spiritual Embryo (Shen Tai, 神胎) at the Huang Ting cavity (黃庭). When it is ready, lead it up to the Upper Dan Tian to be born (opening the third eye). To achieve this, first build up a high level of Water Qi (Shui Qi, 水氣, Original Qi) at the Real Lower Dan Tian. Lead it up, and lead Fire Qi (Huo Qi, 火氣, Post-Heaven Qi) down from the Middle Dan Tian, so they meet at the Huang Ting (黃庭). This process is called intercourse of dragon and tiger (Long Hu Jiao Gou, 龍虎交媾), the interaction of Yin and Yang, commonly called Kan and Li (坎離). This results in the conception of life. Then, you lead Shen down to meet this life, until a new Shen develops in the embryo. This process is called Mutual Dependence of Mother and

Son (Mu Zi Xiang Yi, 母子相依). Mother means Qi and Son means Shen. From this process, a Spiritual Embryo is conceived (Figure 6-2).

When the Spiritual Embryo is ready, lead it up through Chong Mai to the brain. When the energy reaches a high level, the third eye (Tian Yan, 天眼) opens.

**Theoretical Foundations of Embryonic Breathing** 胎息之理論基礎. Here we review the role and function the Eight Vessels (Ba Mai, 八脈) play in Qigong practice, especially in Nei Dan (內丹) Qigong.

1. The Eight Vessels comprise four Yin and four Yang vessels which balance each other. These eight vessels comprise the major framework of the body's Qi network and regulate the Qi in the Twelve Primary Qi Channels (Shi Er Jing, 十二經).

2. They are Qi reservoirs that store Qi, but like Yin and Yang primary channels, the Yang vessels manifest Qi, while the Yin vessels preserve it.

3. The Conception Vessel (Ren Mai, 任脈) in front is a Yin vessel that balances the Yang Governing Vessel. It regulates the Qi in the six primary Yin channels (Qi rivers) while the Governing Vessel (Du Mai, 督脈) governs the Qi of the six primary Yang channels. Since these Twelve Channels distribute Qi through the body, the two vessels control Qi distribution throughout the body.

4. The physical structure of the vessels is very likely constructed of various layers of tendon sandwiched between fasciae. Tendons are better conductors than muscles, while fasciae are insulators (poor conductors). This structure comprises a sort of battery to store Qi, which flows better in tendons than muscles. The Governing Vessel exhibits various layers of tendons attached at the center line of the spine, sandwiched by fasciae.

5. The Girdle Vessel (Dai Mai, 帶脈) is extreme Yang and counterbalances the Thrusting Vessel (Chong Mai, 衝脈) which is extreme Yin. The Girdle Vessel's Qi expands horizontally, providing physical and mental balance, while the Thrusting Vessel centers your body and mind (Figure 6-3). These are the two most vital vessels of the Qi network. When Qi expands in the Girdle Vessel, Guardian Qi (Wei Qi, 衛氣) manifests strongly, as does the immune system. When Qi is abundant in the Thrusting Vessel, the central energy line is strong, and Shen is raised up. The glands along the central energy line, the pineal, pituitary, adrenals, and testicles (or ovaries), are nourished and their hormone production stimulated. Marrow Qi is also abundant, so healthy blood cells are produced. We will discuss this in more detail in a future publication, *Spiritual Enlightenment Meditation*.

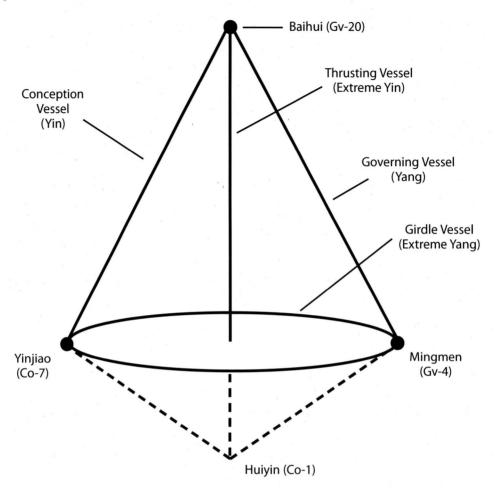

Figure 6-3. Thrusting Vessel and Governing Vessel

6. When you wake up in the morning, you start using your body. Your exhalation is longer than inhalation, since your mind is outside the body. Qi is led out to be manifested. The Conception and Governing Vessels regulate the Qi in the Twelve Primary Qi Channels, so it circulates aggressively in the Conception and Governing Vessels. But at night you sleep, with your body relaxed and your inhalation longer than exhalation. Qi is led inward to the central energy line, and Guardian Qi shrinks. Hormones are produced by the glands, and the brain obtains Qi nourishment. This promotes dreaming, as the brain cells readjust their energy.

This is no different from the Qi cycle of a fish. During daytime, Qi circulates strongly along the upper and lower contours of the fish, so the fins and tail move aggressively. At night, this Qi circulation weakens and Qi is focused at the center line. Electromagnetic waves are emitted from the third eye of the fish, enabling it to swim without colliding with obstacles or other fish (Figure 6-4).[6]

During daytime, a tree's energy spreads up and out from the root, which is its biobattery, to exchange Qi with that of the sun. At night, its Qi returns to its center and back down to the root (Figure 6-5). All living things are part of the Dao, which remains the same throughout nature. If you comprehend one clearly, you can interpret others easily.

7. The other four vessels exist in pairs. They are the Yin Heel Vessel (Yinqiao Mai, 陰蹻脈), Yin Linking Vessel (Yinwei Mai, 陰維脈), Yang Heel Vessel (Yangqiao Mai, 陽蹻脈) and

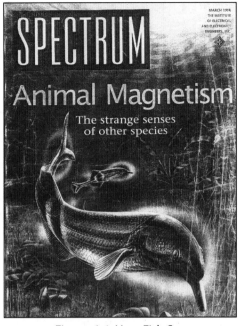

Figure 6-4. How Fish See Things in the Dark

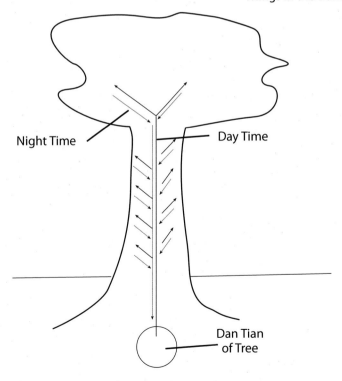

Figure 6-5. The Tree's Energy Moves Upward and Outward in the Daytime, and Moves Downward and Inward at Nighttime

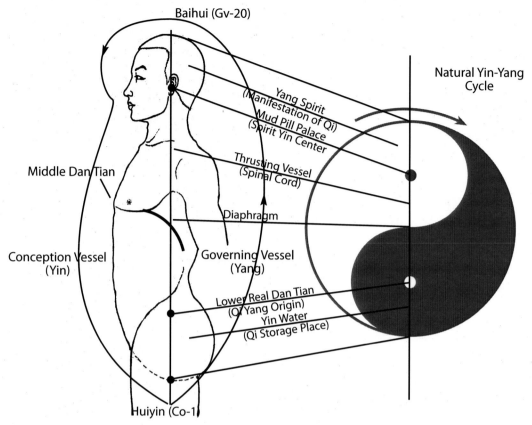

Figure 6-6. The Body's Yin and Yang, and the Two Polarity Centers

Yang Linking Vessel (Yangwei Mai, 陽維脈). The two Yin vessels connect at the Huiyin, where they meet the other two Yin vessels, the Conception and Thrusting Vessels. The perineum is called Huiyin, the gate which connects all four Yin vessels in the body. When this gate opens, Qi manifests, and when it closes, Qi is preserved. For example, when you are happy and excited, exhalation is longer than inhalation, and the body turns Yang which leads excess Yang to the internal organs, especially the heart. Then you automatically balance it by making a sound of "Ha" while pushing the perineum out. By contrast, when you are sad or scared, inhalation is longer than exhalation and you feel cold. To preserve Qi, you hold up the perineum automatically to close the gate. Using the perineum to control Qi in the body is one of the hidden keys in Qigong practice.

**Illustration of the Body's Yin and Yang Polarities** 人身陰陽兩儀解. Here we compare the natural Taiji Yin-Yang symbol with the body's Yin-Yang energy structure to discover the correspondences between them. Since one's body is part of nature, one should be able to interpret its Qi manifestation using the Yin-Yang symbol (Figure 6-6).

1. The direction of Qi circulation along the Conception and Governing Vessels is the opposite of the natural Yin-Yang cycle, so Yin and Yang in the body can be balanced by natural Yin and Yang.

2. Shen is considered Yang, and the term Yang Shen (陽神, Yang Spirit) is commonly used in Chinese Qigong documents. Shen is the general who controls the manifestation of Qi. When Shen is high, Qi is controlled and manifests effectively. Once you raise Shen to a high level, your vital force is enhanced. Normally, Shen is raised through the Baihui, the place of extreme Yang at the top of the Yin-Yang symbol. Baihui means 'hundred meetings', the meeting place of all the body's Qi. It is the pivotal point controlling all the body's energy, the most Yang place in the body.

3. Huiyin is the most Yin place in the body. It is sometimes called Haidi (海底, sea bottom), because Qi is similar to water, with the intestines as the ocean which stores it. While Qi remains here, the body is calm and peaceful, but when it is consumed through manifestation, mind and body are excited and Shen diverges. Keep calm by inhaling deeply and leading Qi down to the abdomen, then exhale while relaxing. In this way tension dissipates and blood pressure is lowered.

4. The body's Yin and Yang are connected by the Thrusting Vessel. The Spirit Yin Center in the Mud Pill Palace, controls, governs, and restrains the Yang Shen's manifestation. If Shen stays here, it is focused and centered. To bring Shen to this Yin center, first calm the mind, and avoid emotional disturbance and desire.

5. The Real Lower Dan Tian produces Qi and stores it, supplying it to the body and brain. The Upper Dan Tian controls the quality of Qi. With the Girdle Vessel (Extreme Yang Vessel) and Thrusting Vessel (Extreme Yin Vessel), it forms a spiritual cultivation triangle (Figure 6-7). The more Guardian Qi there is, the higher the Shen can be raised. The base of the triangle represents physical life, while the center line represents spiritual life.

**Interaction of Yin and Yang (Intercourse of Dragon and Tiger)** 龍虎交媾
Keep your Shen and Qi at their centers to Embrace Oneness (Bao Yi, 抱一). These are two poles of the same life, which synchronize and correspond with each other. Physically they are two, but in function they are one. One is for physical life and the other for spiritual life, but they are indivisible.

The first definition of Embryonic Breathing is to unite Shen and Qi at the Real Lower Dan Tian, to return to the source of life. Here, life is initiated and developed.

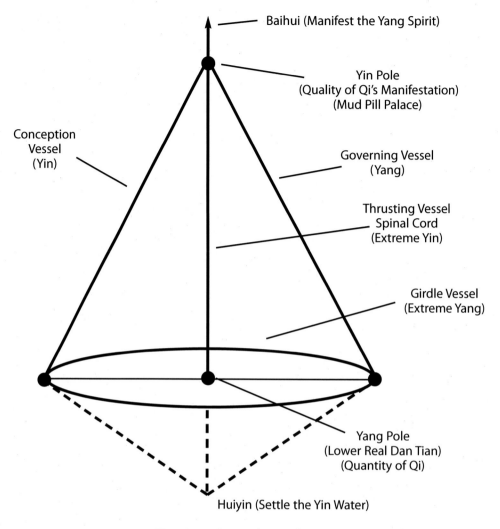

Baihui (Manifest the Yang Spirit)

Yin Pole
(Quality of Qi's Manifestation)
(Mud Pill Palace)

Conception
Vessel
(Yin)

Governing Vessel
(Yang)

Thrusting Vessel
Spinal Cord
(Extreme Yin)

Girdle Vessel
(Extreme Yang)

Yang Pole
(Lower Real Dan Tian)
(Quantity of Qi)

Huiyin (Settle the Yin Water)

Figure 6-7. Spiritual Triangle

To many Daoists, the first goal of Embryonic Breathing is to find this center to unite Shen and Qi (Figure 6-8). Since the goal of this practice is to return to the Wuji center, I call this Wuji Breathing (Wuji Xi, 無極息).

The second definition of Embryonic Breathing is to conceive a Spiritual Embryo (Shen Tai, 神胎) at the Huang Ting. Concentrate the wisdom mind (Yi, 意), lead Fire Qi down from the Middle Dan Tian and Water Qi up from the Real Lower Dan Tian to meet at Huang Ting (Figure 6-9). This interaction of Yin and Yang is called intercourse of dragon and tiger (Long Hu Jiao Gou, 龍虎交媾), or Kan and Li (坎離). Then you lead Shen down from the Upper Dan Tian to unite with Qi and conceive the Spiritual Embryo.

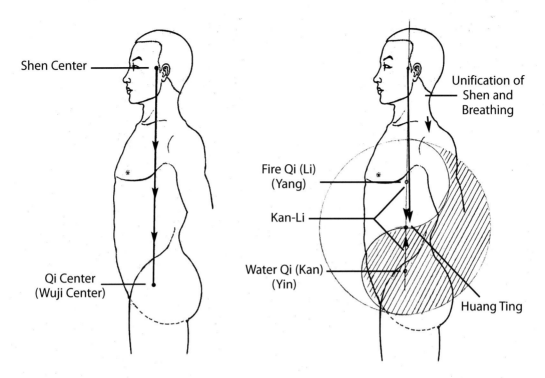

Figure 6-8. Unification of Shen and Qi at the Wuji Center

Figure 6-9. Conceiving the Spiritual Embryo

## Summaries

1. *The Complete Book of Principal Contents of Human Life and Temperament, About Large and Small Tripod and Furnace,* (性命圭旨全書, 大小鼎爐說) says, "Huang Ting (黃庭) is the tripod, Qi Xue (氣穴, Qi cavity) is the furnace. Huang Ting is just on top of Qi Xue, interconnected with numerous Luo (絡). It is the meeting place of hundreds of Qi vessels in the body. Original Qi (Yuan Qi, 元氣) is dense between these two cavities and is called Small Tripod Furnace (Xiao Ding Lu, 小鼎爐). If the Qian (乾, brain) is the tripod and the Kun (坤, abdomen) is the furnace, then Ni Wan (泥丸, Upper Dan Tian) is the tripod and the Lower Dan Tian is the furnace. This is called Big Tripod Furnace (Da Ding Lu, 大鼎爐)."[7] This document explains the large Yin-Yang and Small Yin-Yang symbols and how they relate to the body (Figures 6-10 and 6-11).

2. In the Small Tripod Furnace (Xiao Ding Lu, 小鼎爐), you search for the Wuji state of Kan and Li. Then the Spiritual Embryo (Shen Tai, 神胎) is conceived. Later, when it is mature, it is led up for cultivation of spiritual enlightenment.

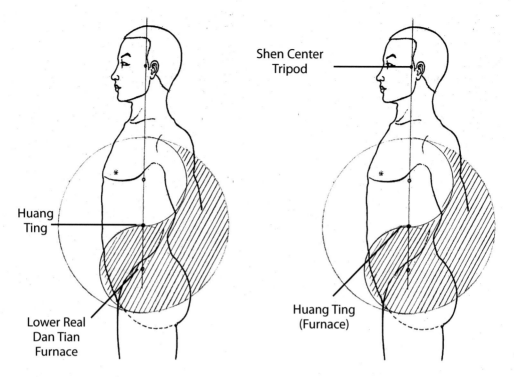

**Figure 6-10. Small Tripod and Furnace**  **Figure 6-11. Large Tripod and Furnace**

3. In the Big Tripod Furnace (Da Ding Lu, 大鼎爐), you look for the Wuji state of your original being, returning life to its very origin. Bring Shen down to the Real Lower Dan Tian to unite with the Qi.

## 6-3. Methods of Embryonic Breathing 胎息法

Here we discuss the practice of Embryonic Breathing. First, your mind must locate the Upper Dan Tian and the Real Lower Dan Tian. Next, you condense the spirit to a higher level of focus and produce more abundant Qi. Then lead the spirit and the Qi to their residences, and keep them there. Finally, you unite the spirit and the Qi at the Real Lower Dan Tian.

We briefly discuss the method of the Qi's Kan and Li and how to unite it with the Shen at the Huang Ting (黃庭) to conceive the Spiritual Embryo. The method of leading Qi up to nourish the brain and Shen will be discussed in the forthcoming book, *Grand Circulation and Enlightenment Meditation*.

**Times to Practice.** The best times to practice are dawn, noon, dusk, and midnight, but this is not easy to achieve. I recommend dawn and right before you go to sleep. If your time schedule allows you to take an afternoon nap, use this time to practice Embryonic Breathing. Your body is most Yang during early afternoon, and Embryonic Breathing stores the surplus Qi inside.

When your mind and body are very calm and relaxed, you may allow yourself to fall asleep. Embryonic Breathing is not the same as other Nei Dan meditation in which you lead the Qi. In Nei Dan you should not fall asleep since Qi will enter the wrong path. However, in Embryonic Breathing your mind is not leading the Qi, so falling asleep will not cause any problem.

You should not be restricted to the suggested times. Once you have mastered Embryonic Breathing, you can practice anytime and anywhere.

**Orientation of Practice.** Embryonic Breathing takes advantage of natural Qi, the most significant being the Qi of the sun, moon, and earth. So orient your meditation accordingly. (Table 6-1) For a detailed exposition, refer to *The Root of Chinese Qigong*, by YMAA.

### Table 6-1. Meditation Orientation and Times

| Timing | Purpose | Orientation | Natural Qi Source |
|--------|---------|-------------|-------------------|
| Dawn | Nourishing | Face east | Sun |
| | Retreating* | Face west | Sun |
| Noon | To calm down | Any direction | —— |
| Dusk | Prevent retreating | Face east | Sun |
| Retreating | | Face west | Sun |
| Night** | Nourishing | Face south | Earth's magnetic field |
| | Retreating | Face north | Earth's magnetic field |

*Retreating means to remove some Qi from your body to make it more Yin.

**To absorb Qi from the moon, meditate two to three days before full moon, facing the moon. Not recommended after full moon, since the moon then drains your Qi.

## Recognize the Yin Center of the Upper Dan Tian and the Yang Center of the Real Lower Dan Tian

(Shang Xia Dan Yin He Yu Xian Dan Tian Yang He Zhi Ren Shi, 上丹田陰核心與下丹田陽核心之認識, Xue Wei Ren Tong, 穴位認同)

The first step is to recognize the Yin center of the Upper Dan Tian (Yin Shen, 陰神) and the Yang center of the Real Lower Dan Tian (Yang Quan, 陽泉)(Figure 6-6). The only way to locate these two centers is through inner feeling.

The Upper Dan Tian (Shang Dan Tian, 上丹田) is at the center of the Spiritual Valley (Shen Gu, 神谷), where the pineal and pituitary glands are located. This is the Mud Pill Palace (Ni Wan Gong, 泥丸宮), the central spiritual residence (Shen Shi,

神室, Upper Dan Tian). It lies where the line joining the tops of the ears meets the line joining the Yintang (M-HN-3, 印堂) with the Qiangjian (Gv-18, 強間). The Yin Shen is at the center of the Dan Tian, and has a different quality of feeling than the rest of the Dan Tian itself. To recognize this point through feeling, be free of emotional disturbance and external attraction, so your mind is clear. Search for the place sincerely, and you will soon find it.

The Yang Quan is the Yang center of the Real Lower Dan Tian (Zhen Xia Dan Tian, 真下丹田) where the large and small intestines are located, a couple of inches above the center of gravity. The whole digestive system constitutes the Real Lower Dan Tian. If you can find its center, you can keep the Qi there, storing it to an abundant level. It is located behind Yinjiao (Co-7, 陰交) and in front of Shiqizhuixia (M-BW-25, 十七椎下) below the 17th vertebra, at the center between these two cavities. Search for this point through feeling when you meditate, and you should find it in a short time.

## Condensing Shen and Qi into Their Centers

(Regulating the mind, spirit, and Qi)(Tiao Xin, 調心)(Tiao Shen, 調神)(Tiao Qi, 調氣)

Having located the Yin center of the Upper Dan Tian, you raise up the spirit and keep it there. Calm your emotional mind (Xin, 心), cut off external distractions and the material attractions of desire and ambition. Concentrate your mind in raising your spirit, and condense it at the Yin spiritual center. Whenever you encounter difficulties in this, simply focus on your breathing. Keep the inhalation soft, long, and slender. Exhale naturally and allow carbon dioxide to be released by itself. In this way you stabilize and calm your mind. Focus your spirit at the Yin spiritual center. In this way the Yang spirit (陽神), the manifestation of Qi by the spirit, is brought under control. On one hand you aim to raise your spirit to a high level, but on the other you need to bring it under the control of the Yin spirit.

To condense Shen at this Yin spiritual center, simply imagine your head as a ball, with the Mud Pill Palace (Ni Wan Gong, 泥丸宮) as its center. Inhale deeply, softly, and slenderly, using Reverse Abdominal Breathing (Ni Fu Hu Xi, 逆腹呼吸) while holding up the Huiyin gently. Imagine the ball shrinking and condensing inward to the Mud Pill Palace. When you exhale, relax, and allow the abdomen and Huiyin to return to their normal state. So you pay more attention to the inhalation, and the Yi of inhalation is strong, which leads Shen and Qi inward to condense at their centers.

## Conditioning the Biobattery (Real Lower Dan Tian)

(Zhen Xia Dan Tian Zhi Gai Liang, 真下丹田之改良)

To store abundant Qi at the Real Lower Dan Tian, first condition it extensively to improve the storage capacity significantly. You cannot expect exceptional Qi capacity from an average biobattery.

The ancient classic of *Muscle/Tendon Changing and Marrow/Brain Washing Qigong* (Yi Jin Jing; Xi Sui Jing, 易筋經・洗髓經) describes the most efficient way of conditioning this biobattery (False and Real Lower Dan Tians), namely through massage and stimulation. Massage gets rid of the fat hidden inside, so the circulation can be smooth, and stimulation conditions the nerves to store a significant amount of Qi there. The conditioning process is long and arduous, and you need a clear grasp of its theory. It is impossible to explain it all here, but it is described in detail in the book, *Qigong—The Secret of Youth*.

A. **Condition your nervous system.**

Conditioning the biobattery requires stimulating the abdomen's nervous system, using abdominal breathing and massage. When enough energy is stored there, it agitates the nervous system, which at first may simply feel warm. After extensive stimulation, the nerves reach their tolerance threshold, and the muscles twitch and vibrate by themselves. No more Qi can be stored, but will simply disperse. It is best to start conditioning practice using massage. Appropriate methods are described in *Qigong—The Secret of Youth*.

B. **Improve the quality of the biobattery's material structure.**

The higher the structural quality of the abdomen and bowels, the better the conditions for storing abundant Qi. There are two ways to reach this goal. One is through massage as described in the last section. The second is through pounding the area with special tools. The force reaches deeper and stimulates the whole system, qualitatively changing the area. Naturally you must be patient, using correct techniques to avoid injury.

C. **Reduce the thickness of fat (insulators).**

To increase the charge of a battery, the insulator between the conductive area must be thin, but with high insulating capability. Fat and fasciae act as insulators in the body, sandwiched between good conductors (muscles). To store more Qi at the Real Lower Dan Tian, you need to reduce the thickness of the fat and improve the insulating capacity of fasciae. This is achieved through massage and pounding, and also through abdominal exercises. Correct methods of exercise reduce the fat and condition the fasciae effectively.

**Increase the quantity of Qi** (Qi Liang Zhi Jia Qiang, 氣量之加強)

Having conditioned your biobattery, you need high quality Qi to store in it. There are three ways to increase the quantity of Qi in the body:

### A. Qi Furnaces.

About two inches below the navel is an area called Qihai (Co-6, 氣海, Qi Ocean) in medical society. In Daoist society it is called Dan Lu (丹爐) (Elixir Furnace) or Dan Tian (Elixir Field), the place which produces Qi. Move the abdomen in abdominal breathing, facilitating conversion of fat into Qi.

### B. Herbs.

Different diets affect the body's Qi, and Chinese medicine uses herbs extensively, some of which increase the body's Qi. Appropriate herbal prescriptions are listed in *Qigong—The Secret of Youth*, although some ingredients are difficult to find, not being in common use. I recommend consulting a qualified Chinese doctor, since these prescriptions have been passed down over fifteen hundred years, and their accuracy is in doubt. Be very cautious when you use them.

### C. Increase hormone production.

Hormones are called Original Essence (Yuan Jing, 元精) in Chinese Qigong. They act as catalysts to facilitate biochemical reactions in the body's metabolism. When hormones are abundant, Qi from biochemical reaction is enhanced. Hormone therapy can extend our lifespan significantly. Qigong practice targets the adrenals, the gonads, and the pituitary and pineal glands.

#### a. Adrenals (Kidneys).

Adrenal glands fit like small cups on top of the kidneys. Each is divided into two parts, the cortex or outer portion, and the medulla, or central section. The cortex and medulla produce different hormones. The cortex, absolutely essential to life, secretes about thirty hormones and regulates several metabolic processes. The medulla produces the hormone epinephrine, commonly called adrenaline.

There are three ways to stimulate hormone production.

i. Massage. This includes circular rubbing and tapping the kidneys. Please refer to the YMAA book, *Qigong Massage*.

ii. Spinal movement. Correct movement of the lower back and spine massages the kidneys, maintaining health and stimulating hormone production. Please refer to the YMAA book, *Back Pain Relief*.

iii. Deep abdominal breathing. This lowers the diaphragm and accesses the adrenal glands, enhancing hormone production.

#### b. Testicles or ovaries (Gonads).

The testicles produce the male hormone testosterone, while the ovaries produce estrogen and progesterone. When these hormones are adequate, the life force is strong and activity is vigorous. There are two ways to stimulate production.

    i. Massage. Traditional techniques for men are described in *Qigong—The Secret of Youth*. To massage the ovaries is more difficult, and the most common way is to circle and rub them gently with the palms.

    ii. Testicle or ovary breathing. Lead the Qi to the sex glands, in coordination with abdominal breathing, to stimulate hormone production. Alternatively one may use imaginary sexual activity, but this can lead you into the domain of illusion and I do not recommend it.

**c. Pituitary and pineal glands.**

These glands are located in the Mud Pill Palace (Ni Wan Gong, 泥丸宮) where the spirit resides. This area can raise your spirit and increase your life span.

The pituitary gland produces growth hormone and stimulates, regulates, and coordinates the functions of the other endocrine glands. For this reason it is called the master gland. Scientists know little about the function of the pineal gland. It produces melatonin and is related to the body's time clock.

    i. Massage. The Mud Pill Palace is connected to the sacrum through the spinal cord and to the bottom of the feet through the two Yin vessels (Yin Heel and Yin Linking Vessels, 陰蹻脈・陰維脈). When the sacrum or the bottoms of the feet are massaged, hormone production of the pituitary and pineal glands is stimulated.

    ii. Brain Washing Qigong practice. Lead the Qi up through the spinal cord to nourish the brain around the Mud Pill Palace, using Embryonic Breathing.

### Store the Qi in Abundance—Embryonic Breathing (Cavity Breathing, Wuji Breathing) ( 胎息 )

These techniques enable you to produce more Qi. You need to store it in the Real Lower Dan Tian, otherwise it flows out to be consumed in manifestation.

Keep your mind in the Real Lower Dan Tian, then Qi will not be led away from its residence. Move the navel (Yinjiao) and the lower back at the same time. The navel is called Sheng Men (生門), the door of life. The lower back is called Bi Hu (閉戶), the closed door, or Mingmen (Gv-4, 命門) cavity between L2 and L3 (Figure 6-12). Through synchronized movement of the front and back, you can locate the Yang water center easily. Your mind initially focuses on both front and back. But later, when you reach the stage of regulating without regulating, the mind will find the center. *The Secret of Embracing Oneness and Containing Three* (抱一函三秘訣) said, "Between the two kidneys is the root, called the elixir foundation of the ancestral herb."[8] This emphasizes the importance of the Mingmen cavity, located between the two internal kidneys.

When you synchronize moving the two doors up and down, extra Qi is produced in both places. Also coordinate with movement of Huiyin. Soon you feel Qi in the Girdle Vessel expanding and contracting (Figure 6-13).

These movements stimulate the glands and enhance production of insulin hormone in the Islets of Langerhans in the pancreas, DHEA (dehydroepiandrosterone) in the adrenal glands, and testosterone (male), or estrogen and progesterone (female), in the sex glands.

In addition to focusing your mind at the Yang center of the Real Lower Dan Tian, also focus it at the Yin center

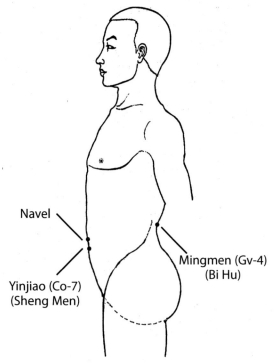

Figure 6-12. Sheng Men (the Door of Life) and Bi Hu (the Closed Door)

of the Upper Dan Tian. These are the Two Polarities of the central energy line, and they correspond and synchronize with each other. They are two aspects of the same thing and cannot be separated. Shen and Qi are like son and mother which cannot be separated when you practice Embryonic Breathing.

When the mind concentrates at the Yin center of the Upper Dan Tian, production of melatonin (pineal gland) and growth hormone (pituitary gland) is also enhanced. These hormones smooth the biochemical reactions, and regulate and improve the metabolism.

The final stage of Embryonic Breathing is to bring Shen down to the Real Lower Dan Tian, to unite with Qi. Qi stays at its residence and is stored to a very high level. This is called harmonization of Shen and Qi (Shen Qi Xiang He, 神氣相合). The two poles unite and become one, embodying the Wuji state, the beginning of life. I call this stage Wuji Breathing (Wuji Xi, 無極息). Lead the Shen down to the Real Lower Dan Tian through the concentrated mind in coordination with breathing.

## Two Ways of Leading Qi and Shen to the Real Lower Dan Tian

There are two types of breathing that enable you to lead Qi and Shen to the Real Lower Dan Tian for effective unification. When Qi is raised up to the brain, the Shen

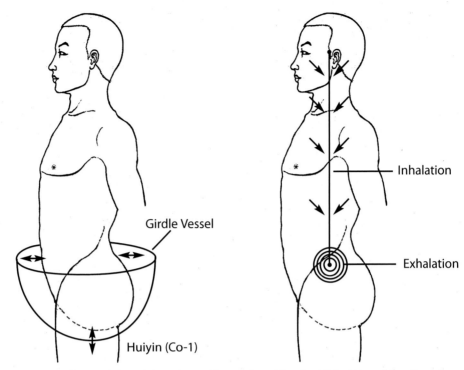

Figure 6-13. Embryonic Breathing

Figure 6-14. The Buddhist Way of Leading the Qi Down to the Real Lower Dan Tian

is excited, and the mind becomes scattered. Blood pressure and heartbeat rise as the manifestation of Qi is enhanced. But when Qi is led down to the Real Lower Dan Tian, it is stored and stays there, and the mind is calmed and relaxed. The body cools down and blood pressure goes down. Shen is also led down by the calm mind.

**Buddhist Way:** Inhale deeply using the mind to lead Qi down through the Thrusting Vessel to the Real Lower Dan Tian. Then exhale, keeping the mind there. When you inhale, the abdomen expands, while the Huiyin gently pushes down. When you exhale, relax the abdomen and Huiyin, and allow them to return naturally (Figure 6-14). Then a lot of Qi is led down to stay at its residence. The more you practice, the faster you can make it happen. This Buddhist technique is used to lower blood pressure, ease the excited mind and also slow down the heartbeat. It effectively relaxes both body and mind.

**Daoist Way:** Inhale to condense Qi into the center as you pull in your abdomen and Huiyin. Guardian Qi (Wei Qi, 衛氣) shrinks and enhances Marrow Qi (Sui Qi, 髓氣). Once Qi is led to the Thrusting Vessel, exhale deeply while leading Qi down (Figure 6-15). While exhaling, push your abdomen and Huiyin out gently, as you store Qi at the Real Lower Dan Tian. This Daoist technique effectively cools the excitement of the body.

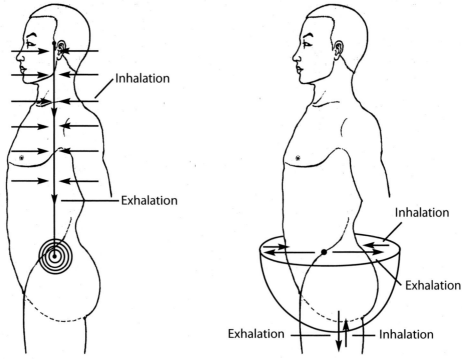

Figure 6-15. The Daoist Way of Leading the Qi Down to the Real Lower Dan Tian

Figure 6-16. Girdle Vessel Breathing

**Two Suggested Approaches:**

1. Buddhist way first and then Daoist: This calms the mind and Shen first, then the calmed mind leads Qi inward.
2. Daoist way first and then Buddhist: This leads Qi inward to calm down the body and then the mind.

    Each has advantages and disadvantages, depending on individual preference.

Having led the Qi down and stored it inside the Real Lower Dan Tian, you must then keep your mind there, using two Embryonic Breathing practices. One is classified as Yang and called Girdle Vessel Breathing (Dai Mai Xi, 帶脈息), while the other is classified as Yin and called Marrow Breathing (Sui Xi, 髓息). Since Qi is led laterally when practicing these techniques, it is most effective to use Reverse Abdominal Breathing (Daoist breathing) instead of Normal Abdominal Breathing (Buddhist breathing).

### Girdle Vessel Breathing (Dai Mai Xi, 帶脈息)

In this form you focus strongly on exhalation. When you exhale, the breath is long and slender, and firmly leads Qi outward from the Girdle Vessel. You gently push your abdomen out and Huiyin down (Figure 6-16). The mind leads Qi out horizontally, a few feet or even yards. The body turns more Yang and its Guardian Qi expands. To enhance the expansion of Qi, once you have exhaled completely, hold your breath for a few seconds, and allow Qi to reach wherever the mind wishes. For even greater effect, also make the sound "Ha" while exhaling. When you inhale, relax, and allow the abdomen and Huiyin to return to normal.

Qi manifestation in the Girdle Vessel is Yang and makes your body and mind Yang. Qi manifestation in the Thrusting Vessel is Yin and calms down your body and mind. Using Girdle Vessel Breathing you can change the body's Qi from Yin to Yang. That strengthens your Guardian Qi and rids you of the feeling of cold. It is suitable for winter time or when you are depressed. Naturally, it consumes your Qi.

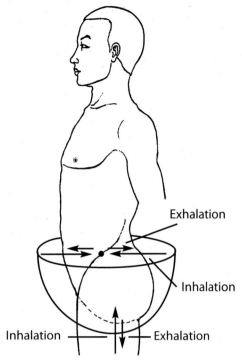

Figure 6-17. Marrow Breathing

## Marrow Breathing (Sui Xi, 髓息)

Here you focus strongly on inhalation. When you inhale, the breath is long and slender and firmly leads Qi inward from the Girdle Vessel, as you draw your abdomen in and Huiyin up (Figure 6-17). The mind continues to lead Qi in until it reaches the Yin center of the Real Lower Dan Tian. The body turns more Yin, and the Guardian Qi shrinks. To lead the Qi in more effectively and keep it at the Real Lower Dan Tian, once you have inhaled completely, hold your breath for a few seconds, and allow the Qi to reach the Yang center within the Yin. When you exhale, relax, and allow the abdomen and Huiyin areas to return to normal.

You are storing the Qi at the Real Lower Dan Tian and also leading it into the bone marrow for marrow washing. Your Guardian Qi shrinks, weakening your resistance to cold, so you should not practice this in the winter. Instead, start in the spring and enhance the practice in the summer. When fall comes, change to Girdle Vessel Breathing to strengthen your Guardian Qi for the winter.

### Conceiving the Spiritual Embryo, the Initiation of Enlightenment (Shen Tai Zhi Yun Yu, 神胎之孕育)

Here is a brief description of the method of conceiving the Spiritual Embryo (Shen Tai, 神胎) and leading it up to the Upper Dan Tian to be born (enlightenment). Please also refer to the forthcoming book about Spiritual Enlightenment Meditation.

Lead Fire Qi (Huo Qi, 火氣, Post-Heaven Qi) down from the Middle Dan Tian (Zhong Dan Tian, 中丹田) and Water Qi (Shui Qi, 水氣, Pre-Heaven Qi) up from the Real Lower Dan Tian to meet at the Huang Ting (黃庭), the inner space between the diaphragm and the Real Lower Dan Tian. This is called Kan and Li. Yin and Yang Qi interact with each other, and the Spiritual Embryo (life) is conceived in the presence of the Shen, which is also led down to meet the Qi at the Huang Ting.

### Summary of Embryonic Breathing:

1. Reversed Abdominal Breathing is more effective.

2. If inhalation and exhalation are of equal length, the body remains neutral.

3. If exhalation is longer than inhalation, it is Girdle Vessel breathing. Qi expands horizontally to build up Guardian Qi. It is also called Skin Breathing (Fu Xi, 膚息) or Body Breathing (Ti Xi, 體息). The spirit is raised and the body energized. You should not practice this too much in the summer or when your body is already energized, as it can make your body too Yang and become harmful. You should practice it in the winter so the Guardian Qi can expand against the cold.

4. If inhalation is longer than exhalation, it is Wuji Breathing. Qi is led to the Real Lower Dan Tian and stored there, charging the biobattery. You should not practice this in the fall or winter, when you need stronger Guardian Qi to defend against the cold. Practice it in the summer and store the excess Qi.

# Breathing's Yin and Yang 呼吸陰陽圖

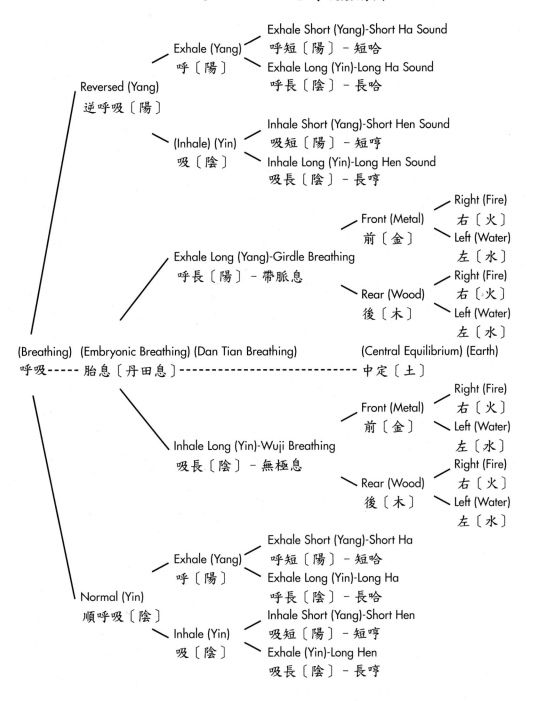

Table 6-2. Breathing's Yin and Yang

# References

1. 《道德經・十六章》：〝致虛極，守靜篤。〞

2. 《道德經・十六章》：〝致虛極，守靜篤；萬物并作，吾以觀其復。夫物芸芸，各復歸其根。歸根曰靜，靜曰復命。〞

3. 《道德經・六章》：〝谷神不死，是謂玄牝。玄牝之門，是謂天地根，綿綿若存，用之不勤。〞

4. 《道德經・十章》：〝載營魄抱一，能無離乎？專氣致柔，能如嬰兒乎？滌除玄鑒，能無疵乎？愛民治國，能無為乎？天門開闔，能為雌乎？明白四達，能無知乎？生之畜之，生而不有，為而不恃，長而不宰，是謂玄德。〞

5. 《靈劍子導引子午記注》：〝胎息者，抱一守中之法也。〞

6. "Animal Magnetism, The Strange Senses of Other Species," P. 32, *IEEE Spectrum,* March, 1996.

7. 《性命圭旨全書 》（大小鼎爐說）：〝黃庭為鼎，氣穴為爐。黃庭正在氣穴上，縷絡相連，乃人身百脈交會之處。〞元氣氤氳二穴之間，謂之〝小鼎爐。〞〝乾位為鼎，坤位為爐。〞即泥丸宮為鼎，下丹田為爐，謂之〝大鼎爐。〞

8. 《抱一函三秘訣》注云：〝兩腎之間，為我之根本，名曰藥祖丹基。〞

## CHAPTER 7

# Important Points in Meditation
# 靜坐要點

## 7-1. INTRODUCTION 介紹

From the previous chapters, you have a sound map of how to practice Small Circulation without doubt and confusion. This can save you years of searching for the correct way. By preparing your journey both physically and psychologically, you lay a smooth path for your expedition. Before a long journey, first check your oil, map, flashlight, spare tire, weather report, and your first aid kit to eliminate possible obstacles which may prevent you from completing your journey.

The first step is psychological preparation. Do you trust the theory? Do you have confidence you can complete the practice to its conclusion? Can you cope with the obstacles you will encounter? Most important of all, do you recognize why you want to practice? Are you aiming just for a peaceful mind, or for ultimate enlightenment? You should test yourself first. Sit quietly, keeping your mind calm and clear for thirty minutes a day, for a month, and see how you cope. This is not easy, and your greatest challenge is dealing with your mind, which is at the same time the most important factor in success. Without a clear, calm, and concentrated mind, you cannot lead the Qi, or accomplish the training. There are also important physical preparations for establishing a peaceful mind and making the practice flow smoothly.

Here we discuss some important preparations, such as choice of location, timing of meditation and orientation, common experiences one may encounter, and possible deviations and how to correct them. The traditional twenty-four rules of meditation are reviewed in the last section.

## 7-2. PREPARATIONS 準備

Preparation has mental and physical aspects. Are you forcing yourself to meditate? If so, it could take a long time to calm down. Be prepared for it. Do you have ego or expectations? You will probably be disappointed. When you meditate, you cannot set up a schedule of progress, else you will be under pressure, and the mind will hinder the whole process. Is your mind peaceful before meditation? Do you get upset or excited before meditation? The point is to calm the mind before you meditate. You should meditate just to regulate your mind, if anything will stimulate it and lead it away from calmness and peace. Do not try to circulate Qi with a troubled mind.

**Take a shower.** Dirt and sweat seal the pores of your skin, making you uneasy and uncomfortable. It is best to shower or bathe half an hour before you meditate, to assist physical relaxation. Afterwards let your body return to normal after the stimulation of the water temperature.

**Bowels.** Go to the toilet before meditating. Tightness in the abdomen and bowels affects Qi flow at the Real Lower Dan Tian, and your mind will be scattered and bothered. You should not go to the toilet directly after meditation, but should wait at least ten minutes. This gives your body time to digest Qi you have built and stored in your Real Lower Dan Tian, which would otherwise be lost.

**Clothing.** When practicing Qigong meditation, don't wear artificial fibers such as polyester or rayon. These new artificial products were developed only in recent decades and our bodies have not adapted to them, having used natural materials for millions of years. Artificial fibers generate static, and this interferes with normal Qi circulation. This traps your energy, clouds your judgment, and makes you feel uneasy and impatient, depressed, or excited without reason. You may have a similar feeling before it rains, with low clouds and humidity, and a strong electric field between the clouds and the earth. Our emotions are also affected by the full moon, when the electromagnetic field between the moon and the earth is at its strongest.

So wear natural materials such as cotton or silk. Wear loose clothes, especially pants, for a comfortable, natural feeling, and to help Qi flow through the Real Lower Dan Tian. This assists accurate sensing of your body's Qi.

**Keep warm.** In profound meditation, you are in the semi-sleeping state. Your body relaxes while your mind is awake, regulating the Qi circulation. Your heartbeat slows down and breathing becomes slower and deeper. As in sleep, inhalation is longer than exhalation, which shrinks Guardian Qi (Wei Qi, 衛氣) and lowers skin temperature. You can catch cold easily, so you should keep warm and comfortable. Cover your knees and ankles with a blanket of natural fibre. In relaxation, the joints are open, which allows cold Qi such as wind or moisture to enter them. This weakens the immune system and can generate arthritis.

**Meditation cushion.** When you meditate, you should prepare a meditation cushion. To prevent excess Qi from entering the legs, it is very important that you cross them when sitting, which narrows the Qi path. Start with a cushion about six inches high, made from natural material like cotton, sitting for thirty minutes. Adjust the height for comfort, so you can sit for thirty minutes, using it for a week or so until you are satisfied with the height. Pay attention to your sitting posture, as wrong posture can also generate discomfort.

**Floor.** The floor where you meditate is very important, and should not be too hard. Sit on a mat to ease pressure on the legs.

**Light.** If possible, sit in the dark. Uneven light can affect your judgment. For example, if the light to your right is stronger than to your left, you will feel stronger energy there. This can mislead your feeling and judgment. If you cannot sit in the dark, sit where the light is evenly diffused. Sitting under fluorescent light is not a good idea, as its strong electromagnetic radiation can affect your body's energy.

**Electric field.** You should sit away from any strong electric field, such as an electric outlet, especially one in use. Use a sensitive compass to find a good spot in the house, where the needle aligns with the earth's magnetic field. Do not use an electric blanket at all, as the electromagnetic field it generates is strong and harms Qi circulation, especially in your heart.

**Humidity.** Humidity can also affect your emotional mind. Too much can make you feel sticky and uncomfortable. Too little can cause static to build up around you. The most comfortable humidity for meditation is around 50-60%.

**Temperature.** Temperature is one of the main concerns. Extremes of heat or cold can affect your feelings during meditation. Avoid sitting close to a heater or air conditioner, as they affect your temperature significantly.

**Noise.** Most important of all during meditation is to prevent noise. Sudden loud noise can disturb your meditating mind and lead the Qi into the wrong path, which is dangerous and harmful. In meditation, your mind and body are extremely relaxed, and any slight noise can disturb you, tensing both mind and body. If you are leading Qi circulation, it can be led into the wrong path, damaging your nervous system or internal organs. Unplug your telephone, turn off your mobile phone, and place a sign at the entrance for people to see. Make sure the alarm clock is off, and keep noise out of your meditation place.

## 7-3. MEDITATION PLACE 靜坐地點之選擇

For profound Qigong practice, one needs four things: money, partner, techniques, and place. So an appropriate location is important, not only for a peaceful mind for your cultivation, but also to obtain Qi from the natural surroundings. Choosing a good location for living, for burying the dead, and for Qigong practice is an important profession known as Feng Shui (風水, wind-water).

Mountains are classified as fire (Li, 離) and provide Qi, while water (Kan, 坎) soothes and cools your Qi, bringing you to a calm and harmonious state. To have harmonious Qi, live next to water, such as the ocean, rivers, or lakes. However, to obtain more Qi to nourish your body for Qi circulation and enlightenment meditation, find a suitable mountain.

The earth cooled down from a liquid state, spinning towards the east, so heavier materials such as metals tended to accumulate in the west. Large mountain ranges in North and South America, and in Asia are located to the west (Figure 7-1). Qi is generally stronger in the mountains and more harmonious near the sea.

Finding the best place for spiritual cultivation has been a major challenge in establishing Buddhist and Daoist monasteries. An appropriate location shortens the time needed to reach the final goal of cultivation.

## 7-4. BEST TIME FOR MEDITATION 靜坐之最佳時刻

In general, you may meditate at any time. But at specific times, you benefit from it more, and Qi circulation will be more efficient. If you meditate when natural Qi is changing from Yin to Yang and vice versa, it enhances the achievement significantly, because the Qi in your body is also changing at this time. We age quickly and get sick due to irregular Qi being exchanged during these periods. *The Complete Book of Principal Contents of Life and Human Nature* (性命圭旨全書), says, "Zi (子, 11 P.M. to 1 A.M.), Wu (午, 11 A.M. to 1 P.M.), Mao (卯, 5 to 7 A.M.), and Qiu (酉, 5 to 7 P.M.), these four periods are the time gates for entrance and exit of Yin and Yang."[1] These are the best times for meditation. When your practice is well established however, you can adjust the body's Yin and Yang at any time and gain the same benefit, with a smooth and vital Qi flow. Huo Zi Shi (活子時) means time of vital Zi. Zi (11 P.M. to 1 A.M.) is the best time of all for marrow/brain washing.

The Qigong dictionary describes Huo Zi Shi as "When practicing Qigong, shape and spirit are peaceful and calm, condense the spirit to the Qi cavity (Real Lower Dan Tian). When you feel Qi moving there, then it is time to generate Yin and Yang."[2] The Daoist book, *Observing Vessels* (脈望) says, "When you begin to build the foundation of generating Dan (Elixir or Qi), do not be restricted in the timing of Zi (11 P.M. to 1 A.M.) and Wu (11 A.M. to 1 P.M.). As long as there is movement in the calmness, then it is the time of Gui (end of calmness), which is the time of vital Zi."[3] Gui (癸) is the last of the Ten Celestial Stems (Tian Gan, 天干), meaning that Yin is ending, and Yang is just starting.

Although the times for meditation are not very strict, it is advisable as a beginner to meditate according to natural Yin and Yang. Other than Zi, the best time is early morning until sunrise, the second best is sunset, and the third is at noon. Noontime meditation is only used to calm the body's Yang and to lead the Qi downward and inward for storage, since our body is extremely Yang at this time. This is the best period for Embryonic Breathing, from noon until 2 P.M., when natural Qi and the body's Qi have passed extreme Yang and are just begin to cool down. Instead of sunset, you may also practice about one hour before sleeping.

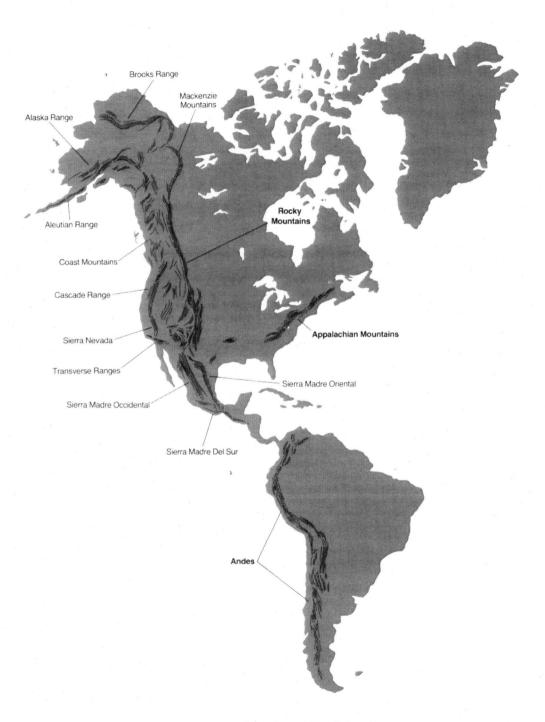

Figure 7-1. Map of South and North America

## 7-5. MEDITATION ORIENTATION

Our body's energy is always influenced by nature, especially cosmic energy, solar energy, lunar energy, and earth energy. Earth energy includes the earth's magnetic field, the heat concealed below, electric charge in clouds, air energy, and all objects both living and inanimate. In choosing your location, consider the landscape, trees, water, and climate. This earth Qi directly affects the body's energy. Here we also discuss how to absorb Qi from the sun, moon, and the earth's magnetic field. Since we do not understand cosmic Qi, it is not discussed here.

Chinese medicine classifies the front of the body as Yin, and the back as Yang. Qi is stored in front while it manifests at the back. External Qi is more easily absorbed by the front, while the back repels and rejects it. To exchange Qi with outside, the Yin side absorbs, while the Yang side rejects. This is important when working with energy from the sun, the earth, and the moon.

**Sun (Daytime).** The early morning sun is gentle, soft, and nourishing, and easily absorbed by the body. Later in the day, its energy is stronger, and the body instinctively rejects it so as not to absorb too much. The sun's rays at sunset are also gentle and soft, but take energy with them, so it is a good time for cooling down instead of nourishing.

**Earth (Nighttime).** The Qi from the Earth's magnetic field starts at the geographic south pole (magnetic north pole) and returns to earth at the geographic north pole (magnetic south pole). If you face the south, you will be nourished by earth Qi, while if you face north, the earth Qi will reduce your Qi and therefore help you to calm down. This is discussed at length in the YMAA book, *The Root of Chinese Qigong.*

**Moon (Nighttime).** Facing the moon between three days before full moon until the full moon itself is a good time to absorb moon Qi for nourishing. The three days after full moon are good for reducing or releasing Qi when facing the moon. To absorb more Qi from nature for your cultivation, you need to nourish (Bu, 補) or add fire. However, if you are already excited and energized and need to calm down, then simply maintain your Qi level or even allow nature to take some away. This is called releasing (Xie, 洩) or adding water.

To summarize:

For Qi nourishment (Bu, 補)(Li, 離)
1. Sunrise—face east to absorb Sun Qi
2. Noon—face south to absorb Earth Qi
3. Sunset—face east to stop the Qi from being drained by the sun
4. Night—face south to absorb Earth Qi
5. Night (3 days up to full moon)—face the moon to absorb its Qi

**Preventing Qi nourishment or for releasing it** (Xie, 洩)(Kan, 坎)

1. Sunrise—face west to stop Qi being nourished by the sun
2. Noon—face north to release Qi to the earth
3. Sunset—face west to release Qi to the sun
4. Night—face north to release Qi to the earth
5. Night (2-3 days after full moon)—face the moon to release Qi to it

## 7-6. COMMON EXPERIENCES FOR QIGONG BEGINNERS 初學氣功之一般經驗

There are common phenomena experienced in practice. Some are caused by improper posture, timing, or training methods. Since most beginners cannot generate significant Qi, they are usually harmless. But if you ignore them and continue to train incorrectly, you build bad habits which may eventually bring you harm. It is important to attend to them and understand their causes.

**The mind is scattered and sleepy** (散亂與昏沉). The Daoist Ni Wan Zu (泥丸祖) said: "For one hundred days, banish sleepiness. Sleepiness and confusion make the mind scattered and disordered, and you lose the real practice."[4] Having a scattered and disordered mind is one of the most common experiences of beginners, with their Yi (意) unable to control Xin (心). Though Yi is strong, Xin is even stronger, so first strengthen Yi and regulate Xin, and analyze the causes and possible results of the disturbance.

If sleepiness is the result of fatigue, it is best to stop practicing, and relax or take a nap. Lie down comfortably, and pay attention to deep breathing as you bring your mind to the deep places of your body. Smoothly and slowly release the carbon dioxide, and every time you exhale, relax deeper. Breathing and heart rate slow down, and you feel rested, with your mind clear and your spirit fresh. Now raise your spirit, and keep it at its residence, centered and balanced.

Sleepiness can also result from relaxation and a scattered mind. Keep your mind inside and observe your inner self. Bring your mind back to the third eye, and raise your spirit. After a few minutes, bring your mind back to the Real Lower Dan Tian for Embryonic Breathing. If you are sleepy, do not use your mind to lead the Qi, which can be as dangerous as driving a car in that condition.

**Feeling cold** (發冷). Feeling cold during still meditation is very common. In moving Qigong you energize your body, so it is warm and more Yang. But in still meditation you calm your mind and slow your breathing, reducing your heart rate and making your body more Yin. In the winter, your body releases energy into the surrounding air more quickly than in the summer, and feeling cold can be more of a problem. So when you meditate in the early morning or in the winter, wear warm clothes and cover your legs, especially your knees, with a blanket.

Sometimes you feel cold even when warmly dressed and with the room at a comfortable temperature. This is most likely caused by your mind, which significantly influences Qi circulation in your body. Sometimes you may feel cold when nervous tension, emotional upset, or fear send a sudden chill through your body. Since your mind has such an effect on you, it is important to regulate it through meditation. You may also feel some part of the body suddenly colder or warmer. This is a common experience as Qi redistributes during deep relaxation, so do not be too concerned about it.

**Numbness** (麻木). Numbness is very common in Qigong still meditation. When you sit for a long time, your circulation slows down, reducing the blood supply to your legs. This is very common with beginners. You should not continue your meditation once concentration is affected. Stretch your legs and massage the bottom of your feet, especially the Yongquan (K-1, 湧泉), to speed the recovery of circulation. If you meditate regularly, you will find you can sit longer and longer without your legs becoming numb. Your body adjusts the blood supply to fit the new situation. After six months of regular practice, you should be able to sit at least thirty minutes without any problem. If your lower back feels stiff, adjust your posture by sitting on a higher cushion or a chair with back support.

**Discomfort (Soreness and Pain)** (酸痛). Discomfort is frequently caused by incorrect posture. Common places are the lower back, hips, and shoulders, caused by wrong sitting height or posture. Correct the problems before they affect your concentration or cause injury, and regulate your body to a comfortable and natural state.

**Part of the body feels hot** (半邊身熱). Sometimes part of your body may feel hot, or just one portion feels cold while the rest feels hot. This usually happens when you are emotionally upset, sick, or recovering from illness. When you circulate unbalanced Qi, you may interfere with the body's efforts to achieve Qi balance. Simply relax and meditate on your Real Lower Dan Tian, and be aware of your body and emotions.

**Headache and eye ache** (頭痛眼痛). A common cause of headache during Qigong practice is failure to breathe smoothly. You may hold your breath without noticing it, causing Qi and blood flow to stagnate, which reduces oxygen supply to the head.

Eye ache is also common, for two main reasons. "The eyes watch the nose, and the nose watches the heart."[5] To keep your mind inside without being distracted by what is going on around you, restrain your vision. Focus your mind in your heart and regulate Xin, your emotional mind. You do this with your mind, not your body. Don't actually stare at your nose, a major cause of eye ache.

Your eyes may also ache when you focus the spirit (Shen) at its residence. Do this without using force. Lead the spirit back to its center firmly but gently. Mental force will cause not only eye ache but also headache.

**Trembling body** (身體抖動). Body trembling occurs spontaneously, mostly in the limbs, though sometimes also in the torso. During deep relaxation, extra Qi flows easily to activate muscles and causes them to tremble. Your upper body may sway by itself, following your breathing. These are good signs, indicating success in regulating your body, breathing, and mind, but you should not make it happen intentionally.

**Warmth and sweating** (溫熱出汗). In still meditation, even though you are not moving externally, you are exercising internally. When Qi increases significantly, it will manifest at the surface of your skin as warmth, even making you sweat. Be sure not to expose your sweaty body to a cold draft.

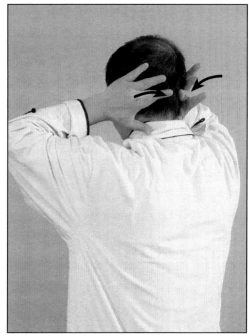

Figure 7-2

**Fright** (受驚). This is one of the worst things that can happen during Qigong meditation. It generally occurs for two reasons. Sometimes your mind is very clear but you cannot center it, and it may start to generate fantasy or illusion. This is called entering the demon, or being bewitched (Ru Mo, 入魔). You may feel a cold draft and think it is an evil spirit, as your imagination generates thoughts to disturb you.

Unless you regulate your mind right away, you may start to believe the illusion and become very scared. The danger is that Yi no longer leads your Qi, disturbing your Qi circulation. If this happens during very deep meditation, it may cause you serious injury, so it is very important that your mind should be clear and calm, with emotions completely controlled.

If you experience this kind of fright, your Yi is too confused to lead your Qi correctly, so you should discontinue practice. There are several ways to help you collect yourself. The first is to cover your ears with your palms and tap the back of your head by snapping your index fingers off the middle fingers (Figure 7-2). This is called beating the heavenly drum (Ming Tian Gu, 鳴天鼓) and is one of the most common ways for your mind to find its center. You may drink some hot tea or coffee, wash your face with warm water, or take a shower. Alternatively, generate an An (唵) sound in your brain, vibrating in the Spiritual Valley. This can often lead your mind into the spiritual center and stop the illusion. This is called righteous sound (Zheng Yin, 正音), commonly used to stabilize the spirit and keep it at the Mud Pill Palace.

The second type of fright happens when you realize your Qi has gone into the wrong path, called entering the fire, or entering the wrong path (Zou Huo, 走火). For example, suddenly your heart starts beating fast or your head starts to ache. Your mind is disturbed, and you are confused and scared. If this happens, calm your mind and move it away from trouble. The more you focus on the area of concern, the more Qi will flow there and stagnate, worsening the situation instead of helping it. Once your mind is calm, lead the Qi back to your Real Lower Dan Tian. Sit still for a few minutes and gradually bring your mind back to your surroundings. Do not resume practice, but instead wait until the next session.

**Difficulty sleeping** (反易失眠). It is common to have difficulty sleeping for a while, because when you practice Qigong, your mind is energized and your spirit raised. This keeps you from falling asleep. Pay attention to your breathing, thinking every time you exhale that your body is becoming more and more relaxed. Inhale longer than you exhale to make the body more Yin. Don't use Yi to lead Qi, but just breathe and relax, and soon you will fall asleep. You may also practice Embryonic Breathing, leading excited Qi down from your head to the Real Lower Dan Tian. Then the mind becomes calm and the body relaxes.

**Coughing** (咳嗽). Beginners sometimes cough during practice. The most common reason is that breathing is not being regulated smoothly. You may be breathing too fast or holding your breath. Use Yi to regulate the breathing until it is no longer necessary.

The second possibility is that your body is not regulated correctly. For example, if you push your head too far back, the front of the throat will tense and cause you to cough.

The third possibility is that when you are in deep meditation, your heart beat slows, and body temperature drops. You feel cold, which may also cause coughing, so keep your body warm during meditation.

**Sexual arousal** (性衝動). It is normal to have sexual feelings and even to become aroused during meditation. Abdominal breathing increases Qi circulation in your lower body, stimulating the sexual organs. While this increases sexual desire, remember you are practicing Qigong to increase production of hormones to raise your spirit. You need to regulate your mind and not waste this extra supply through sexual activity.

Sexual arousal is a great problem in Marrow/Brain Washing Qigong. This trains methods of stimulating hormone production, so that hormonal essence can be converted into Qi to nourish the spirit and brain. People who do not understand the training or whose will-power is weak, waste the achievement of their practice.

## 7-7. COMMON SENSATIONS IN STILL MEDITATION 静坐之動觸與景象

When you practice still meditation, regulating your body, breathing, and mind, you enter into deep meditation. Qi readjusts and balances itself, reaching even the smallest place in your body. You have feelings and visions, which cannot be experienced when you are not in meditation. The Chinese call them Qi scenery or Qi view (Jing Qi, 景氣), and when you reach this point, it is called enter the scenery (Ru Jing, 入景). Don't expect to experience all of these sensations, as they depend on the individual, the time of day, how deep you are in meditation, and even the environment in which you are sitting.

**The Eight Touches (Physical and Sensory Phenomena, 八觸).** The Eight Touches (Ba Chu, 八觸) felt during Qigong practice, such as sensations of heat, someone touching you, or heaviness, are also called Touch Feel (Chu Gan, 觸感) or Moving Touch (Dong Chu, 動觸). Some practitioners list them as moving (Dong, 動), itching (Yang, 癢), cool (Liang, 涼), warm (Nuan, 暖), light (Qing, 輕), heavy (Zhong, 重), harsh (Se, 澀), and slippery (Hua, 滑). Others list them differently as shake (Diao, 掉), ripple (Yi, 猗), cold (Leng, 冷), hot (Re, 熱), float (Fu, 浮), sink (Chen, 沈), hard (Jian, 堅), and soft (Ruan, 軟).

These are normal sensations in Qigong practice, even in the beginning. If you experience something, determine its cause. If it is the result of Qi redistribution, let it happen and don't worry about it. Otherwise, correct the circumstances causing them. For example, if you feel cold because the room temperature is too low, either put on more clothing or turn up the thermostat.

Don't expect these phenomena or look for them, and don't worry about them. Simply follow nature and let it happen, and continue your practice. Keep your mind clear and calm, and don't be distracted.

**Sensations of movement or vibration** (動盪景). This is different from the above where one part of the body spontaneously starts to move or tremble. This sensation occurs in the False Lower Dan Tian, and you might feel warmth there. After a couple of weeks, the area may start to vibrate by itself. This means Qi is becoming abundant there and it is time for your Yi to lead it through small circulation. This is often the first sensation, and it gives you confidence you are practicing correctly and making progress.

**Sensations inside the abdomen** (小腹內景). Once you feel warmth and vibration in your Real Lower Dan Tian, the abundant Qi spreads out through your abdomen. The movement as you breathe increases circulation in your intestines and sometimes causes sounds and the release of gas. After a while, you feel warmth and other sensations throughout your abdomen, and the Qi flows smoothly and strongly. Sometimes you sweat. Afterwards, these sensations disappear as all the channels in the abdomen open up, and Qi moves without stagnation.

**The feeling of lightness** (飄然之景). During deep meditation, with Qi circulating smoothly, your body may feel light and airy, and seems to disappear. This is very comfortable, but don't be distracted by it. Be aware of what is happening, but don't pay attention to it. To reach this stage, your body must be in deep relaxation, where breathing and heartbeat slow down to the minimum, and your mind is extremely calm and peaceful.

**White clouds in the empty room** (虛室生白). You may suddenly feel your physical body disappear and blend with the surrounding Qi. It seems the room is empty, filled with a white cloud or fog. If you pay attention to this scenery, it disappears immediately, because your mind is not familiar with emptiness and generates an image of familiar, physical scenery to fill the void.

If you experience this white emptiness, be aware of it, but don't pay attention to it. It happens only when your mind is completely regulated in a highly concentrated and relaxed state. The Daoist Wu Yi Zi (悟一子) said, "If you wish to fill the abdomen with Qi, first empty the Xin. If you wish to generate the White, first empty the room."[6] To accumulate Qi in your abdomen, first empty the emotional mind (Xin). Only then can Yi (wisdom mind) start the fire (Qi Huo, 起火) to build up the Qi. White here means simple, pure, light, and clean, like fog or cloud, and represents the disappearance of the physical body. To unite with surrounding Qi, first let go of all objects, including your physical body.

**Six other sensations** (六景). At a higher level of Qigong meditation, there are six other sensations you may experience. These are a). the False Lower Dan Tian is hot as though it were on fire; b). the kidneys feel as though boiling in water, c). the eyes emit a beam of light, d). winds are generated behind the ears, e). an eagle is shouting behind your head, and f). your body is energized and your nose trembles. These are called Six Verifications (Liu Zhong Ying Yan, 六種應驗), because they verify correct meditation.

**Six Transportations** (六通). When you regulate and raise your spirit (Shen), it will be high and its supernatural Ling (靈) power will reach farther than any ordinary person's. Your mind will be able to communicate with the six natural powers:

- **Seeing the present.** Your mind is so clear it can analyze and understand events clearly and thoroughly. You see things from a neutral point of view, without being confused by Xin, something most people cannot do.

- **Understanding the past and seeing the future**. You understand the past and predict the future. Since your mind is clear, you can analyze what happened, understand its causes and see the results. As your experience accumulates, you can predict the future, since people remain the same and history repeats itself.

- **Viewing the whole universe.** At the highest stage, your spirit senses the whole universe, including mountains, rivers, oceans, and the heavens. Your Qi unites with that of the universe, and you can exchange information freely.

- **Hearing the sounds of the universe.** Your spirit listens to and understands the sounds generated by variations of natural Qi, including wind, rain, waves, and many other things. You can also hear spirits and communicate with them.

- **Seeing a person's destiny.** After all this, you will be able to look inside a person's mind, personality, and true nature, and see his destiny. You will even be able to see his spiritual future, whether it involves enjoyment (heaven) or suffering (hell).

- **Knowing a person's thoughts.** Since you have energized your spirit and brain significantly, they are open to a much wider range of wavelengths. You will be able to match wavelengths with other people's minds and know their thoughts.

Daoist Wu Zhen Ren (伍真人) said, "Return to emptiness to combine with the Dao. After you reach steadiness and can leave your body, you can communicate with the powers of nature and transform into thousands of changes and ten thousand variations; nothing cannot be done."[7] This stage is Buddhahood or Enlightenment, where you can separate your spirit from your body and unite with nature, and have already reopened your third eye (Tian Yan, 天眼). Your spirit and the natural spirit have been unified as one (Tian Ren He Yi, 天人合一).

## 7-8. DEVIATIONS AND CORRECTIONS 偏差與矯正

Once you accumulate Qi, especially at the False Lower Dan Tian, be careful lest Qi deviate from the correct path and bring you into danger. This is caused by lack of knowledge, misunderstanding, or wrong training. Deviations are called Zou Huo Ru Mo (走火入魔), which means Mislead the Fire and Enter the Devil. Mislead the fire means to lead the Qi into the wrong path, and Enter the Devil means the mind enters the domain of evil. Serious problems or injury usually result. Here we discuss the causes of common Qigong deviations and how to correct them.

### Causes of Deviations:

**The Qigong style trained does not fit the individual or the circumstances.** Every style of Qigong has its own special training methods and objectives. Each Qigong set was created by a knowledgeable Qigong master to train a specific group of people. When you choose a Qigong style for your training, first know your body's condition, the purpose of your training, and whether the Qigong style chosen is appropriate.

For example, Iron Shirt (Tie Bu Shan, 鐵布衫) Qigong is used to train people whose bodies are already stronger than average. If you are weak and force yourself to train Iron Shirt, you encounter difficulties and deviations. With Qigong styles for improving general health, such as The Eight Pieces of Brocade (Ba Duan Jin, 八段錦) and Five Animal Sports (Wu Qin Xi, 五禽戲), you do not have to worry too much about deviations caused by choosing the wrong style. Such styles were created for average people, so you are safe so long as you follow the instructions.

**Lack of a firm mind or a knowledgeable teacher.** Find a knowledgeable teacher and stay with him, else there is a good chance you may be taught incorrect practices. Don't lose patience or confidence and change to another teacher, which may only increase your confusion. If you train Qigong without patience, perseverance, confidence, and strong will, sooner or later confusion and deviations occur.

**Anticipating phenomena.** One common cause of deviation is expecting phenomena that you have heard about. Just because someone else has experienced something doesn't mean that you will experience it too. If you try to make it happen, you are likely to fall into wrong practices, and be misled by the wrong sensation or by illusion.

**Body and mind are not regulated.** Many practitioners encounter serious deviations caused by body tension. If your body is tired and your muscles tense, first calm down and regulate your breathing to help your body relax and recover from fatigue. Any attempt to circulate Qi when you are tired is dangerous.

Deviations are also common when people circulate Qi before their minds are regulated. If you are excited or angry, your Yi is unsteady and it is dangerous to lead your Qi. If you cannot regulate your mind, you should not practice.

If you practice under these circumstances, your Qi can stagnate or enter wrong channels. It is very common to experience headache or various pains. Regulating your body, breathing, and mind are basic requirements before you regulate Qi.

**Losing patience.** Don't lose patience during practice and use Yi aggressively to lead the Qi. This is very dangerous, especially for beginners. Take your time, be patient and confident. Your understanding and experience grow with practice, until the time is right. Some beginners circulate Qi in Small Circulation before they really know what Qi is, or can move their abdomens easily. This only causes problems, like a child playing with fire.

**Mixing imagination with Qigong exercises.** Qigong is a science, not a religion or superstitious belief. Imagination will lead you to the wrong path. It is a major cause of fear and of entering the domain of the devil. Most people who have imagination lack scientific knowledge and understanding. They are confused and wonder what they are doing.

**External interference.** Some of the worst deviations are caused by external disturbances during Qigong meditation. For example, you are meditating when suddenly you are shocked by the telephone ringing, a loud noise, or a friend talking to you. Such things can cause serious injury, especially when you are circulating Qi in Small Circulation or practicing other higher levels of practice where great concentration is necessary. Before you practice, you should prevent all possible disturbances.

**Believing non-professional opinions.** A common failing is to believe and trust other people's judgment more than our own. We are especially open to advice from our friends. When you encounter a problem during practice, do not discuss it with anyone who is not experienced with Qigong. You can discuss it with your teacher or fellow students, but it is best not to talk about it with friends not practicing Qigong. You are likely to be much better qualified to evaluate things than they are.

**Not following advice and rules of the Masters.** At the end of this section, we discuss twenty-four rules you should observe while practicing Qigong, to avoid the most common and serious problems.

Though we have pointed out many possible sources of deviation and danger, you should not let this scare you away from practicing Qigong. Every practice always has some level of risk. For example, you would not ban swimming simply because some people drown, and you shouldn't refuse to drive a car even though many people are killed or injured by them. The proper approach to any of these things is to understand what you are doing, know the source of potential problems, define the training rules, and proceed cautiously.

Most deviations happen to those who generate a strong Qi flow, yet still do not understand and master the regulation of the body, breathing, and mind. Once you generate strong Qi in your body, you must know how to lead it, otherwise it may move into the wrong paths and affect normal Qi circulation. This is harmful and even dangerous. That is why they are called deviations rather than phenomena, the term used earlier to refer to common experiences.

### Deviations and corrections:

**Headache.** Earlier we discussed the headaches beginners have. Here we discuss the potentially serious headaches caused by excess Qi and blood, or lack of oxygen in the brain. Excess Qi and blood is usually caused by forced concentration, which means the mind is not regulated properly. Even when concentrating, Yi and body should be relaxed. If you force yourself to concentrate, your mind leads Qi and blood to the head, and you will become more tense and get a headache. If you can't sleep, it's no good trying to force yourself to sleep, just relax and let it happen.

The headache caused by lack of oxygen usually occurs when your breathing is not regulated properly. Beginners frequently concentrate Yi so hard that they unconsciously hold their breath. This reduces oxygen supply to the brain and causes headaches or dizziness. So regulate the breath until it is smooth and natural, which is regulating the breath without regulating. Only then concentrate on leading Qi.

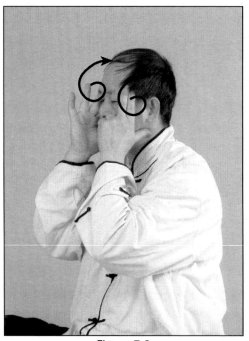

Figure 7-3

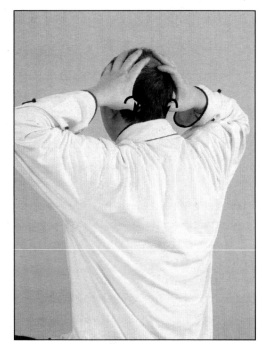

Figure 7-4

If you get a headache while practicing Qigong, immediately lead the Qi to the Real Lower Dan Tian, and stop training after a few breaths. With your breathing smooth, relax your body deeply. This opens the Qi channels in the neck, and excess Qi and blood in your head can disperse. Massage your temples (Figure 7-3), the Fengchi cavity (GB-20, 風池, Wind Pond)(Figure 7-4), and the muscles at the back of your neck, pushing downward to lead the blood and Qi out of your head. Finally, place the center of your palm on the Baihui cavity, lightly circle a few times and then follow the muscles down the back of the neck (Figure 7-5). Tap the head gently from the center to the sides and from the front to the back. This leads stagnant Qi out to the surface of the skin (Figure 7-6). Then use the palms to smooth the hair back from the forehead to the back of the neck (Figure 7-7). Naturally, you may also brush it forward and down the Fire Path with your palms (Figure 7-8).

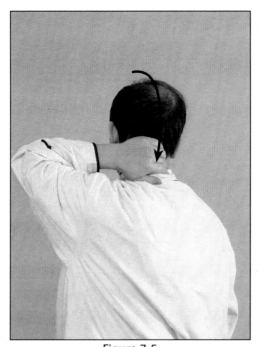

Figure 7-5

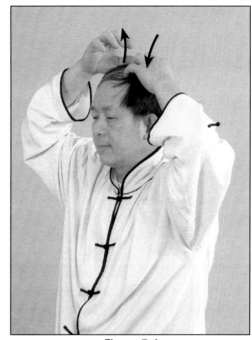

Figure 7-6

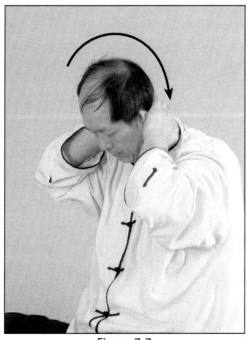

Figure 7-7

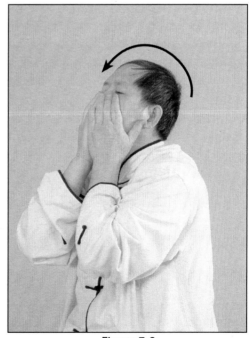

Figure 7-8

**Stagnant Qi in the Upper Dan Tian.** When Qi stagnates in your Upper Dan Tian, it feels like fly paper stuck to your third eye. This usually happens when you concentrate there very intensely. When you concentrate your spirit, your Upper Dan Tian usually feels comfortably warm. If you feel uncomfortable, it means the Qi is stagnant. When this happens, massage your third eye and lead the Qi past the temples and down the sides of the neck (Figure 7-9).

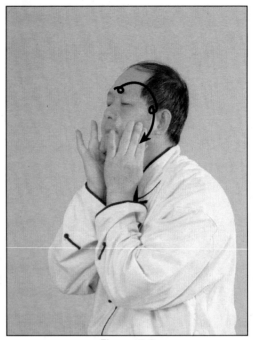

Figure 7-9

**False Lower Dan Tian feels distended and uncomfortable.** This is more common with beginners and usually happens when you force your abdominal muscles in and out. When the muscles are tired, you can't control them. When training abdominal movement, remain soft and relaxed so Qi does not stagnate there. If your abdomen feels uncomfortable and Qi stagnates, massage it in a circular manner (follow bowel system)(Figure 7-10), then open your hands and brush the Qi down to the thighs (Figure 7-11).

**Pressure and discomfort at the diaphragm.** This usually happens if you don't regulate your breathing correctly. Reverse Abdominal Breathing can cause a feeling of pressure and discomfort, so start the session on a smaller scale, with smaller movements of the abdomen. There is a limit to how far you can move your abdomen without feeling pressure on your diaphragm. Discomfort means Qi is stagnant from pressure around the diaphragm. Stop training, fold your hands, and gently press in on the solar plexus a few times (Figure 7-12), then brush down and to the sides (Figure 7-13).

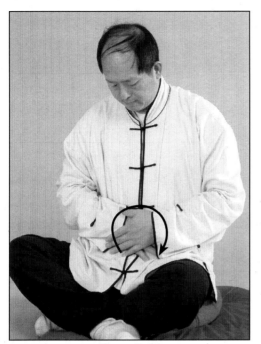

Figure 7-10

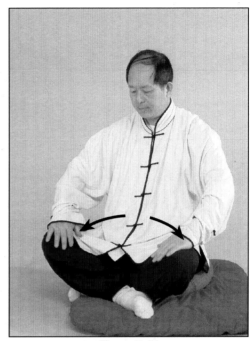

Figure 7-11

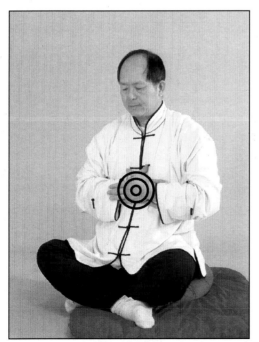

Figure 7-12

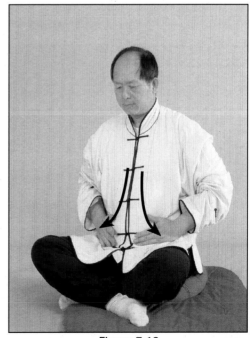

Figure 7-13

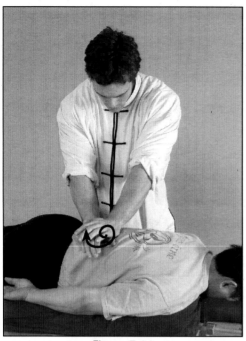

Figure 7-14

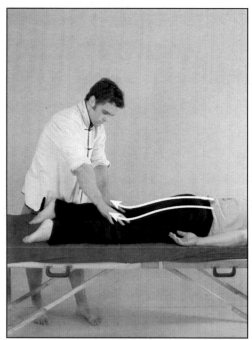

Figure 7-15

**Back pain**. Back pain in Qigong is usually caused by incorrect posture, especially during sitting meditation, causing Qi circulation to stagnate and increasing pressure on the muscles. If you have back pain, stop practicing immediately, else you only disturb your mind and make things worse. If possible, have someone massage the painful area (Figure 7-14), following the spine down to the hips (Figure 7-15). Spread the Qi to the sides of the body and down to the legs. You may gently lean your back against some support during meditation, but not against a wall or something that can drain your Qi. A comfortable couch can serve the purpose.

**Nocturnal emissions**. This happens when you accumulate Qi without keeping and circulating it. If you do a lot of Lower Dan Tian exercises, Qi is abundant, your sexual organs are energized, and your body produces more hormones. This increases sexual desire and causes frequent erections, often without apparent cause. Without being sexually active, internal sexual pressure builds which your body automatically releases through nocturnal emissions. If you practice Qigong and semen is released automatically more than twice a month, it means you are not converting essence into Qi and circulating it properly. You need to coordinate the movement of your Huiyin with your breathing.

This can also occur when Qi is depleted, due to illness, excessive walking, or incorrect Qigong training. There is not enough Qi to keep the muscles functioning normally, and you occasionally experience nocturnal emissions. Massage your abdomen after practice until warm.

**Qi circulates strongly by itself.** Some people build Qi faster than their Yi can control it, which can be very dangerous and cause serious injury. Many Qigong students are impatient and try to regulate Qi before regulating body, breathing, and mind. When you feel Qi move by itself in Small Circulation, you are elated at the sign of progress. But if the Qi builds so much you cannot control it, you should stop practicing completely for a while. Practice regulating body, breathing, and mind until you are confident and understand what you are doing before you start regulating Qi. It is wisest to consult an experienced master. Qi may circulate by itself on a small scale, usually not for too long before it stops by itself. This is nothing to worry about, and you should simply continue your practice with a calm and peaceful mind.

**Qi entering the wrong path.** This happens when your Qi is strong but your mind is scattered, and the Qi may go anywhere. It might make your internal organs too Yang or too Yin, and you could become ill. Qigong without a regulated mind is as dangerous as a car with a drunken driver. Always remember to regulate body, breathing, and mind before regulating Qi. If you are already ill because of Qigong practice, stop practicing immediately. Relax and get enough rest, and wait until the Qi regains its balance. You usually do not need to see a doctor, and if you keep calm and relaxed, it will balance itself. When you start again, begin with the most basic regulating exercises first, so that you do not repeat the problem.

If the Qi stagnates or enters the wrong path at the Three Gates (San Guan, 三關) during Small Circulation, the situation can be very dangerous. You should treat it seriously and pay attention to avoiding injury. I urge you to read section 5-5 again about these three gates and the dangers involved, and understand the remedies for the problems.

**Stiff tongue.** When the tongue is stiff in Qigong practice, Qi can stagnate in the Small Circulation. Practice relaxing your tongue as the tip lightly touches the roof of your mouth. Do this naturally and comfortably before practicing Small Circulation.

## 7-9. TWENTY-FOUR RULES FOR QIGONG PRACTICE 氣功練習二十四則

The twenty-four rules which have been passed down are based on study and experience by generations of Qigong masters, and you should observe them carefully. Where they do not fit today's lifestyle, judge wisely. They are summarized here for your reference and consideration.

**Don't be stubborn about plans and ideas (Yu Zhi Wang Nian)** 預執忘念. This is one of the easiest mistakes for beginners to make. When we take up Qigong we are enthusiastic and eager. However, sometimes we don't learn as fast as we would like to and become impatient, and try to force things. Sometimes we set up a schedule for ourselves, such as: today I want to make my Lower Dan Tian warm, tomorrow I want to get through the tailbone cavity, by such and such a day I want to complete the

Small Circulation. This is the wrong way to go about it. Qigong is not an ordinary task you set for yourself. You cannot make a progress schedule for it. This only makes your thinking rigid and stalls your progress. Everything happens when the time is ready. If you force it, it will not happen naturally.

**Don't focus on discrimination (Zhuo Yi Fen Bie)** 著意分別. When you practice, don't focus on the various phenomena or sensations which occur. Be aware of what is happening, but center your mind where it is supposed to be for the exercise you are doing. If you let your mind go where you feel something interesting happening, the Qi will follow and interfere with your body's natural tendency to rebalance itself. Don't expect anything to happen, and don't let your mind wander around looking for various phenomena. Nor should you judge the phenomena, such as asking "Is my Lower Dan Tian warmer today than it was yesterday," or "Where is my Qi now?" When your mind is on your Qi, your Yi is there also, and this stagnant Yi will not lead the Qi. Be aware of what is happening, but don't pay attention to it. When you drive a car, you don't watch yourself steer and work the pedals and shift gears. Simply think of where you want to go and let your body automatically drive the car. This is called regulating without regulating.

**Avoid miscellaneous thoughts remaining on origins (Za Nian Pan Yuan)** 雜念攀緣. This is a problem of regulating the mind. The emotional mind is strong, and every idea is connected to its origin. If you cannot cut the ideas off at their source, your mind is not regulated, and you should not try to regulate Qi. You will also find that, even though you stop the flow of random thoughts, new ideas are generated during practice. For example, when you notice your Lower Dan Tian is warm, your mind immediately recalls where this is mentioned in a book, or how the master described it, and you start to compare your experience with that. Or you may start wondering what the next step is. These thoughts lead you away from peace and calm, and your mind ends up in the Domain of the Devil (Ru Mo, 入魔). It becomes confused, scattered, and often scared, and you will get tired quickly.

**Xin should not follow the external scenery (Xin Sui Wai Jing)** 心隨外景. This is also a problem of regulating the Xin. When your emotional mind is uncontrolled, any external distraction leads it away from your center and toward the distraction. Train yourself so that noises, smells, conversations and such will not disturb your concentration. Be aware of what is happening, but your mind remains calm, peaceful, and firmly on your cultivation.

**Regulate sexual activity (Ru Fang Shi Jing)** 入房施精. A man should not have sexual relations at least twenty-four hours before or after practicing Qigong, especially in Small Circulation. The conversion training is a very critical part of these practices, and if you practice Qigong soon after sex, you harm your body significantly. Sex depletes your sperm and the Qi level in the lower portion of your body. Practicing Qigong under these conditions is like doing heavy exercise right after sex.

When your Qi level is abnormal, your feeling and sensing are not accurate either, and your Yi can be misled. You should wait until the Qi level returns to normal before you resume Qigong practice. Only then will the Essence-Qi conversion proceed efficiently.

One major purpose of Qigong is to increase the conversion and use this Qi to nourish your body. Once a man has built up a supply of Qi, having sex will only pass this Qi on to his partner. Many Qigong masters insist that you should not have sex three days before and four days after practice.

During sexual relations, the woman usually gains Qi while the man loses Qi during ejaculation. The woman should not practice Qigong after sex until her body has digested the Qi she has obtained from the man. There are certain Daoist Qigong techniques which teach men how to avoid losing Qi during sexual activity and how women can receive Qi from the man and digest it. We leave the discussion of this subject to Qigong masters who are qualified and experienced in it.

**Don't be too warm or too cold (Da Wen Da Han)** 大溫大寒. The temperature of the room in which you are training should be neither too hot nor too cold. You should practice in a comfortable environment which will not disturb your mind and cultivation.

**Beware of the five weaknesses and internal injuries (Wu Lao An Shang,** 五癆暗傷**).** Five weaknesses are those of the Yin organs, namely heart, liver, lungs, kidneys, and spleen. When any of them is weak, you should proceed very gently. Qigong practice is an internal exercise directly affecting these five organs. Excessive exertion does not build up strength and may cause serious injury.

Internal injuries disturb your internal Qi circulation. Practicing Qigong may exacerbate your problem and interfere with the natural healing process. Certain Qigong exercises are designed to heal internal injuries, but to use them properly you need a deep understanding of the Qi situation of your body.

**Avoid facing the wind when sweating (Zuo Han Dang Feng)** 坐汗當風. Don't practice facing the wind, especially cold wind. When you practice Qigong you are exercising both internally and externally. With your pores wide open, you are vulnerable and liable to catch cold.

**Don't wear tight clothes and belt (Jin Yi Shu Dai)** 緊衣束帶. Always wear loose, comfortable clothes during practice, and keep your belt loose. The abdomen is the key area in Qigong practice, and anything which limits movement of this area interferes with your practice.

**Don't eat too much greasy and sweet food (Tao Tie Fei Gan)** 饕餮肥甘. Regulate your eating while practicing Qigong. Greasy or sweet food increase Fire Qi, scattering your mind and letting your spirit stray from its residence. Eat more fruit and vegetables, and abstain from alcohol and tobacco.

**Don't hang your feet off the bed (Ba Chuang Xuan Jiao)** 跋床懸腳. In ancient times the most common place for Qigong practice was sitting on the bed. Since most beds were high, if you sat on the edge of the bed your feet would hang above the floor. When you practice Qigong, your feet should touch the floor, else all your body weight presses down on the lower part of your thighs and reduces Qi and blood circulation.

**Don't practice with a full bladder (Jiu Ren Xiao Bian)** 久忍小便. You should go to the toilet before starting your practice. If you need to go during practice, stop your practice to do so. Holding it in disturbs your concentration.

**Don't scratch an itch (Sao Zhua Yang Chu)** 搔抓癢處. If you itch for some external reason, such as an insect biting you, do not be alarmed, and keep your mind calm. Let your Yi lead the Qi back to the Lower Dan Tian. Breathe a couple of times, and gradually bring your consciousness back to your surroundings. Then you may scratch or think of how to stop the itching. However, if the itching is caused by Qi redistribution, don't move your mind there. Simply ignore it and let it happen. Once it reaches a new balance, the itching stops. Scratching this kind of itch disturbs your mind, while your hands interfere with the natural rebalancing of your body's Qi.

**Avoid being disturbed or startled (Cu Hu Jing Ji)** 猝呼驚悸. If this does happen, calm down your mind, and refrain from losing your temper. Now prevent it from happening again. Most important is learning to regulate your mind when you are disturbed.

**Don't take delight in the scenery (Dui Jing Huan Xi)** 對景歡喜. It is very common during practice to notice something happening inside of you. Perhaps you feel Qi moving more strongly than ever before, or you sense your bone marrow, and feel elated and excited. This is a very common trap, as your concentration is broken and your mind divided, which is dangerous and harmful. You need to be aware of what is going on inside you without getting excited.

**Don't wear sweaty clothes (Jiu Zhuo Han Yi)** 久著汗衣. Sweaty clothes make you feel uncomfortable, affecting your concentration. It is better to change into dry clothes before resuming practice.

**Don't sit when hungry or full (Ji Bao Shang Zuo)** 飢飽上坐. You should not practice Qigong when hungry or when your stomach is full. When you are hungry, it is hard to concentrate, and when you are full, your practice affects your digestion.

**Heaven and Earth strange disaster (Tian Di Zai Guai)** 天地災怪. Your body's Qi is directly affected by changes in the weather. It is not advisable to practice when there is a sudden change of weather, because it interferes with your body's natural readjustment to the new environment. Nor can you sense and control your Qi flow as you do normally. You should remain emotionally neutral when you do Qigong, and even during a natural disaster like an earthquake, remain calm so that your Qi stays under control.

**Listen sometimes to true words (Zhen Yan Ou Ting)** 真言偶聽. You need confidence when you practice Qigong. You should not listen to advice from inexperienced people who are not familiar with the condition of your body. Some people listen to classmates explaining how they reached a certain level, or how they solved a certain problem and then blindly try to use the same method themselves. Everyone has a different body, with a different state of health, and everyone learns differently. When the time comes to learn something new, you will understand what you need. Play it cool, and always have confidence in your training.

**Don't lean and fall asleep (Hun Chen Qing Yi)** 昏沉傾欹. Discontinue Qigong training when you are sleepy. Leading Qi with an unclear mind is dangerous. Your body will not be regulated, tending to lean or droop, which interferes with Qi circulation. It is better to rest until you regain your spirit.

**Don't meditate when too angry, happy, or excited (Da Nu or Da Le Ru Zuo)** 大怒、大樂入坐. When your mind is scattered, Qigong will bring more harm than peace.

**Don't keep spitting (Tu Tan Wu Du)** 吐痰無度. It is normal to generate a lot of saliva while practicing Qigong, which should be swallowed to moisten your throat. Spitting wastes it and disturbs concentration.

**Don't doubt and become lazy (Sheng Yi Xie Dai)** 生疑懈怠. You need confidence in the methods of practice. Doubt leads to laziness and discontinuing the practice. Then you will not be successful.

**Do not ask for speedy success (Bu Qiu Su Xiao)** 不求速效. Qigong practice is time consuming and progress is slow. To reach your goal, you need patience, a strong will, and confidence. Let your practice proceed naturally.

## References

1. 《性命圭旨全書·王子喬胎息訣》：〝子、午、卯、酉四時，乃是陰陽出入之門戶。〞
2. 習煉氣功中，形神安靜，凝神入氣穴，覺丹田氣動，陰陽生發之時。
3. 《脈望》：〝下手立丹基，休向子午推，靜中才一動，便是癸生時，謂之活子時。〞
4. 泥丸祖曰：〝百日之中忌昏，昏迷散亂失卻真。
5. 眼觀鼻，鼻觀心。
6. 悟一子曰：〝欲實其腹，先虛其心，欲生其白，先虛其室。〞
7. 伍真人云：〝還虛合道，出定以後，倏出倏定也可，六通十通皆能，千變萬化，無所不能。〞

## CHAPTER 8

# Small Circulation Meditation Practice

小周天靜坐練習

## 8-1. INTRODUCTION 介紹

After studying the theory of Small Circulation, practice it with caution. Always go back and ponder it. During practice, you may have new questions or doubts, and the best way to find a solution is pondering the theory which has been derived from past experience. After finding a possible answer, go back and put it into practice. From repeating this process, you become wiser and more proficient. Theory is like a map. The more you understand it, the easier and more safely you can approach your goal.

Often, theory alone is not enough, and you need guidance from an experienced teacher. There are different approaches to a problem, and many paths can lead to the same goal. The more you open your mind, the more you learn and experience on the way to becoming a real expert of Small Circulation. You should not be concerned with dignity and pride, but remain humble and learn from experience. Filter ideas and adopt those which are appropriate for you.

Since Small Circulation is so important for spiritual cultivation, different practice methods have been developed by different cultures. It is called Microcosmic Orbit in Indian Yoga, where its methods are different from those used by Chinese. The methods used in Buddhist and Daoist monasteries also differ from each other. Although the methods differ, the theory and the goal remain the same.

The most important factor for successful practice is training your feeling. *Deep feeling leads to profound communication between your spirit and body.* It connects with the subconscious mind and raises up the spirit.

There was a wise king in Korea who had a fifteen-year-old son. This son had grown up comfortably in the palace, with all of the servants' attention. This worried the king, who believed his son would not be a good king to care for his people. So he summoned a wise old man living deep in the woods.

In response to this call, the old man came to the palace. He promised to teach the prince to be a wise, good king and took him to the deep woods. After they arrived there, the old man taught him how to find food, cook, and survive in the forest. Then he left him there alone, but promised to return a year later.

A year later, when the old man came back, he asked the prince what he thought about the forest. The prince replied, "I am sick of it. I need a servant. I hate it here. Take me home." The old man said, "Very good. That is good progress, but not enough. Please wait here for another year, and I will be back to see you again." Then, he left again.

Another year passed, and the old man came back to the woods, asking the same question. This time the prince said, "I see birds and trees, flowers, and animals." His mind had started to accept his environment, and he recognized his role in the forest. The old man was satisfied and said, "This is very good progress, but not enough, so you must stay here for another year." This time, the prince did not even seem to mind.

Another year passed, and the old man returned. This time, when the old man asked the prince what he thought, the prince said, "I feel birds, woods, fish, animals, and many things around me here." This time, the old man was very happy and said, "Now I can take you home. If you can feel the things happening around you, then you will be able to concern yourself with the people's feelings, and you will be a good king." Then he took him home.

When you do anything, you must put your mind into it, feel it, taste it, and experience it. Only then may you say that you understand it. Without this deep feeling and comprehension, the arts you practice or create will be shallow and lose their essence.

In this chapter, we finally reach the keys of practice. From section 8-2 to 8-6, we discuss the methods of regulating the body, breathing, mind, Qi, and spirit in Small Circulation. Because the Original Essence (Yuan Jing, 元精) is one of the keys to success, we review the concept of regulating it in section 8-7. Then we summarize how to recover from deep meditation, in section 8-8. Finally we discuss how to use meditation to heal yourself, in section 8-9.

## 8-2. REGULATING THE BODY 調身

The first step is to sit correctly, comfortably, and naturally for at least thirty minutes. If you cannot sit still that long, you may have difficulty leading the Qi safely. When you lead the Qi in Small Circulation meditation, your mind must be comfortable and focused. If it is disturbed by an uneasy posture, it can scatter, so you should not advance further. First learn to sit correctly and patiently. Most important is to cultivate the mood and joy of meditation. You regulate the body to establish a very relaxed, comfortable, natural feeling, so your mind can concentrate on regulating. Start with only five minutes, and gradually increase it.

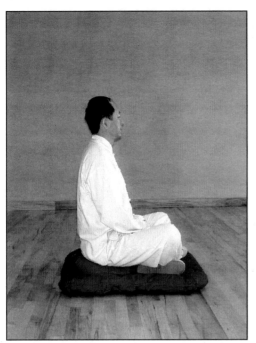

Figure 8-1. Sitting Meditation Posture

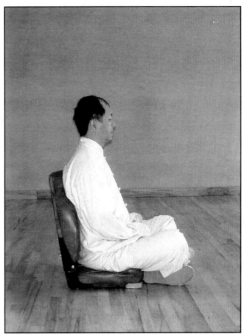

Figure 8-2. Sitting Meditation on a Fishing Chair

**Torso.** The correct posture of the torso is very important to make the body balanced, centered, and relaxed. Only then can the Qi circulate smoothly without stagnation, and the mind can easily lead the Qi to circulate naturally.

This also applies to the neck and the head. The neck must relax to allow Qi and blood to flow easily to the brain. It is the junction where Qi and blood are exchanged between the head and torso, and when it relaxes, the brain obtains ample nourishment. The head must also be comfortable. First relax the mind, then the head can relax too.

In meditation, keep the torso upright and the head as though suspended from above. You should not lean forward, backward, or sideways. Improper posture makes the torso tense and scatters your mind. This is especially true for beginners who may easily lean forward and fall asleep, leading to lower back pain and blocking Qi circulation. You should not stiffen the torso when you keep it upright. It should be relaxed so the Qi can circulate smoothly.

Practice for some time on a meditation cushion (Figure 8-1). If you continue to experience tightness in the torso, especially your lower back, sit on a chair which supports your back (Figure 8-2). Alternatively, sit on a couch or sofa which provides good support while not restricting your Qi flow and which is not so comfortable that you fall asleep (Figure 8-3). If you are too tired to practice, simply lead the Qi to the Real Lower Dan Tian, and take a short nap. Don't keep struggling, which may bring more harm than good.

**Hands.** The hands should be placed comfortably on your legs in front of your abdomen. It does not matter which hand is on top as long as they feel comfortable and natural. Some teachers claim a man should place the right hand on top while women place the left hand on top. The most important thing is to feel balanced. The Qi circulating on either side of the body is not perfectly balanced, nor is the body itself. Heart and spleen are on the left, while the liver is on the right. Hands, legs, and feet are not the same length. Due to this imbalance, Qi circulation is not balanced either. The mind adjusts the feeling of unbalanced Qi in the body, so body and mind can coordinate with each other. If you force left-handed people to change to using the right hand, they experience emotional and mental imbalance, and children often develop a stutter.

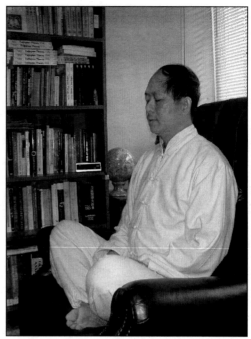

Figure 8-3. Sitting Meditation on a Couch

Placing the hands in front of the lower abdomen is called Wo Gu (握固) which means to hold and to firm. In *Dao De Jing*, Chapter 55 (道德經・五十五章), it says, "When the bones are weak and the tendons soft, then Wo Gu."[1] When your body is weak, the first thing you should do is to store abundant Qi at the Real Lower Dan Tian. Wo Gu helps keep your mind there. Then Qi is not led outward, and can be preserved and stored.

To enhance the feeling of firming the Qi, various ways of holding the fingers were taught. *The Thesis on the Origins and Symptoms of Various Diseases* (諸病源候論) said, "What is Wo Gu? It is to use the four fingers of both hands to hold the thumb."[2] That means holding the thumb in the four fingers in front of the Lower Dan Tian (Figure 8-4). *The Necessary Book of Entering the Daoist Religion* (道門通教必用集) said, "Wo Gu is using the thumb to nip the middle of the middle finger and the four fingers are gathered at the center."[3] The finger nail of the thumb presses the middle of the middle finger while the other four fingers are holding it (Figure 8-5). In fact, this is only a trick to help beginners concentrate the mind at the Lower Dan Tian.

Various hand forms are used in Buddhist meditation. These are called hand stamps (Shou Yin, 手印). In Daoist society, it says, "There are two different purposes for hand posture. First, concentrate the mind and spirit on the Shou Yin, persevere and finally obtain the steadiness of Chan. Second, after forming the Shou Yin,

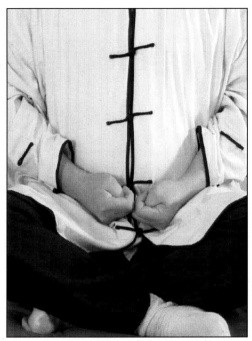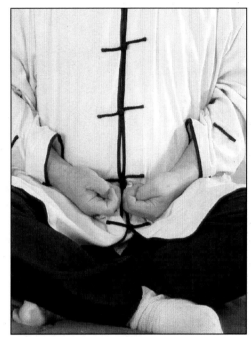

| Figure 8-4 | Figure 8-5 |

the mind and spirit are on the breathing, to reach the highest level and become the Buddha."[4] Hand posture or Shou Yin helps one calm down the mind and concentrate on the Lower Dan Tian and breathing. Again, this is a trick to regulate the mind and breathing. The Buddhist classic, *The Classic of Tuo Lo Ni* (陀羅尼集經) said, "There are various body stamping techniques in chanting, if using hands to make Shou Yin and chanting, it can easily be effective."[5] Chanting is very common in different religions, to achieve the state of hypnosis and harmony. Meditation is considered self-hypnosis in Chinese Qigong practice. Through chanting and different hand stamps, Buddhists reach a high level of meditation.

**Legs.** When you sit for Small Circulation, the legs should be crossed comfortably (Figure 8-6). This prevents stronger Qi flow to the legs. Since man has walked for millions of years, the Qi naturally flows there strongly, instead of in the Small Circulation path. To prevent the stronger Qi flow from injuring the legs, they should be crossed, blocking it at the hip area. In this way, Qi flow is stronger and more efficient in the Governing and Conception Vessels. Another way of restraining the strong Qi flow to the legs, is to stand with the knees bent (Figure 8-7). This is how the ancient Shaolin martial monks (Seng Bing, 僧兵) practiced Small Circulation.

Crossed legs are called Jie Jia Fu Zuo (結跏趺坐) in Buddhism.[6] You must keep searching for the most comfortable and stable posture, so your mind can concentrate fully. In the beginning, when you cross your legs, don't place one on top of the other. This pressure causes numbness of the bottom leg. Place them slightly apart. A com-

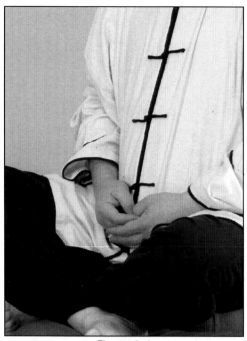

Figure 8-6

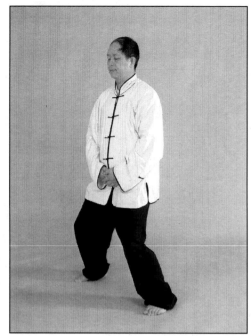

Figure 8-7

fortable cushion of the proper height reduces the problem, and also eases tension in the lower back. You should sit on a thick, comfortable mat to prevent the pressure from the floor generating numbness of the legs. The material used for sitting and wearing should be natural fabrics.

**Eyes and Tongue.** The eyes should be comfortably closed. To keep the thoughts from imagination and fantasy, teachers often have a beginner keep his eyes slightly open. After you have meditated for a long time, it will be easier to lead the Qi if you close your eyes. Then you can feel deeper and more clearly into the deep places of your body.

The tongue should gently touch the palate (Figure 8-8). This connects the Yin Conception Vessel and Yang Governing Vessel and allows Qi to pass. *The Red Wind Marrow* (赤風髓) said, "The secret trick is closing the two eyes, half dropping the curtain (eye lid), and the head (tip) of the red dragon (tongue) touches the palate of the mouth upward."[7] *The Mirror of Cui's (Method) of Entering the Herb* (崔公入藥鏡) said, "The silver river (Milky Way) separates the meeting of Yin and Yang. It must rely on the magpie bridge to cross. Man's tongue is regarded as a magpie bridge". When training Gong, the tongue touches the palate of the mouth to connect Yin and Yang."[8]

You need to provide comfortable and natural conditions for relaxation, Qi circulation, and spiritual cultivation. When you are relaxed, Qi can circulate smoothly. Then you can achieve balance and be centered. When you are centered, you can be

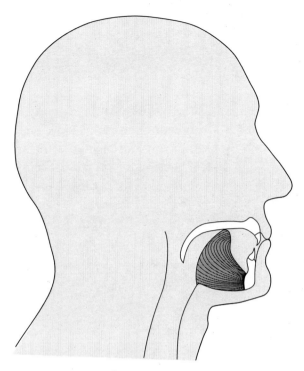

Figure 8-8. Tongue Position

rooted. Only then can you raise up the spirit of vitality for spiritual cultivation. Relaxing, balancing, centering, rooting, and finally raising up the spirit, form a chain of sequential connections.

Once you regulate your mind to a deeper level, regulation of the body can also be more profound. The goal is to feel the bone marrow and internal organs, and relax them. At this level, you feel any Qi imbalance. For example, if you have an injury to your right shoulder or back, you feel the body tends to turn right when you reach a highly relaxed state. This is because the muscles of the right side of the body are tighter. Let the turning happen by itself. Once it reaches its maximum, relax it and allow it to return to its original state. From this practice, you can easily heal your injuries. This kind of mind and body communication is called 'Gongfu of internal vision' (Nei Shi Gongfu, 內視功夫).

Once you reach a good level of regulating the body, you should increase regulation of the breathing. Even then, you continue to regulate your body, because the two are closely related.

## 8-3. REGULATING THE BREATHING 調息

Remember, the goal is to absorb oxygen and expel carbon dioxide efficiently. Then the body has plenty of oxygen for production of new cells and can remove dead cells from the deep places in the body. When you have plenty of oxygen, your energy is high, because it is the vital element for combustion and energy production. To generate strong Qi, you must breathe correctly and efficiently.

To produce abundant Qi, the breathing must be soft and slender, and the body relaxed. Then, oxygen consumption is low and metabolism is efficient. *Dao De Jing*, Chapter 10 (道德經 · 十章) said, "Focusing the breathing to reach softness, can it be soft like a baby?"[9] When breathing is soft, the Qi circulation becomes soft and smooth. *The Complete Book of Principal Contents of Life and Human Nature* (性命圭旨全書) said, "Focus on making the breathing soft and the spirit stays long. The real breathing (Embryonic Breathing) is long, gentle, and slow. Breathe softly to return the Original Qi. Unlimited spiritual fountain will flow naturally."[10] This implies that one produces unlimited Qi flow through correct Embryonic Breathing, where "Exhaling is slender and inhaling is soft and slow."[11]

When you practice correct breathing, you regulate it until regulating is no longer necessary. That means correct breathing has become natural and smooth. *Easy Understanding of Daoist Talking* (道言淺近) said, "Regulating the breathing must regulate until the real regulating is stopped... To condense the spirit and regulate the breathing, you need a peaceful mind and harmonious Qi."[12] *The Complete Book of Principal Contents of Life and Human Nature* (性命圭旨全書) said, "Regulating the breathing, must regulate until the real regulating ceases. Training the Shen, must train until the spirit is no longer necessary for the training."[13] When you regulate your breathing or train your spirit, first use your mind and spirit to make it happen. However, after long practice, everything becomes natural and happens automatically. Then, no more regulating is necessary.

You should follow the following procedures to achieve Embryonic Breathing:

1. **Normal Abdominal Breathing** (Zheng Fu Hu Xi, 正腹呼吸)
   When you inhale, expand your abdomen while pushing your Huiyin (Co-1, 會陰, perineum) out gently and softly (Figure 8-9). When you exhale, withdraw your abdomen and hold up your Huiyin (Figure 8-10). Huiyin is the gate which controls the Qi at the Real Lower Dan Tian, letting it be stored or released. Your tongue touches the palate of your mouth to connect the Conception and Governing Vessels. In Normal Abdominal Breathing, you lead the Qi through the twelve primary channels to the four limbs. This makes you feel natural and relaxed.

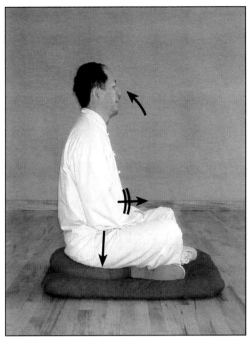

Figure 8-9

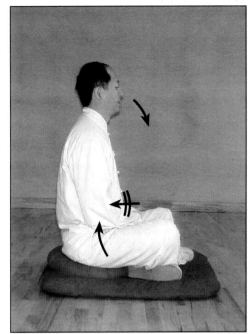

Figure 8-10

Start with small abdominal movement until you feel comfortable, gradually increasing the scale. Do not tense, which causes Qi circulation to stagnate. After long practice, your mind can control the abdominal muscles, so they stay relaxed even though the abdominal movements are big. This accomplishes the first step of Embryonic Breathing.

2. **Reversed Abdominal Breathing** (Fan Fu Hu Xi, 反腹呼吸 )(Ni Fu Hu Xi, 逆腹呼吸)

When you can control the abdominal muscles easily and naturally from Normal Abdominal Breathing practice, you begin Reversed Abdominal Breathing. When you inhale, withdraw your abdomen and hold up your Huiyin (Figure 8-11). When you exhale, push your abdomen and Huiyin out, gently and softly (Figure 8-12). Reversed Abdominal Breathing leads Qi from the twelve primary channels laterally through the muscles to the skin to strengthen Guardian Qi, and also to the bone marrow to enhance marrow Qi and to nourish and clean the marrow.

As with Normal Abdominal Breathing, start with small abdominal movements to keep the area relaxed, proceeding gradually and carefully. When you can control the movement, you increase its scale while remaining relaxed. Then you can lead the Qi in from the body to the Dan Tian and out from the Dan Tian to the whole body.

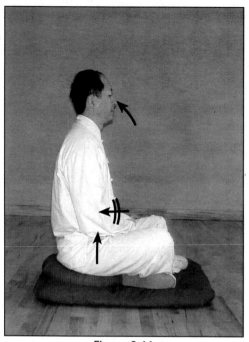

Figure 8-11

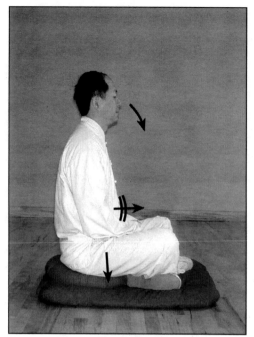

Figure 8-12

### 3. Embryonic Breathing (Tai Xi, 胎息 )

Embryonic Breathing is used to store Qi in the Real Lower Dan Tian and to strengthen the Guardian Qi through Girdle Vessel Breathing (Dai Mai Hu Xi, 帶脈呼吸 ). This is achieved by keeping the mind there. It is commonly called Yi Shou Dan Tian ( 意守丹田 ) which means to keep the mind at the Dan Tian. When the mind is there, the Qi is led there and stays in its residence (Qi She, 氣舍 ). When the mind's focus is elsewhere, Qi is led away and consumed. To store the Qi, the inhalation should be longer than exhalation, and done in the spring and summer. If you strengthen Guardian Qi through Girdle Vessel Breathing, your exhalation should be longer than inhalation. The Girdle Vessel Breathing should be done in the fall and winter time, when strong Guardian Qi is important to protect against the cold.

Since you are leading Qi laterally to the skin and bone marrow, you must use Reversed Abdominal Breathing. The only difference is that when you inhale, the abdomen and lower back withdraw at the same time, while holding up Huiyin. When you exhale, the abdomen and lower back expand, at the same time pushing your Huiyin down, softly and gently.

Again, you start from a small scale of movement, until you control the muscles efficiently, then increase it. After long practice, every movement becomes natural, easy, and automatic without too much mental effort, as you achieve real regulating. Slowly and gradually your mind shifts to the Real Lower Dan Tian and remains there at the center of your body.

Before Small Circulation, practice Embryonic Breathing for a few minutes. If you inhale longer than exhaling, you lead Qi to the Real Lower Dan Tian and calm yourself down. This calms down your mind and stores Qi for the circulation practice.

In Nei Dan Qigong practice, the Real Lower Dan Tian is called Qi Cavity (Qi Xue, 氣穴). Above it is the Yellow Yard (Huang Ting, 黃庭), the tripod (cooking utensil) in which the herb is cooked. When Kan Water Qi from the Real Lower Dan Tian is mixed with Li Fire Qi at the Huang Ting, the Spiritual Baby Embryo (Shen Tai, Sheng Tai, or Ling Tai, 神胎、聖胎、靈胎) is conceived. This interaction of Water and Fire is called Kan and Li (坎離). Once this Spiritual Baby Embryo is ready, it is led to the spiritual residence (Shen Shi, 神室, Upper Dan Tian) for further cultivation and later leaves through the third eye to unite with the natural spirit.

*The Complete Book of Principal Contents of Life and Human Nature* (性命圭旨全書) said, "Huang Ting is the tripod and the Qi cavity is the furnace. Huang Ting is right above the Qi cavity and they are connected with each other by Luo. This is the meeting place of hundreds of channels in the body." The Original Qi condenses between the two cavities in the Small Tripod Furnace (Xiao Ding Lu, 小鼎爐). "The position of Qian (乾) is tripod while the position of Kun (坤) is furnace." If this concept is applied in the Circulation Meditation, the brain (Ni Wan Gong, 泥丸宮 or Upper Dan Tian, 上丹田) is Qian (tripod) while the Lower Dan Tian (Xia Dan Tian, 下丹田) is Kun (furnace).[14] *The Verification Thesis of Golden Immortal* (金仙証論) said, "Those who pick up the herb (Qi) to transport the cyclic heaven (Small Circulation) should start the fire at the Kun furnace (Real Lower Dan Tian). Ascend to the Qian head (tripod) and descend to the Kun abdomen (furnace). This is what the ancients meant by using Qian Kun as the cooking tools. Whenever Shen and Qi rise and fall, the tripod's Qi exists." When there is Shen and Qi, you have furnace and tripod. Without Shen and Qi, there is neither furnace nor tripod.[15]

Therefore, when you start the fire in the False Lower Dan Tian and accumulate it in the Real Lower Dan Tian, breathing significantly influences how the Qi builds up. If you build it up slowly with long, gentle technique, it is called scholar fire (Wen Huo, 文火). If you build it up quickly with short, fast, heavy breathing, it is called martial fire (Wu Huo, 武火). *Anthology of Daoist Village* (道鄉集) asked, "What is scholar fire? It is to keep and to exist. Do not extinguish and do not assist."[16] In scholar fire cultivation, it seems the breathing is there but not there. It is like cooking with a very small fire to simmer the food.

The Daoist book, *The Record of Reaching the Mystic with Heavenly Nature of Wind and Moon* (性天風月通玄記), said, "Among the calmness, there is movement of the fire. This is the right time to refine the large returning (Da Huan, 大還, nourish the Shen with Qi). When Qi is picked up, it is the herb, and within the herb, there is fire. If asked for martial fire, raise up the wind strongly, if asked for scholar fire, Embryonic Breathing slow and soft."[17] When you meditate, your body is in an extremely calm state. You build up the fire at the Real Lower Dan Tian, then lead it up to the brain to nourish the spirit. Martial fire is generated from quick, heavy breathing, while scholar fire is produced from slow, gentle Embryonic Breathing.

Since Embryonic Breathing is vital in storing Qi for spiritual cultivation, you should study this subject first, as described in the previous YMAA book, *Qigong Meditation—Embryonic Breathing*.

## 8-4. Regulating the Emotional Mind 調心

The way you regulate your mind depends on your purpose. But no matter what the purpose is, the general rule is simple. When the mind is calm and peaceful, it can be centered at the Qi residence, leading Qi to stay there. When the mind is elsewhere, it leads Qi out to be manifested and consumed.

You regulate your mind according to your purpose. The first purpose for regulating the mind in Small Circulation is to store abundant Qi at the Real Lower Dan Tian. Qi in the eight vessels is raised, and the twelve primary Qi channels are regulated, so the whole body's vital energy is strong, healthy, and in high spirits. The second main purpose of practicing Small Circulation is to lead the Qi to circulate smoothly in the Conception and Governing Vessels. This strengthens the body and is crucial to the Muscle/Tendon Changing practice.

In Small Circulation meditation, first lead your mind from the Third Eye to the Mud Pill Palace. This calms down random thoughts and leads it into the state of emptiness. You are regulating your emotional mind to set it free from the bondage of the seven emotions and six desires described earlier. If you have difficulty regulating this emotional mind, by paying attention to your third eye and leading it to the Mud Pill Palace, you may simply focus on your breathing.

The normal procedure of taming the emotional monkey mind has three steps. "The eyes observe the nose, and the nose observes the Xin (emotional mind)."[18] Focus your vision inside by closing your eyes, then pay attention to the breathing. The breathing gradually regulates the Xin.

Make the inhalation long, soft, and slender, and allow the exhalation to happen slowly by itself. This calms down your mind and body. With clear inner feeling, you bring your mind to the Jiuwei (Co-15, 鳩尾, Middle Dan Tian) and continue regulating your mind, assisted by the breathing. To cool down the body's emotional and physical fire, you must first cool down the Middle Dan Tian, which is the center of the Post-heaven fire Qi. Once you cool down this fire center, you can lead your physical and mental bodies to a very calm and peaceful state.

After this, shift your mind to the Real Lower Dan Tian. This is Embryonic Breathing, which slowly leads Qi to its residence. The physical body will not be energized further, and it starts to cool down. Continue Embryonic Breathing for a while until you feel Qi has accumulated to a comfortable level. Then it is said you have grown the herb (Chan Yao, 產藥), meaning you have built up a fire.

Producing the herb at the Real Lower Dan Tian depends on the movement of the tricky gate, Huiyin. Huiyin can lead the Qi to the Real Lower Dan Tian and store it there (Yin), and can also lead it to the physical and mental bodies to manifest it (Yang). Reversed Abdominal Breathing leads the Qi to store it at the Real Lower Dan Tian. Then your mind can circulate it. This is picking up the herb (Cai Yao, 采藥).

Set yourself free from lingering emotional bondage, which confuses the present and sows doubt about the future. This is caused by lack of understanding of the meaning of life. Recognize yourself, be aware of yourself and your environment, and let your mind awaken to comprehend occurrences. Then you can set yourself free from bondage. Confucius (Kong Zi, 孔子) said, "Once the knowing (self-recognition) has stopped, then there is steadiness. After steadiness, then it can be calm. When it is calm, then it can be peaceful. When it is peaceful, then you can think. Once you can think, then you will gain."[19] This is the process of building up self-confidence in life or in any study. Without it, your mind will wander and be confused, nor will your emotional mind be governed by the wisdom mind.

The final goal is called the righteous mind (Zheng Nian, 正念), the mind of no mind (Wu Nian, 無念), or the real mind (Zhen Nian, 真念). The mind is completely separated from emotional thoughts. It is said in the book, *The Complete Book of Principal Contents of Life and Human Nature* (性命圭旨全書), "If one desires to cease the initiation of the Xin (emotional mind), one must start from the thought of no thought."[20] To reach this stage, body and mind must be extremely calm and empty. *Dao De Jing*, Chapter 16 said, "Reach the extreme emptiness, and keep the profound calmness."[21] When this stage is reached, the Yin and Yang in the body interact in harmony with each other, generating the Yang essence of life. *The Complete Book of Principal Contents of Life and Human Nature* (性命圭旨全書) said, "(When) there is nothing in your mind, it is emptiness. When no more thought arises, it is calmness. Reaching emptiness to its extremity, keeping calmness to its profundity. Yin and Yang interact naturally. Then the Yang essence is generated."[22]

In *Anthology of Daoist Village* (道鄉集), it is said, "When Xin (desire) is generated, then observe its crux. When no Xin (Wu Xin, 無心) is generated, then observe the marvelousness. These words describe the applications of the Dao. The saying that 'if desire is generated, then observe the crux,' is actually the application of the saying that 'if no desire is generated, then observe the marvelousness.' The saying that, 'if desire is generated, then observe the marvelousness (of the Dao),' is, in fact, the core of the saying that, 'if desire is generated, then observe the crux.' 'If there is desire, then observe its crux,' means having an intention of doing. It is the time when the spirit and Qi return to the body. 'There is no desire, and observe the marvelousness (of the Dao),' means there is no intention of acting. This is the state of no others, no self, no mountain, no river, grass, or trees, mixed and indistinguishable, no sense and no feeling."[23]

This paragraph discusses the two states of meditation, the state of desire and the state of no desire. In the state of desire, or intention, your emotional mind leads Qi to fulfill your desire and to nourish and raise your spirit. Then, you are paying attention to the methods (crux) of leading and cultivating. The other state is the state of no desire. This is the state of Wuji, of no extremity and no thought. When you reach a profoundly calm state, it is "the thought of no thought." In this state, you are part of nature and forget yourself and nature, both becoming indistinguishable. Your spirit blends and unites with the natural spirit. This is the state of Unification of Heaven and Man (Tian Ren He Yi, 天人合一), the end and the origin of life.

When you practice Small Circulation in the state of Embryonic Breathing, your mind is at the center. If you have a desire to store Qi at the Real Lower Dan Tian or expand it to the Girdle Vessel (Dai Mai, 帶脈), you have an intention. However, once you have reached a very deep level, the stage of "regulating of no regulating," then you have the "thought of no thought." You are in the extremely calm Wuji state, which allows you to be in harmony with nature.

However, when you are in the state of using the mind to lead Qi in the Conception and Governing Vessels, you have an intention. Once you reach the state of "regulating of no regulating," everything becomes natural and you enter "the thought of no thought."

## 8-5. REGULATING THE QI 調氣

Regulating the Qi in Small Circulation practice can be divided into two parts. The first part is, through Embryonic Breathing, to build up abundant Qi and to store it in the Real Lower Dan Tian. The second part is using the mind to lead the Qi to circulate smoothly in the Conception and Governing Vessels. Here we focus on methods of circulating the Qi in the Conception and Governing Vessels.

There are many paths of Small Circulation, but here we only focus on the path of circulating the Qi in the Fire Path. This is the safest and most important path, and most favored by beginners and experienced practitioners alike. It follows the natural path of Qi circulation and strengthens the Qi circulation in the body. Most Small Circulation practitioners follow the Fire Path exclusively.

There are also many ways of circulating the Qi in the Fire Path. Buddhists accumulate Qi at the Lower Dan Tian and lead it to circulate using Normal Abdominal

Breathing. However, Daoists prefer using Reversed Abdominal Breathing. The Daoist method is more aggressive, since the mind is more actively involved in leading the Qi, so it is classified as Yang method, compared with the Buddhist method which is classified as Yin. I only practiced the Buddhist method for three years, starting when I was 16 years old. After more than thirty years of practicing the Daoist method, I have more experience in that technique. Here, I share with you what I have experienced of Daoist Small Circulation techniques.

The most important point in Small Circulation practice is that there are three dangerous gates (San Guan, 三關) which, according to

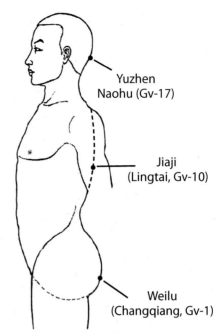

Figure 8-13. Three Gates (San Guan): Yuzhen, Jiaji, and Weilu

experience, could cause serious injury, especially for beginners. They are called 1). Changqiang (medical society) or Weilu (Tailbone, Daoist society), 2). Lingtai (medical society), Mingmen (Life Door, martial society), or Jiaji (Daoist society), and 3). Fengfu (medical society) or Jade Pillow (Daoist society)(Figure 8-13). How to lead the Qi past these three gates was kept secret in ancient practice. Next, I share what I believe is the safest and most natural ways to do so.

To start, you should keep the mind at the False Lower Dan Tian and start the fire for at least five minutes. Not only is the fire built, but your mind also gradually moves from outside the body to internal feeling. If you inhale longer than exhaling, you can easily calm down. However, if you know Embryonic Breathing, then you may use it instead, paying more attention to the inhalation.

After five to ten minutes of False Lower Dan Tian Breathing or Embryonic Breathing, you should notice a distinct feeling of warmth in the area. You may also feel vibration if the False Lower Dan Tian is used. Don't be alarmed, as all of these phenomena are very common.

Keep your tongue touching the center of your palate gently. This is called Da Que Qiao (搭鵲橋, build the magpie bridge,) which allows you to connect the Conception (Yin) and Governing (Yang) Vessels in your mouth. Daoists call this place Shang Que Qiao (上鵲橋, Upper magpie bridge), while the Huiyin, which also connects the two vessels, is called Xia Que Qiao (下鵲橋, Lower magpie bridge).

To help beginners lead Qi past the first gate, Changqiang or tailbone, I teach what I call Small Small Circulation (Xiao Xiao Zhou Tian, 小小周天). *The key is to lead the Qi by keeping the mind ahead of it.* When the mind is on the Qi, then it stagnates. The mind should not be on the Qi.[24] Place the mind one or two cavities ahead of the Qi, then it can be led.

In Small Small Circulation, you inhale keeping your mind at the Lower Dan Tian, then exhale to lead the Qi to the Huiyin. Inhale, and lead the Qi upward from Huiyin to Mingmen (Gv-4, 命門), and then return to the Lower Dan Tian or Real Lower Dan Tian (Figure 8-14). Repeat the cycle.

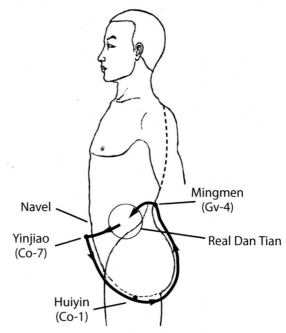

Figure 8-14. Small Small Circulation

When you practice, you should ignore the existence of the Changqiang cavity. The more you focus on this gate, the more the Qi stagnates there.

You may experience that your Qi moves faster than your mind. In this case, it is just like leading a cow with a rope, but instead the cow walks ahead of you. This means your mind is not leading the Qi, so practice until you can do it effectively. Slow down your breathing, and move your Huiyin up and down slowly. Your mind needs to be calm, peaceful, and concentrated. You should practice for a few months until you are proficient in it.

Next, you circulate Qi in the regular path of Small Circulation. You lead it up the spine step by step, advancing a few cavities at a time. When you reach a certain point, you must turn and lead the Qi back to the Real Lower Dan Tian. There are various turning points which you can use, which are normally kept secret in different styles. If you choose the correct point, the danger can be significantly reduced. Do not push to make it happen, but take your time, otherwise your ego and anxiety can obstruct and endanger you. Take it easy and enjoy the practice. The following turning points are considered the safest for practice:

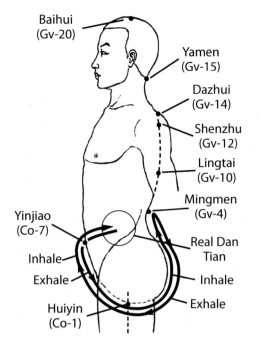

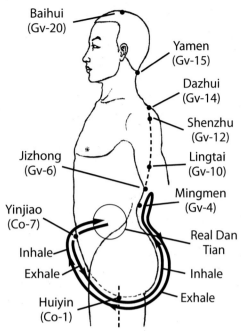

Figure 8-15. Real Dan Tian-Yinjiao-Huiyin-
Mingmen-Huiyin-Yinjiao-Real Dan Tian

Figure 8-16. Real Dan Tian-Yinjiao-Huiyin-
Jizhong-Huiyin-Yinjiao-Real Dan Tian

1. **Mingmen** (Gv-4, 命門). Use Mingmen as the first turning point. Since Mingmen connects to the Real Lower Dan Tian, if there is any stagnation, Qi can easily return through this cavity.

   First exhale and lead the Qi to the Huiyin, then inhale and lead it up to the Mingmen. Exhale again to lead Qi back to the Huiyin, and finally inhale and lead it back to the Real Lower Dan Tian (Figure 8-15). There is a simple rule to coordinate your breathing with leading the Qi. *Whenever you lead Qi out from the Dan Tian, you exhale, and whenever you lead it back to the Dan Tian, you inhale.*

2. **Jizhong** (Gv-6, 脊中). Once you can lead the Qi to the Mingmen easily, you extend the path by leading it up to the Jizhong, which means spinal center. Use this cavity for a turning point because it is away from the vital cavity Lingtai (Gv-10, 靈台), the second tricky gate. First exhale and lead Qi to the Huiyin, then inhale and lead it up to the Jizhong. Exhale and lead it down to the Huiyin, and finally inhale and lead it back to the Dan Tian (Figure 8-16).

3. **Shenzhu** (Gv-12, 身柱) or Dazhui (Gv-14, 大椎). Again, after you have practiced for a while and feel comfortable leading the Qi to the Jizhong, then can you proceed to lead it to the Shenzhu or Dazhui cavity. These cavities are chosen because if the Qi is stagnant there after practice, it can easily be dispersed into the arms to prevent any problem. Between Jizhong and these two cavities is the dangerous Lingtai cavity. The method of dealing with this gate is to ignore it. The more you focus on it, the more Qi is led there and enters the heart. Ignore it and pay attention to the Shenzhu or Dazhui cavities. First exhale and lead the Qi to the Huiyin, then inhale and lead it up to Shenzhu or Dazhui. Exhale and lead it back to Huiyin, and finally inhale and lead it back to the Dan Tian (Figure 8-17).

4. **Yamen** (Gv-15, 啞門). The next step is leading the Qi to the Yamen, or Mute Door, located at the rear center of the neck. One moves the neck all the time, so any Qi stagnation there can be removed easily before it causes harm. First exhale and lead the Qi to Huiyin, then inhale and lead it up to the Yamen. Exhale and lead it down to Huiyin, and finally inhale as you lead it back to the Dan Tian (Figure 8-18).

5. **Baihui** (Gv-20, 百會). Above Yamen is the Fengfu (Gv-16, 風府) or Jade Pillow (Yuzhen, 玉枕), the third tricky gate, which you ignore. The more you pay attention to it,

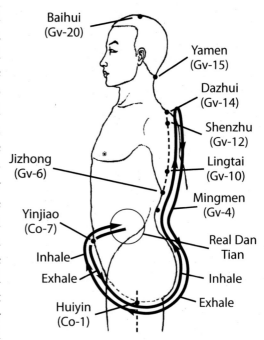

Figure 8-17. Real Dan Tian-Yinjiao-Huiyin-Dazhui-Huiyin-Yinjiao-Real Dan Tian

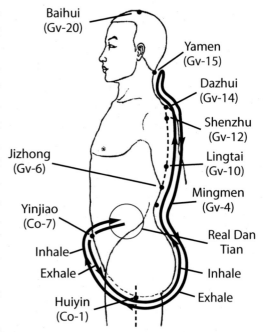

Figure 8-18. Real Dan Tian-Yinjiao-Huiyin-Yamen-Huiyin-Yinjiao-Real Dan Tian

the more Qi stagnates there. Simply lead the Qi to Baihui, the "hundred meetings" which is connected to the central energy line. When the spirit is raised up at this cavity, the whole body's Qi can be governed efficiently, and any stagnation easily led away. First exhale and lead the Qi to Huiyin, then inhale as you lead it up to Baihui. Exhale and lead it down to Huiyin, and finally inhale and lead it back to the Dan Tian (Figure 8-19).

6. **Palate** (Shang E, 上顎). The palate of the mouth is the Qi junction of the Yin (Conception) and Yang (Governing) vessels. There you change your inhalation to exhalation and lead the Qi down the front of the body to Huiyin to complete the cycle. You first exhale and lead Qi to Huiyin, and then inhale to lead it up past Baihui and down to the palate of the mouth. Exhale and lead the Qi down the front of the body to Huiyin (Figure 8-20). While leading it down past Yinjiao (Co-7, 陰交), you are also leading more Qi from the False or Real Dan Tian to join the Qi flow to enhance its circulation.

Now you have completed the Small Circulation. You should continue circulating for twenty minutes or more, depending on your condition. How fast should the Qi be led by the mind? This depends on each individual's technique. Ancient documents described three ways of leading the Qi in Small Circulation,

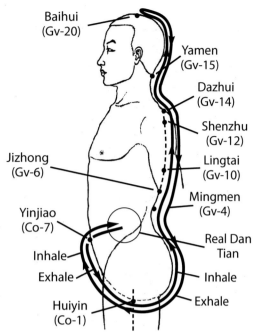

Figure 8-19. Real Dan Tian-Yinjiao-Huiyin-Baihui-Huiyin-Yinjiao-Real Dan Tian

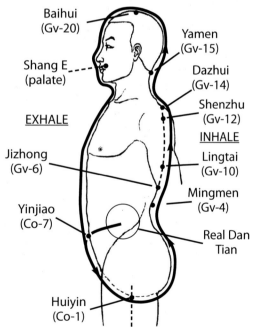

Figure 8-20. Small Circulation

called He Che (河車, River Vehicles). From Weilu to Jiaji was classified as "Sheep vehicle" (Yang Che, 羊車), and its Qi movement should be slow. From Jiaji to Yuzhen was classified as "Deer vehicle" (Lu Che, 鹿車), and the Qi movement should be fast. Finally, from Yuzhen to Niwan is classified as "Bull vehicle" (Niu Che, 牛車), and the Qi movement should be strong. These three ways of Qi's transportation are commonly called San Che (三車) which means three vehicles.[25] This is only for your reference. The most important of all is your feeling.

If you enjoy it and feel comfortable, you may meditate for a couple of hours. However, if you feel uneasy even just for a short time, you should stop and try again later. You should not force yourself to sit long, if it causes you more tension and discomfort. I would like to remind you of a few important points:

1. When you lead Qi to a cavity, do not focus on its exact location. Simply pay attention to the area. This is different from acupuncture, in which the accuracy of the needling is very important. In meditation, if you pay too much attention to the exact location, your mind stagnates together with the Qi. Simply pay attention to the area, and the Qi will be led smoothly.

2. The Conception Vessel is Yin, while the Governing Vessel is Yang. They regulate the six Yin and six Yang primary channels independently. To prevent the Yin vessel from becoming more Yin, when you lead Qi in it, you exhale (Yang) to balance the Yin. Similarly, when you lead Qi in the Governing Vessel, you inhale (Yin) to stop it becoming too Yang. This balances the Qi status when you meditate. Huiyin is used as the turning point when you change the breathing from exhalation to inhalation, and the palate is the turning point as you change it from inhalation to exhalation.

3. Often, to make the breathing more smooth and natural, a master teaches his student two-cycle breathing. If one-cycle breathing for Small Circulation is too urgent and uncomfortable, you may add another inhalation and exhalation. From my personal experience, the best place to add this extra breath is in front. That means when you exhale to lead the Qi down from the palate, instead of leading it to the Huiyin directly, first exhale to Yinjiao (Co-7, 陰交), then inhale and lead the Qi into the Real Lower Dan Tian. Finally, exhale again and lead the Qi to Huiyin to complete the cycle (Figure 8-21).

4. Remember a simple rule. When you practice Small Circulation, do not hold your breath. Inhale and exhale smoothly and naturally. Whenever you hold your breath, you tense your body and mind, and this causes Qi stagnation.

5. If you cannot yet control the abdominal area, don't lead the Qi, as it means your mind is still regulating your abdominal breathing. If you lead the Qi regardless, your stomach and abdominal area will be tense and uncomfortable. This hinders the meditation process. You should practice abdominal breathing for a

while until it becomes very natural, smooth, and comfortable.

6. While meditating, pay attention to your back. It can become tense after meditating for a while. First regulate your body until it is regulated. Then regulate your breathing until it is regulated. Only then have you provided good conditions for your mind to lead the Qi. Take it easy and be natural. Whenever your body is tense, the Qi circulation becomes stagnant.

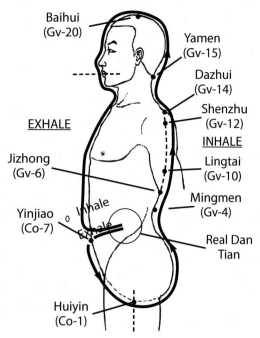

Figure 8-21. Small Circulation (Two Respirations)

## 8-6. REGULATING THE SPIRIT 調神

Regulating the spirit is the final stage of Qigong regulating. According to different schools, the purposes of spiritual regulating are also different. For example, for medical Qigong, regulating the spirit is simply for raising the spirit of vitality for healing purposes. For the scholar group, it regulates the spirit until it reaches extreme calmness and peace. To martial arts Qigong, regulating the spirit raises up the awareness and fighting morale.

To reach this state of peace, scholar Qigong practitioners strive to be free from emotional bondage. *Dao De Jing*, Chapter 1, said, "Always maintain the state of no desire, so can see its marvelousness."[26] Chapter 16 said, "Attain the insubstantial extremity, and maintain true calmness."[27] What is the insubstantial extremity? It is what is defined as spirit. *All Application Secrets of Real Holy Embryonic Spirit* (諸真聖胎神用訣) said, "What is spirit? It is the application of insubstantiality and nothingness."[28] Spirit is invisible, empty and intangible. It is the master of being, residing in our physical form.

However, in religious society, regulating the spirit is intended to give birth to the Spiritual Embryo, to open the third eye for enlightenment or Buddhahood. Buddhists and Daoists also strive for emotional emptiness, or freedom from emotional bondage. The Buddhist classic, *Sixth Ancestor's Lecturing Classic* (六祖壇經) said, "Bodhi does not have a tree originally, nor is there a shining mirror in front. There are no objects there originally, so how can they be contaminated by dust or mud (objects or emotions)?"[29] Bodhi is a special Buddhist term which refers to the ultimate wisdom, developed from a high level of spiritual cultivation. Tree means all the physical objects around us and mirror reflects the emotional reactions to events. If there is neither object nor emotional disturbance in your mind, how can you be disturbed by the emotional dust or mud?

Spirit is called Yuan Shen (元神, Original Spirit). This spirit was born originally in physical form and resides in the brain. The book, *A Detailed Outline of Basic Herbs* (本草綱目) clearly points out, "brain is the residence of Original Spirit."[30] The brain is also called Upper Dan Tian (Shang Dan Tian, 上丹田) by Daoists. The book, *Observing Vessels* (脈望) said, "The brain is the Upper Dan Tian, the palace where the Original Spirit resides. If one firms the Original Spirit and keeps it residing in its original residence, then the golden Qi is raised and the real breathing steady automatically. This is what is said, when one knack opens, a hundred knacks will open. When the big gate is passable, then hundred gates are passable."[31] The Original Spirit resides at the Mud Pill Palace, the center of the brain where the pineal and pituitary glands are situated. These two glands are shaped like small mud pills. The Daoist book, *Further Study of Can Tong Qi* (參同契發揮) said, "Follow the real breathing's to and fro, allow the real Qi to ascend and descend freely. From morning till evening, the Original Spirit should always reside in Mud Pill."[32] Again, it is first very important to read and understand the book *Qigong Meditation—Embryonic Breathing*.

Original Spirit is also called Valley Spirit (Gu Shen, 谷神), because the space between the two hemispheres of the brain forms a valley which generates echo and resonance. This space is also called Spirit Valley (Shen Gu, 神谷). *Dao De Jing*, Chapter 6 said, "Valley spirit does not die, it is called Xuan Pin. The door of Xuan Pin is the root of heaven and earth. It is as though it were existing. When used, it will not be exhausted."[33] Daoists believe the spirit does not die with the physical body. The spirit finds a new body and enters it for reincarnation. Xuan Pin (玄牝) means the creation of life from the combination of the physical object and the invisible spiritual energy. From Xuan Pin, millions of lives are born. Therefore, Xuan Pin is the root of the physical world. If we know how to keep this spiritual force strong, it will last forever. Spirit is called Original Spirit or Valley Spirit and its residence is the brain, Upper Dan Tian, Spiritual Valley, or Mud Pill Palace.

To Buddhists and Daoists, the final goal of regulating the spirit is to open the third eye and allow the spirit to communicate with the external spiritual world. This is called the unification of heaven and man (Tian Ren He Yi, 天人合一). The third eye is also called heavenly eye (Tian Mu, 天目), as explained in the Daoist book, *The Illustration of Cultivating the Truth in Wudang* (武當修真圖): "Under the Mingtang, the upper mid-place of the line between the two eyebrows, there is a spiritual light emitted here; it is called heavenly eye."[34] Mingtang (明堂) means the forehead. The third eye is called Yintang (M-HN-3, 印堂) by medical society and heavenly yard (Tian Ting, 天庭) by the general public.

The third eye is the door for the spirit to exit and enter the Spiritual Valley. The Daoist book, *Seventh Bamboo Label of Bookcase* (云笈七签) said, "The place between the two eyebrows is the (precious) jade door of Mud Pill."[35] The third eye is the door to the Mud Pill Palace, the residence of Original Spirit.

There is an ancient document which describes the cultivation of spirit in Small Circulation:

### Anthology of Daoist Village
### 《道鄉集》

*Small Circulation should be practiced after the real seed enters the furnace, at the time the Yang fire (Qi) just starts to produce. Follow the opportunity (timing) of this production and growing, use the spirit to lead, and use the breathing to blow (fan the flames). When the fire receives the leading of the spirit and the blowing of the breath, it ascends naturally. But you need not be confined by the diagrams for divination (in Bagua) or restricted by the time. When there is an opportunity to ascend, then lead it up. When there is an opportunity for steadiness and calmness, then allow it to be steady and calm. It does not matter how, always lead when there is movement (of Qi), and stabilize when there is calmness. If there is no movement and you lead, it is useless. If there is no calmness and you stabilize, it is harmful. It does not matter whether it is movement or calmness, each must follow its opportunities. In this case, it is coordinating with the natural (Dao). Though using the spirit to lead, yet you should not observe (concentrate), and though using the breathing to blow, it should not be stagnant. When Qi starts to move and ascend, the Original Spirit condenses in Xuan Guan (tricky gate, Real Lower Dan Tian). Then use some spirit (mind) to lead the ascending Yang fire, and use the breathing to enhance it. It is not because the breathing can (make Qi) ascend by following the Yang fire. It is just using the function of inhalation (to lead Qi to ascend). When exhaling, then follow the natural way. Though the function of the exhaling breath is downward, however, when the Yang fire receives the pressure of the real breathing, it will turn and ascend. It is only when using spirit and breathing. I follow its (Qi's) ascending and descending. Therefore, the Yang fire begins from Xuan Qiao (Huiyin) and ends at Xuan Qiao to complete a cycle. This is called the heavenly cycle.*

小周天，行于真種入爐之後，陽火發生之時，順其生發
之機，以神而引，以息而吹，火受神息引吹，自然上升。
但不必論其爻象，限其時刻，有上行之機，則引上行，
有定靜之機，則聽其定靜。總是動而后引，靜而后定。
不動，引之無益；不靜，定之有損。無論動靜，均須順
其機而為之，方合乎自然也。雖有神引，亦不可看，雖
以息吹，亦不可滯，當升機發動之時，元神仍凝玄關，
稍分其神，以引上升之陽火，息之吹逼，非息能隨陽火
上升也。不過稍作用于吸機，呼則順其自然，息機雖向
下，而陽火受真息壓迫，反轉而上升也，用神用息，不
過如是，餘則聽其自升自降而已。因此，陽火發于玄竅，
止于玄竅，經過一周，故曰周天。

In Small Circulation practice, first you build up the Qi (Fire) through abdominal breathing. You focus your mind and spirit at the False Lower Dan Tian to initiate the seed fire. Through abdominal breathing for some time, abundant Qi accumulates. The abdomen first feels warm and later starts to vibrate by itself. This state is called Chan Yao (產藥). Next, you lead this Qi to circulate in the vessels. This stage is called Cai Yao (采藥) and means picking up the herb. Herb here means Qi or elixir. When you reach this stage, the Qi will have an intention to move. Use your mind and spirit to lead Qi to the Huiyin, and then up the Governing Vessel to reach the Upper Dan Tian. When your mind leads the Qi, you should coordinate it with the breathing. Breathing is regarded as the strategy of Qigong practice, which significantly enhances the leading of the Qi.

When you use your mind to lead the Qi, you should not concentrate but simply pay attention and lead it gently. When your breathing enhances Qi circulation, it should be smooth and natural, otherwise it becomes stagnant. Though you are using your mind to lead the Qi, do not forget that mind and spirit should always be kept in the Real Lower Dan Tian. It is the same as travelling away from home; your mind should always be concerned for your family at home.

Xuan Guan (玄關) means Lower Dan Tian, and Xuan Qiao (玄竅) means Upper Dan Tian. Though you are inhaling, you are leading the Qi upward, and after passing the Upper Dan Tian, you allow Qi to flow down the Conception Vessel in coordination with the natural exhaling. Finally, complete the Small Circulation circuit.

When you reach a profound meditative state, you are as though asleep and as though awake. It seems you are sleeping but your conscious mind is still aware in a drowsy state, and the Qi in the brain is strong. The Daoist document, *A Comparative Study of the Zhou's Yi* (周易參同契) said, "When a truthful person reaches the stage of marvelousness, it seems to be there and seems not to be there. It is like a great deep gulf, suddenly sinks and suddenly floats. When it retreats, it spreads and maintains its position."[36]

When you reach this stage after long practice, you open your third eye and reach enlightenment. We will discuss this more in the forthcoming book, *Spiritual Enlightenment Meditation*.

## 8-7. REGULATING THE ESSENCE 調精

In Qigong and medical society, Jing ( 精 , Essence), Qi ( 氣 ), and Shen ( 神 , spirit) are three precious treasures of life. If you preserve Original Essence (Yuan Jing, 元精 ), inherited from your parents and absorb Post-Birth Essence (air and food) correctly, you have a firm foundation to generate abundant Qi. When this Qi nourishes the brain, the spirit is raised to a high level, and you will have a long, healthy life. This process is necessary to attain Buddhahood or enlightenment.

What is the Original Essence? It is the foundation of one's life ( 生命之本 ). It is formed from the Original Qi of nature. Through the mother's body, a new life is born, and the Original Essence is carried with it. The document, *Discussing Extraordinary Balance* ( 論衡・超奇 ) said, "Heaven has the natural endowment of Original Qi; when man absorbs it, it becomes Original Essence."[37] *Comparative Study of Ancient Documents* ( 古文參同契 ) said, "The Original Qi that is abundant and refined is called Original Essence."[38]

Original Essence also means the hormones or sperm stored in a man's testicles. When a man abuses his sexuality, he loses too much Original Essence. This weakens the function of his kidneys because the Original Essence is stored there. The kidneys with adrenal glands are called Internal Kidneys, while testicles are called External Kidneys. These internal and external kidneys are connected and closely related. When the Qi level in one is weakened, the other is affected as well. So techniques to preserve and control the ejaculation of sperm are a major task in Qigong training. *The Complete Book of Principal Contents of Life and Human Nature* ( 性命圭旨全書 ) said, "Those who refine the essence, it is to refine the Original Essence. It is to draw the original Yang from Kan. When the Original Essence is firmed, then sperm is not released during intercourse."[39] The groin area is considered Yin, as water, and called Kan (Water). The penis is considered Yang within Yin in the groin area.

One method of firming this essence right after meditation, has been recorded and passed down to us:

## Original explanation of not using herbs
## (Secrets of Golden Elixir)
《勿藥元詮・清・汪昂輯》
金丹秘訣

*One rubs and one holds, left and right change hands. The achievement of Nine-Nine (81 times), the real Yang will not be released. Shu (7 to 9 P.M.) and Hai (9 to 11 P.M.) two periods, the Yin strengthens, while the Yang weakens, one hand holds up the External Kidneys, one hand rubs under the navel. Left and right change hands, eighty-one times each. Half month, the sperm is firmed. The longer the better.*

一擦一兜，左右換手，九九之功，真陽不走。戌、亥二
時，陰盛陽衰之候，一手兜外腎，一手擦臍下，左右換
手，各八十一，半月精固，久而彌佳。

Use one hand to hold the testicles. Hold up your Huiyin throughout the process. Inhale and exhale normally with deep relaxation. Then use the other hand to rub the area between navel and groin with a circular motion. Circle for eighty-one times and then change hands and repeat in the other direction. This firms the essence and increases hormone production.

Qigong emphasizes techniques of increasing hormone production in the adrenal glands, sex glands, and pituitary and pineal glands. When the production of Original Essence (hormone) is strong and healthy, the life force Qi is strong and the spirit high. We describe methods of producing growth hormone and melatonin in another book. For ways to increase hormone production in the adrenal glands, please refer to the YMAA book, *The Root of Chinese Qigong*.

## 8-8. RECOVERY FROM THE MEDITATIVE STATE 靜坐後之恢復

The correct way to recover from meditation is most important. If you don't do it correctly, you may experience headache (mental imbalance) or some physical tightness, especially in the spine. Correct recovery methods remove Qi stagnation caused by meditation.

The methods of recovering from meditation are both mental and physical. The trick is to reverse the normal regulating process of meditation. First regulate your mind, then your breathing, and finally your body. Here I introduce the general methods of recovery that have been passed down, or gained through my personal experience.

**Regulate the Mind, Qi, and Breathing.** The first step in recovery from meditation is keeping your mind calm. Slowly awaken from your semi-hypnotic state. It seems that you have just woken up from a deep sleep, yet your conscious mind is still in control.

Bring your mind to the Real Lower Dan Tian. This is very important. Your mind leads your Qi back there, removing it from the path of Small Circulation, where it could otherwise stagnate. Real Lower Dan Tian is the residence of the Qi, so the first step is to return it there to prevent disturbance. This is the same as the treatment in case of shock, if suddenly awakened from deep meditation.

Keep your mind in the Real Dan Tian, and resume Embryonic Breathing for a couple of minutes until you feel that Qi has returned. After Embryonic Breathing, you may practice a few minutes of skin breathing, if you know it well. Try to exhale longer than you inhale. This leads the Qi to the skin surface and rouses the body from the sleeping state.

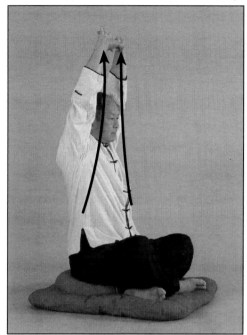

Figure 8-22

Then move your mind to the Upper Dan Tian, and relocate your spiritual center. Sit there for a couple of minutes. When you do this mentally, you wake yourself up completely and comfortably.

Remember, when you recover from your meditative state mentally, you should not resist or speed up the process. You should take it easy, be natural and comfortable. From this, you obtain great satisfaction, peace, and harmony.

**Regulate the body.** After bringing your mind back to the concrete world, you should then regulate your body and arouse it from sleep. Through correct movement, you disperse stagnant Qi that may be caused by long sitting or improper posture. Next, some effective movements and stretches are recommended.

**Upward torso stretching.** First stretch your torso. Interlock your hands and push upwards (Figure 8-22). This stretch loosens any tightness of the torso or spine caused by long sitting. After your hands have reached the highest position, stay there, inhale deeply and then exhale. Inhale again and lower your arms. Repeat twice.

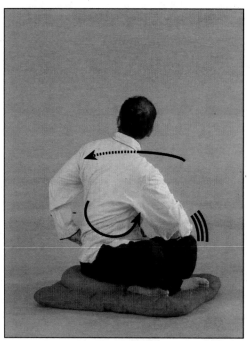

Figure 8-23

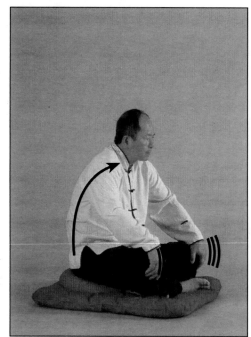

Figure 8-24

**Sideways torso twist.** After the upward stretch, twist your torso sideways. Turn your body to the left first, and use your right hand to pull your left thigh while pushing your left shoulder backwards (Figure 8-23). Stay in this position, inhale and then exhale. Next, repeat on the other side.

**Spine waving.** Next, loosen your vertebrae, section by section, from the sacrum up to the neck. Place your hands on your knees, and pull them to generate a waving spine motion (Figure 8-24). When you begin to pull, the lower torso is thrust forward, and you inhale deeply. When the waving motion reaches the upper spine, you exhale. Move comfortably and naturally, with the spine movement of a sigh. When you are depressed or feel great emotion stuck in your body, you generally inhale deeply, with the "Hen" sound, and generate a waving motion from the lower back. When the motion reaches the upper torso, you exhale. This is the most natural torso movement and it allows you to relax the torso and release any trapped emotional energy.

**Loosening the shoulders.** Next, loosen the upper spine, and remove any stagnant Qi there. Slowly move your shoulders clockwise in a big circle at least six times (Figure 8-25). When they circle forward, inhale deeply, and when they circle backward, exhale deeply. After you complete the clockwise circling, reverse direction and repeat for the same number of times. However, this time you should inhale deeply when you circle backward and exhale when you circle for-

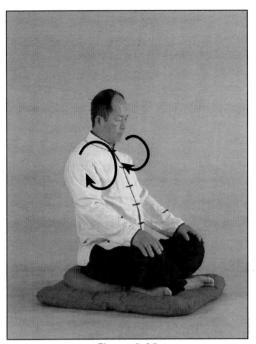

Figure 8-25

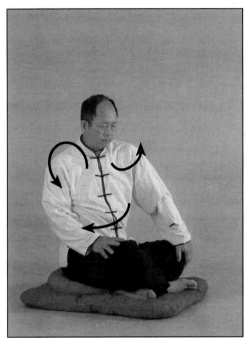

Figure 8-26

ward. To lead stagnant Qi down and loosen up the torso, you may circle one shoulder forward and the other one backward (Figure 8-26). Repeat six times, then reverse direction. In this case, you may coordinate your breathing any way you choose.

**Turning the head.** To loosen the neck, slowly turn your head to the sides (Figure 8-27). Exhale deeply, and inhale when it turns forward. Turn to each side at least six times.

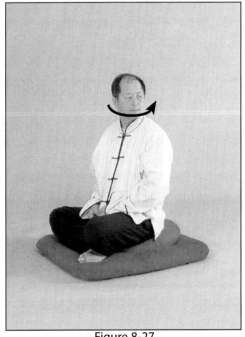

Figure 8-27

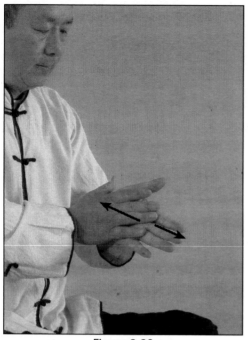

Figure 8-28

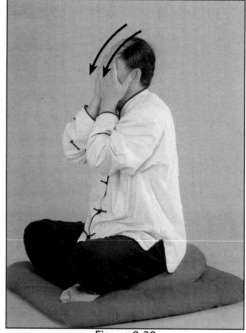

Figure 8-29

**Massage the head.** After loosening the neck, rub your hands until they are warm (Figure 8-28). Then brush the face downwards twenty-four times, using the palms (Figure 8-29). This massage is called washing the face (Xi Lian, 洗臉 ). It rejuvenates the skin with enhanced Qi and blood circulation.

Immediately after washing the face, use the palms to brush the hair from the forehead backward to the neck twenty-four times (Figure 8-30). This is called combing the hair (Shu Tou, 梳頭 ). It keeps your hair healthy and looking young.

Next, rub your hands until they are warm again and use the base of your thumbs to cover your eyes (Figure 8-31). This is called ironing the eyes (Tang Yan, 燙眼 ), which nourishes degenerating eyes. Also massage your eyes with a circular motion to improve the Qi circulation.

Next use your thumb and index fingers to massage the ears for a few minutes (Figure 8-32). Different parts of the ears are related to different organs (Figure 8-33). Massaging them keeps the internal organs healthy. Then cover your ears with

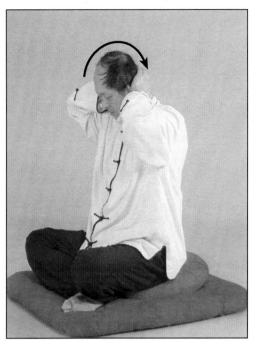

Figure 8-30

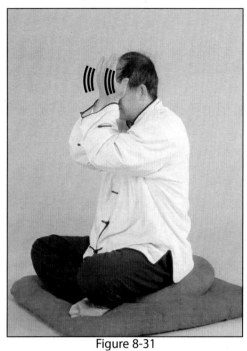

Figure 8-31

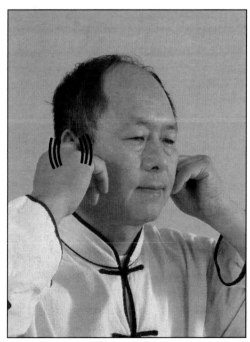

Figure 8-32

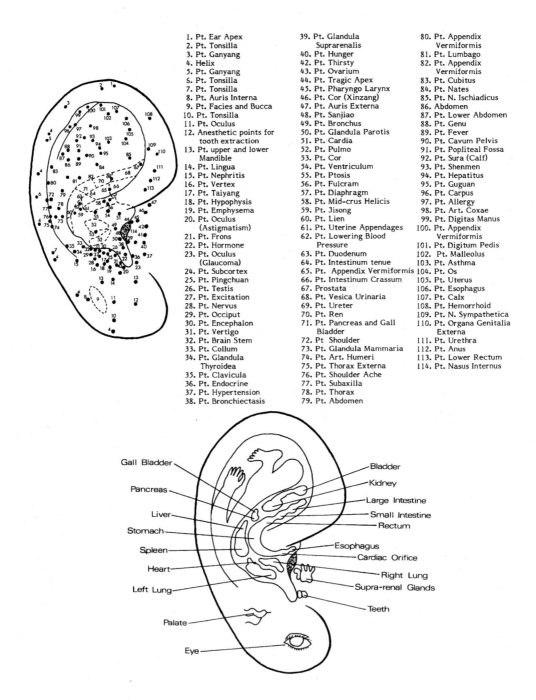

1. Pt. Ear Apex
2. Pt. Tonsilla
3. Pt. Ganyang
4. Helix
5. Pt. Ganyang
6. Pt. Tonsilla
7. Pt. Tonsilla
8. Pt. Auris Interna
9. Pt. Facies and Bucca
10. Pt. Tonsilla
11. Pt. Oculus
12. Anesthetic points for tooth extraction
13. Pt. upper and lower Mandible
14. Pt. Lingua
15. Pt. Nephritis
16. Pt. Vertex
17. Pt. Taiyang
18. Pt. Hypophysis
19. Pt. Emphysema
20. Pt. Oculus (Astigmatism)
21. Pt. Frons
22. Pt. Hormone
23. Pt. Oculus (Glaucoma)
24. Pt. Subcortex
25. Pt. Pingchuan
26. Pt. Testis
27. Pt. Excitation
28. Pt. Nervus
29. Pt. Occiput
30. Pt. Encephalon
31. Pt. Vertigo
32. Pt. Brain Stem
33. Pt. Collum
34. Pt. Glandula Thyroidea
35. Pt. Clavicula
36. Pt. Endocrine
37. Pt. Hypertension
38. Pt. Bronchiectasis
39. Pt. Glandula Suprarenalis
40. Pt. Hunger
42. Pt. Thirsty
43. Pt. Ovarium
44. Pt. Tragic Apex
45. Pt. Pharyngo Larynx
46. Pt. Cor (Xinzang)
47. Pt. Auris Externa
48. Pt. Sanjiao
49. Pt. Bronchus
50. Pt. Glandula Parotis
51. Pt. Cardia
52. Pt. Pulmo
53. Pt. Cor
54. Pt. Ventriculum
55. Pt. Ptosis
56. Pt. Fulcram
57. Pt. Diaphragm
58. Pt. Mid-crus Helicis
59. Pt. Jisong
60. Pt. Lien
61. Pt. Uterine Appendages
62. Pt. Lowering Blood Pressure
63. Pt. Duodenum
64. Pt. Intestinum tenue
65. Pt. Appendix Vermiformis
66. Pt. Intestinum Crassum
67. Prostata
68. Pt. Vesica Urinaria
69. Pt. Ureter
70. Pt. Ren
71. Pt. Pancreas and Gall Bladder
72. Pt Shoulder
73. Pt. Glandula Mammaria
74. Pt. Art. Humeri
75. Pt. Thorax Externa
76. Pt. Shoulder Ache
77. Pt. Subaxilla
78. Pt. Thorax
79. Pt. Abdomen
80. Pt. Appendix Vermiformis
81. Pt. Lumbago
82. Pt. Appendix Vermiformis
83. Pt. Cubitus
84. Pt. Nates
85. Pt. N. Ischiadicus
86. Abdomen
87. Pt. Lower Abdomen
88. Pt. Genu
89. Pt. Fever
90. Pt. Cavum Pelvis
91. Pt. Popliteal Fossa
92. Pt. Sura (Calf)
93. Pt. Shenmen
94. Pt. Hepatitus
95. Pt. Guguan
96. Pt. Carpus
97. Pt. Allergy
98. Pt. Art. Coxae
99. Pt. Digitas Manus
100. Pt. Appendix Vermiformis
101. Pt. Digitum Pedis
102. Pt. Malleolus
103. Pt. Asthma
104. Pt. Os
105. Pt. Uterus
106. Pt. Esophagus
107. Pt. Calx
108. Pt. Hemorrhoid
109. Pt. N. Sympathetica
110. Pt. Organa Genitalia Externa
111. Pt. Urethra
112. Pt. Anus
113. Pt. Lower Rectum
114. Pt. Nasus Internus

Figure 8-33. Acupuncture Points in the Ear

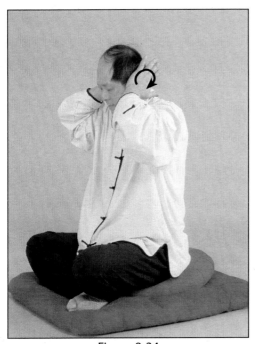

Figure 8-34

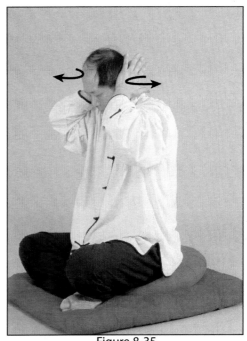

Figure 8-35

the palms and circle ten times on each side (Figure 8-34). This improves the circulation of Qi and blood in the deeper parts of the ears. Finally, press the ears and pop them several times (Figure 8-35). This stimulates the eardrums and improves their circulation. All these are simple ways of maintaining the ears in a healthy condition.

Next, use your index finger and thumb to rub and press down along the sides of the nose and then sideways (Figure 8-36). This releases pressure built up in the frontal sinus.

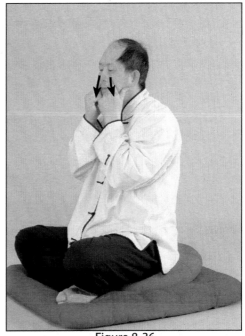

Figure 8-36

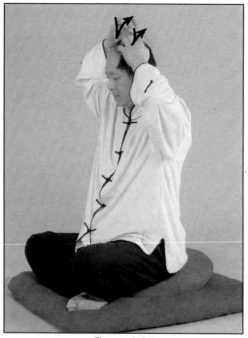

Figure 8-37

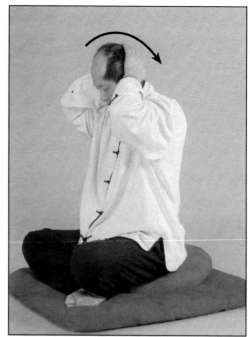

Figure 8-38

Finally, use the fingertips to tap your head from front to back and from the center to the sides for a few minutes (Figure 8-37) This tapping action leads the Qi accumulated inside the head to the skin surface. After tapping, use both hands to brush your head lightly from the front backward (Figure 8-38).

**Massage the three Yin Channels on the legs—spleen, liver and kidneys.** After sitting for a long time, Qi and blood may be stagnant in the hip and knee areas. To remedy this, straighten your legs and bend forward to stretch them out (Figure 8-39). Massage them from the thighs to the bottom of the feet, especially the insides of the legs where the three Yin channels are located. After massaging for a couple of minutes, use your thumb to press the Sanyinjiao cavity (Sp-6, 三陰交)(Figures 8-40 and 8-41). Sanyinjiao means Three Yin Junctions and is the junction of the three Yin channels: spleen, liver, and kidneys. Press in for five seconds, and then release. Repeat three times. This leads Qi down from the hips.

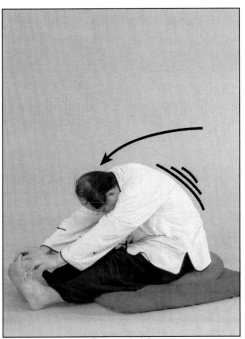

Figure 8-39

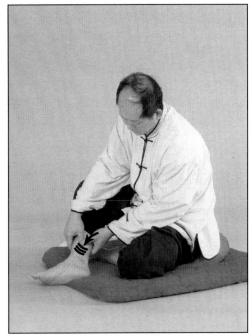

Figure 8-40

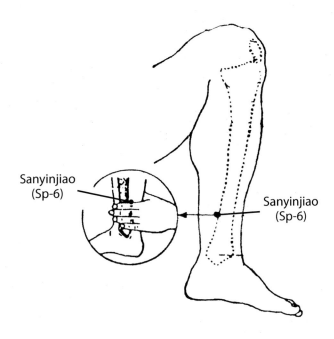

Figure 8-41. The Sanyinjiao (Sp-6) Cavity

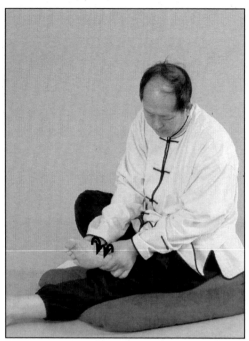

Figure 8-42

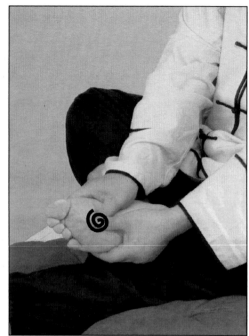

Figure 8-43

Next, massage the inside of the feet where the two Yin vessels (Yin Heel and Yin Linking Vessels, 陰蹻脈・陰維脈) end (Figure 8-42). Finally, massage the Yongquan cavity (K-1, 湧泉) for a few minutes (Figure 8-43).

**Chanting.** Often right after meditation, a meditator makes specific chanting sounds. This leads the Qi down to the Lower Dan Tian. These chanting sounds are commonly used for healing purposes as well. Three of the most common ones used are An (唵), A (阿), and Hong (吽). The use of these three sounds has been recorded in a Buddhist classic, which I would like to translate for your reference.

### Classic of Positioning the Image into the Extreme Calmness[40]
### 《安象三昧儀經》

*After chanting these real words (Buddhist classic), imagine the perfectness of the Buddha's image. Then use An, A, Hong, three words, and place them on the image. Place the word An on the crown, place the word A on the mouth, and place the word Hong in the heart.*

誦此真言已，復想如來如真實身諸相圓滿，然以唵阿吽
三字，安在像身三處，用唵字安頂上，用阿字安口上，
用吽字安心上。

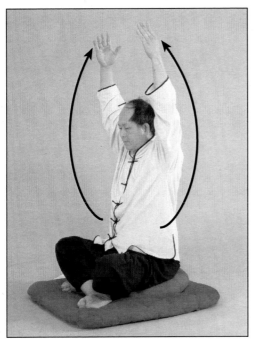

Figure 8-44

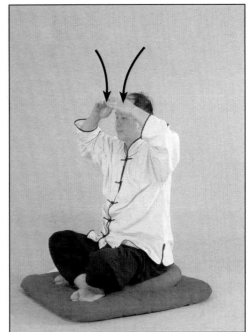

Figure 8-45

It is common for a Buddhist to imagine a likeness of Buddha in his mind and then perform some chanting or meditation. This brings him to a profound level of peace and calmness. The three words, An, A, and Hong, are also commonly used right after chanting of the Buddhist scriptures or deep meditation.

Many meditators use the fourth word to lead Qi down to the Lower Dan Tian. The fourth word does not have sound, and the word itself does not exist. It only exists in the mind right after chanting the third word, as you lead the Qi downward to return to its residence at the Lower Dan Tian. That means returning your being to the Wuji state.

First inhale deeply while raising up your arms from the sides of your body, with the palms facing upward (Figure 8-44). When both hands reach their highest point, start to exhale, lowering the hands with the palms facing downward, while making the sound of An (唵)(Figure 8-45). You feel a strong vibration at the back of your brain when the sound of An is made. Continue to exhale, lowering your hands until they reach the level of the mouth, then change the sound into A (阿), and continue to lower them (Figure 8-46). When the A sound is made, the throat vibrates strongly. Continue exhaling as you lower your hands until they reach the sternum, then

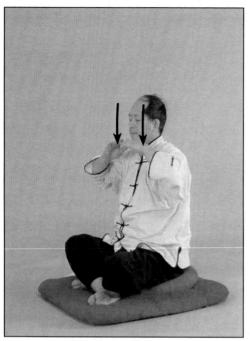

Figure 8-46

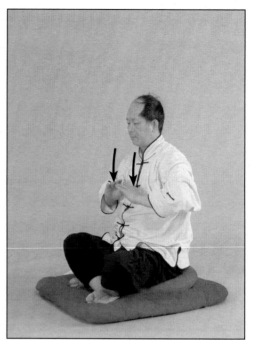

Figure 8-47

change the sound to Hong (吽)(Figure 8-47). When this happens, you feel a strong vibration in your upper chest. Finally, keep quiet while still exhaling, and use the mind to lead the Qi down to the Lower Dan Tian to complete the chanting process. You may repeat the whole process three times.

The positions where you change the words of your chanting are at the Yintang (M-HN-3, Upper Dan Tian), Tiantu (Co-22), Jiuwei (Co-15), and Qihai (Co-6) (Figure 8-48). These four cavities are four of the 7 major corresponding gates of the body.

**If necessary, walk for a few minutes.** If you wish, after you have finished the recovery massage and exercises, you may walk or simply lie down to rest for a few minutes.

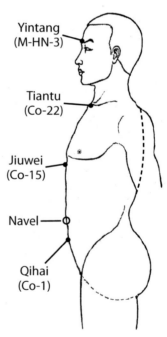

Figure 8-48. Yintang (M-HN-3), Tiantu (Co-22), Jiuwei (Co-15), and Qihai (Co-6)

## 8-9. MEDITATION AND HEALING 靜坐與自療

There are a few ancient documents which record how you can use Small Circulation Meditation for effective self-healing. The theory is very simple. Since your mind can feel and focus on the affected area, it can lead the Qi there to improve circulation of Qi and blood. This is no different from physical massage, which also improves the circulation of Qi and blood. To improve them through meditation is much harder. You need to have reached a high level of meditation to effectively lead the Qi for healing. Next, I translate some ancient documents about healing through meditation. First, one about sealing the breath (Bi Qi, 閉氣 ).

### Vessel Viewing
### 《脈望》

*Sealing the Breath does not mean to hold and choke the breath. It means the spirit is steady and the Qi harmonious, stop thinking and forget about worry, allow the nose breathing to be natural, smooth, and slender, as though it were there and yet as though it were not there.*

閉氣者，非閉噎其氣也，乃神定氣和，絕思忘慮，便鼻息悠悠，若有若無。

This document reassures us that regulating the breathing is not to hold it but to regulate it until it can be natural, smooth, and slender.

### The Secret of Cultivating Original Qi Internally, by Huan Zhen
### 《幻真先生內服元氣訣》

*If there is a sudden uncomfortable feeling in cultivation, or occasional sickness, then immediately go to a secret room. Follow the method of breathing to cultivate the Qi. Once it is abundant, stop and regulate it, and swallow. Think of the place which is in pain, seal your breath, and place your whole mind there, using the Yi to attack the sick place. When inhalation reaches its limit, then utter it. After complete uttering, again swallow. Continue and follow the same method to attack. When the breathing becomes urgent, then stop. After breathing has been regulated, again attack. It may take twenty to fifty times; attack the painful place until sweating and turning a red color, then stop. If there is no improvement, then practice it every midnight or early morning. Practice day and night and use the Yi to attack. It does not matter if the sickness is at the head, face, hands, or feet, just attack wherever there is a problem.*

忽有修養乖宜，偶生疾患，宜速于密室，依服氣法，布
足訖則調氣咽之，念所苦之處，閉氣想注，以意攻之。
氣極則吐之，訖，復咽。相繼依前攻之，氣急則止，氣
調復攻，或二十至五十，攻覺所苦處，汗出通潤即止。
如未損，即每日夜半，或五更晝日頻作，以意攻及。若
病在頭面、手足，但有疾之處則攻之。

Sicknesses here means common uncomfortable feeling, such as the beginning of catching cold, joint pain, internal pain caused by Qi and blood stagnation, or minor injury. Normally, these problems can be corrected through meditation.

First build up Qi in the Lower Dan Tian through abdominal breathing, or the Real Lower Dan Tian by Embryonic Breathing. Then, inhale smoothly and slenderly, and swallow (Yan, 咽) the saliva while using your Yi to lead the Qi to the painful place. Hold the breath until it reaches its limit, and then exhale slowly, and use the mind to lead the Qi away from the painful place. Repeat these processes continuously. If you feel breathing becoming urgent, return to normal breathing until it is comfortable once more. Then repeat the whole process. You may have to do it many times, but it doesn't matter, keep doing it until you start to sweat and become flushed and red, then stop. If it does not ease the pain, repeat day and night until the pain has gone.

## The Important Secret Song of Embryonic Breathing
### 《胎息秘要歌訣》

*If the body is injured or gets sick suddenly, or regularity is abnormal (feeling uncomfortable), condense your Yi, and return to a leisure room (separate and secret room). Strip the body, and lie down on the bed. Face up as though sleeping, and hold firm (place both hands at the Lower Dan Tian). Knock your teeth and burn incense. After swallowing thirty-six times, the Qi in the Dan Tian passes the normal stage. Follow the Xin to lead Qi continuously. Lead it to the injured place. It is adequate when it sweats. This saves the effort of searching for medical prescriptions.*

忽然身染疾，非理有損傷。斂意歸閒室，脫身臥本床。
仰眠兼握固，扣齒與焚香。三十六咽足，丹田氣越常。
隨心連引導，損處最為良。汗出以為度，省求廣利方。

To place the hands at the Lower Dan Tian area is to hold firm (Wo Gu, 握固). Then the mind is in the Dan Tian, and the Qi is stored efficiently. Knocking the teeth (Kou Chi, 扣齒) wakes up the brain and raises the spirit. Burn incense (Fen

Xiang, 焚香) to calm and focus the mind. Other descriptions of training methods are the same as in the previous document.

These two documents about using meditation for self-healing are translated for your reference. The most important way to achieve successful healing is through practice and accumulated experience. Through constant practice and pondering, you soon grasp the secret key of healing.

## References

1. 《道德經・五十五章》：〝骨弱筋柔而握固。〞

2. 《諸病源候論・風身體手足不隨候》：〝握固者，以兩手各自以四指把手姆指。〞

3. 《道門通教必用集》：〝握固以大指掐中指指節，四指齊收于心。〞

4. 指行佛家氣功時，手的姿勢。其作用有二：一精神思維活動專注于手印，持之以恆，穫得禪定。二調節手形成印後，精神思維活動專注于呼吸，達到最高境界，〝即身成佛。〞

5. 《陀羅尼集經》：〝誦咒有身印等種種印法，若作手印，誦諸咒法，易得成驗。〞

6. 《慧林音義》：〝結跏趺坐，略有兩種。一曰吉祥，二曰降魔。凡坐皆先以右趾押左股，後以左趾押右股。此即左押右。手亦左在上，名曰降魔坐。諸禪宗多傳此座。依持明藏教瑜珈法門，即傳吉祥為上，降魔座有時而用。其吉祥座，先以左趾押右股，后以右趾押左股，令兩足掌仰于二股之上，手亦右壓左，安仰跏趺之上，名曰吉祥坐。如來昔在菩提樹下，成正覺時，身安吉祥之座，手作降魔之印，故如來常安此座，轉妙法輪。〞

7. 《赤風髓》：〝訣在閉兌目，半垂簾，赤龍頭胝上齶。〞

8. 《崔公入藥鏡》注：〝銀河阻隔，陰陽之相會，必借鵲橋而渡。人之舌，喻為鵲橋。練功時，舌舐上齶，有溝通陰陽之作用。〞

9. 《道德經・十章》：〝專氣致柔，能嬰兒乎？〞

10. 《性命圭旨全書・亨集》：〝專氣致柔神久留，往來真息自悠悠。綿綿迤邐歸元氣，不汲靈泉常自流。〞

11. 〝吐唯細細，納唯綿綿〞

12. 《道言淺近》：〝調息要調真息息〞，〝凝神調息，只要心平氣和。〞

13. 《性命圭旨全書・蟄藏氣穴，眾妙歸根》：〝調息要調真息息，
    煉神須煉不神神。〞

14. 《性命圭旨・大小鼎爐說》：〝黃庭為鼎，氣穴為爐。黃庭正在
    氣穴上，縷絡相連，乃人身百脈交會之處。〞元氣氤氳二穴之間，
    謂之〝小鼎爐。〞〝乾位為鼎，坤位為爐。〞即泥丸宮為鼎，下
    丹田為爐，謂之〝大鼎爐。〞

15. 《金仙証論》：〝采藥運周天者，當從氣穴坤爐而起火，升乾首
    以為鼎，降坤腹以為爐。即古人所謂乾坤為鼎器者是也。見神氣
    之起伏，而鼎氣在是矣。注：乾在上為鼎，坤在下為爐。有神氣
    即有爐鼎，無神氣即無爐鼎。〞

16. 《道鄉集》：〝何謂文火？若守若存，勿亡勿助。〞

17. 《性天風月通玄記・師徒傳道》：〝靜中一動火正燃，此時正好
    煉大還。采時謂之藥，藥中有火焉。若問武火，大舉巽風；若問
    文火，胎息綿綿。〞

18. 眼觀鼻，鼻觀心。

19. 孔子曰：〝知止而后有定，定爾后能靜，靜而后能安，安爾后能
    慮，慮爾後能得。〞

20. 《性命圭旨全書・玉液煉形法則》：〝欲除生滅心，必自無念
    始。〞

21. 《道德經・十六章》：〝致虛極，守靜篤。〞

22. 《性命圭旨全書・天人合發，采藥歸壺》：〝心中無物為虛，念
    頭不起為靜，致虛而至于極，守靜而至于篤。陰陽自然交媾，陰
    陽一交而陽精產矣。〞

23. 《道鄉集》：〝有心觀竅，無心觀妙等語。乃道之功用也。有欲
    以觀竅，又為無心觀妙之用。無心以觀妙，又為有心觀竅之體。
    要知有欲觀竅有為也，神返氣自回之時也。無欲觀妙無為也，無
    人無我，無山川草木，混混然不知不覺之時代也。〞指〝致虛極，
    守靜篤。〞之意識活動的寧靜，靜而后一陽生，萌發奇妙生機。

24. 意不在氣，在氣則滯。

25. 河車：運載水火之工具。河車搬運水火，由尾閭至泥丸，一撞三
    關。三車：羊車：尾閭關到夾脊關，其行緩慢。鹿車：夾脊關到
    玉枕關，其行宜速。牛車：玉枕關到泥丸關，力大方能過關。

26. 《道德經・一章》：〝常無欲，以觀其妙。〞

27. 《道德經・十六章》：〝致虛極，守靜篤。〞

28. 《諸真聖胎神用訣‧徐神公胎息訣》：〝夫神者，虛無之用。〞

29. 《六祖壇經》：〝菩提本無樹，明鏡亦非台，本來無一物，何處惹塵埃。〞

30. 《本草綱目》：〝腦為元神之府。〞

31. 《脈望》：〝腦為上田，元神所居之宮，人能握元神，棲于本宮，則金氣自升，真息自定，所謂一竅開而百竅齊開，大關通則百關盡通也。〞

32. 《參同契發揮》：〝隨真息之往來，任真氣之生降，自朝至暮，元神常棲于泥丸也。〞

33. 《道德經‧六章》：〝谷神不死，是謂玄牝。玄牝之門，是謂天地根，綿綿若存，用之不勤。〞

34. 《武當修真圖》：〝明堂下，兩眉連線中點上方。有神光出，而曰天目。〞

35. 《云笈七籤》：〝兩眉間為泥丸之玉門。〞指印堂穴。

36. 《周易參同契》：〝真人至妙，若有若無，仿佛大淵，乍沉乍浮，退而分佈，各守境偶。〞

37. 《論衡‧超奇》：〝天稟元氣，人受元精。〞

38. 《古文參同契》：〝元氣之積厚而精英者稱為元精。〞

39. 《性命圭旨全書》：〝煉精者，煉元精，抽坎中之元陽也，元精固則交感之精自不泄漏。〞

40. Chinese Qigong Dictionary (中國氣功辭典), by Lu, Guang-Rong (呂光榮), 人民衛生出版社, Beijing, 1988.

# PART IV

# Questions and Future Human Possiblities

## 疑問與人類之未來

## CHAPTER 9

# Questions and Future Human Possiblities

## 疑問與人類之未來

Many Qigong practices were kept secret in the past and their theories and methods passed down at random. Only recently have many of them been revealed to the general public, so practitioners can learn the secrets of other styles. Even so, because of the long years of secrecy, many available documents remain incomplete or unconfirmed. To compile them and formalize a systematic theory is very difficult. During the course of my study and research, many questions have arisen, the answers to which seem accurate but need scientific verification. Some questions are beyond the scope of any test which could be carried out with current scientific equipment.

Some questions arise due to my limited understanding of Qigong training, others from advances in modern science. In the course of my continuing research, many will be answered. I also await answers from other Qigong masters. Many questions need to be investigated through experiments involving modern equipment. Some may remain unanswered, since I firmly believe that nobody could achieve the very high level of Qigong practice attained by earlier masters.

Personally, I hope these questions help stimulate interest in Western scientific society, and lead to further research. Although the material sciences continue to develop rapidly, our spiritual sciences remain in the same state of stagnation as centuries ago.

**About Essence**

1. Chinese medicine and Qigong society tell us that one's Original Essence is stored in the kidneys. How is it stored?

2. Why is it stored there instead of in other organs? We need a theoretical explanation and experimental proof for this.

3. If Original Essence is stored in the kidneys, what about those people who have only one kidney? Will they die earlier? Will the Original Essence

stored in the single kidney be enough for life? Will its conversion to Qi be reduced?

4. How could we tell a person whose Original Essence is strong from someone whose Essence is weak? Normally, it is judged from one's spirit of vitality and state of health, but there is no standard for this. Is there any scientific way of doing so?

5. Could we see Original Essence? Is it material? Is it the source of hormones? Could we see it in a dead body?

6. Does Original Essence comprise the genes or the hormones? Many sources lead me to believe that genes and hormones are what the ancient Chinese called Original Essence, or at least they are closely related.

7. Could the quantity of Original Essence be increased and its quality improved through modern technology?

8. Could the stimulation of semen production be done in a modern way? For example, through minor electrical stimulation? Would this cause problems, since the one who is stimulated need not regulate his mind?

9. Could the stimulation of semen production through modern technology achieve the same purpose of longevity? Could this be done for an old man without causing problems, such as a heart attack?

10. Could technology enhance the conversion of Essence to Qi, such as using an electromagnetic field to lead Qi from the Real Lower Dan Tian to the brain?

11. Could artificial hormones benefit the body as much as the Essence generated inside the body? What side-effects would there be?

12. What biochemical reaction occurs during the conversion of Essence to Qi? If we knew this, could we enhance it with modern technology?

13. Could we use modern technology to transfer Essence from one person to another, like a blood transfusion?

14. Is it true that Water Qi is converted from Original Essence? How is this done? If Original Essence consisted of the body's hormones, then it could not be converted into Qi. The function of hormones is to regulate the body's metabolism by regulating the biochemical reactions in the body. They act as catalysts which ensure that biochemical reactions occur smoothly, without actively participating in them. Perhaps Original Essence refers to fat being converted to Qi.

**About Qi**

1. Is the traditional concept of human Qi the same as bioelectromagnetic energy, or is it a synthesis of various types of energy? Many practitioners are not convinced that human Qi is merely bioelectromagnetic energy circulating in the body. Many Qigong phenomena cannot be explained satisfactorily by this hypothesis. For example, how does a Qigong master hold a burning coal in his hand without being burned?

2. How do we standardize the measurement of Qi? A unit system is necessary. Many different types of equipment have been designed to measure it in terms of heat (infrared), temperature rise, and electricity. Since human Qi has not been defined, there is no specific equipment which we are convinced is the most accurate method for measuring it. However, if it is proven that Qi is human electromagnetic energy, then we could use an electric unit system to measure it.

3. Since the general definition of Qi is universal energy, how do we relate all kinds of different energy into one, if that were possible? To me, there is no absolute way to relate them. The unit system used to measure heat cannot measure electricity. It may be better to designate Qi, referring for example to Heat Qi or Electric Qi.

4. Qi is transferred from one person to another, what, other than heat and bioelectricity, is transferred? I have often wondered how one person could be more effective in transferring his Qi than another. There must be some extra force transferred emotionally to help the patient build up EMF to cure himself internally. What is this force? Brain waves, emotional touch, or self-confidence, perhaps?

5. If Qi is bioelectricity, how could modern technology increase its circulation in the body and achieve the same results as with Qigong practice? It was not possible to generate electromagnetic fields in ancient times, but very easy to do so today. There should be a way to use external fields to increase circulation, regulate Qi and clean the marrow. Naturally, we must proceed with caution to determine the side-effects. How could an external field duplicate the mental calmness necessary for enlightenment? Even if circulation could be improved, without a disciplined mind there would be fewer benefits. Might other problems arise if people become exceptionally powerful without the discipline of control?

6. How do clouds and fog affect Qi circulation? Low clouds generate an electric field which affects the human energy field. Does fog do this as well? When you are in fog, do the charges surround you uniformly? Can this affect your Qi circulation?

7. Is there any modern way to stimulate and raise fasciae for Qi storage? Would this cause problems if we could not generate enough Qi to keep them full?

8. Since Qi and the brain are closely related, could we adjust the Qi nourishment of the brain to cure mental illness?

## About Spirit (Shen)

1. How do we define spirit? Is it a form of energy? Could a spirit have its own thoughts? If so, how?

2. How do we define spirit and mind? The relationship between them is very confusing. Is Shen generated from mind? If Shen must be generated from mind, how can it exist after physical death? If it can, does this Shen have a mind and can it think independently? How do they relate to brainwaves? Can Shen be measured?

3. Can the spirit and soul exist even if there is no physical life form? It is believed in Chinese religions that the spirit and soul exist even after death. Are spirit and soul in energy form? Are they part of the non-human natural energy, or are they the residues of human energy?

4. Is it true that there is another dimension or world not known to science, yet which can be reached by the spirit or soul? There are many stories of people dying and then coming back. They often say they were outside their physical bodies and could see it. The Chinese believe that the world we live in is the Yang World (Yang Jian, 陽間), and when a person dies, his spirit enters the Yin World (Yin Jian, 陰間). According to the theory of Yin and Yang, Yang must be balanced by Yin. Could this Yin world be reached, other than by energy or spirit?

5. Are events recorded in the spiritual world? Could this spiritual memory be erased? I believe what happens in nature influences its energy, and this influence is recorded in nature. I believe once human science has reached a certain level, we will be able to trace past events through spiritual memory.

6. Is a thought energy or matter? How could it travel from one end of the universe to the other instantaneously? Could it penetrate the past or the future?

7. Is the mind the God (Taiji or Dao) of the human universe (small heaven and earth)? If so, could we then use the model of the human universe to understand the grand universe? Isn't mankind derived from the grand universe, with all spiritual and energy structures being similar to that of the grand universe?

8. How does a human spirit communicate with that of another human or animal? Through the vibrations of the Spiritual Valley? From the structure of the brain, can we regard every brain as a radio transmitter and receiver? Could this spirit communicate with the natural spirit in the same way?

9. Could one person affect another's thinking through brainwave correspondence?

10. Could modern technology increase the flow of bioelectricity to the brain to activate more brain cells? Would there be any side effects? Nowadays, many body builders use electricity to speed up the growth of their muscles to develop the body in a short time. Later they discover that the inner body cannot produce enough bioelectricity to support the muscles, so they degenerate faster than normal. Would we encounter this problem if we activated brain cells in the same way?

11. Could we open the gate of the Upper Dan Tian, the third eye, through external electrical stimulation? What would happen if we opened it quickly, without enough Qi internally to support this wandering spirit? Would we go crazy?

12. When we reach a higher level of spiritual enlightenment, will we then be able to communicate with aliens from outer space? If they are thousands of years ahead of us scientifically, they should have reached a higher spiritual level, so we should be able to contact them somehow.

13. Is the spiritual dimension a new dimension in which we can travel much faster than the speed of light? Would that be how UFOs travel to earth?

14. How important a role will the human spirit play in human history when science leaves its present stage of infancy and enters the stage of its youth?

15. What is the scientific explanation for the halo around the head, or the glow around the body, of a meditator? Though I try to explain it as air de-ionization generated by the body's electrical charge, an experiment needs to be conducted to determine whether this is true.

16. How is spirit generated in a new-born baby? Where does it originate? Does it start when the baby begins to think? Does it exist only in humans?

17. Does a newborn child need an already-existing spirit? Some religions say that it does, in order to form a complete human. If so, where does this spirit come from? From those who died before? If a newborn baby needs this pre-existing spirit, then how does the population keep increasing? Where do the new spirits originate? Do they come from the sun, or from universal energy? Could spirits from other planets immigrate to the earth and be born into human bodies?

18. What are the differences between spirit and soul? Since there is no exact translation from Chinese into English, I would like the exact differences and definitions of these words.

19. How do we generate a "spiritual baby" in Qigong training? In the Qigong tradition, to reach enlightenment you must train until you give birth to this spiritual baby. Only when it has grown to be independent can your spirit survive, and live forever. Is this true? Scientifically, how could this be possible? Could modern science explain it, or is it still beyond what today's science can grasp? If we believe that a highly developed mind could speed up the process of evolution, then it might be able to reach many other things still beyond human understanding.

20. Do the spirits of enlightened people who have died continue to exist? If so, can they help the living? If the answer is yes, do you agree that spirit and soul can exist even after death? When you pray, do you actually receive help from God or the spirits of the dead, or are you helping yourself by building your self-confidence?

21. Does a spirit make its own decisions or is it affected by natural Qi? Can a spirit think? How could it help a living person? Through brainwave communication? Or is the spirit only some human energy residue roaming around in the energy world and being affected by surrounding energy forces?

22. When someone communicates with animals, is this brainwave correspondence? I once saw a woman on a live TV show who seemed able to communicate with all kinds of dogs. The information she learned was verified by the owners. If this were real, would it be brainwave communication? Do the brains of animals and man function on the same frequency band, or just partially overlap?

23. Could a highly concentrated mind make an object move without touching it? What would be the principle behind this? How could brainwave energy become strong enough to do this? Are miracles done with brainwaves or through the spiritual dimension?

24. Could the spirit really leave the body and travel, or is it only that the brainwaves sense something and match its frequency so that you can be aware of it? When someone is hypnotized, he can sense many things beyond his ordinary capability. Is this similar to what happens when a person seems to leave his body during meditation?

25. Could modern technology create an electromagnetic wave whose wavelength is equivalent to the human brainwave? Our technology seems to have progressed that far already. If so, could a brainwave machine generate a wave to affect our thinking and judgment? That would truly be brain-

washing. Could we create a machine to generate brainwave white noise, to act as a shield against such a weapon? Could the wars of the future be fought using brainwave machines?

26. If it is possible to make a brainwave machine, could we determine what frequencies are associated with crime, and somehow block them? Is it possible to really brainwash criminals? Of course, if such a machine fell into the hands of criminals, they would have a powerful tool for evil. Could we accept the moral responsibility for changing an individual's brainwaves?

27. Could a good Qigong meditator avoid being controlled and affected by a brainwave machine? Personally, I believe that one who regulates his mind effectively would be able to avoid the effects, but how long would he be able to do so?

28. What is the bandwidth of the brainwave? What existing materials could shield them out? Metal is usually a good insulator against radiowaves, but could it also keep out brainwaves? If not, is there any material which could be used to shield against them?

29. What is the relationship between spirit (Shen) and brainwaves? I personally believe that when your Shen is high, your brainwaves are stronger, and probably more focused and sensitive in different wavelengths. Is this true?

30. Since our spirit is so closely related to Qi or the energy field, how much has our spirit been affected by energy pollution such as radio waves?

## About Channels, Vessels, and Cavities

1. How did the ancients find out about, and locate the Qi channels, vessels, and cavities? How did they find them with such accuracy? How did they discover they could use them to cure illness?

2. How do blocked channels interfere with the Qi flow? This is a simple question, but one without an easy answer. It will take the most advanced technology to find out exactly how the Qi channels become blocked. Is it caused by an accumulation of fat which significantly reduces electric conductivity, or by some defect in the electrically conductive tissues?

3. How do the channels conduct Qi? How much stimulation can make it move? If Qi is bioelectric energy, then the question is, how much EMF can make the energy move, and where is it?

4. How do the vessels store Qi? If Qi is bioelectric energy, then is a Qi vessel like a battery or a capacitor, which can store and release energy when necessary?

5. What do the Qi channels and vessels actually look like? If they are areas where electrical conductivity is different, then experiments should determine how they are shaped.

6. How could we design a machine sensitive enough to accurately locate all the Qi channels and cavities? This would be very helpful for acupuncture practice.

7. Why are there four vessels in the legs and none in the arms? Is it because people use their legs more than their arms? I believe the vessels in the legs evolved to supply extra Qi to the legs and help regulate them more efficiently.

8. Are there any other vessels which have not yet been discovered? It is possible that there are other, smaller vessels in the body which remain undiscovered. For example, I believe there should be extra vessels in the arms, to serve much the same purposes as those in the legs.

9. What actually happens when we open a channel (gate) in Qigong practice? Does the channel recover its conductivity? What is the best way to do this?

10. Could we use modern bioelectric technology to open the channels and smooth the Qi circulation?

11. Could we use technology to fill up the Qi reservoirs? If they are bioelectric capacitors, we might be able to use external electromagnetic methods to refill them. We would then have enough Qi to nourish the whole body and slow down the aging process significantly.

12. What actually happens when an experienced Qigong master helps a student open his channels? Does he really transport his Qi into the student's body to do the job, or does he only offer stimulation and confidence to the student, allowing him to open them by himself?

13. Exactly what are cavities? Do all cavities have higher electric conductivity, and do they differ in capacity? Is increased electrical conductivity the only factor for locating cavities, or did the ancients have additional criteria?

14. Why are there cavities? Do they just circulate Qi to the skin surface to nourish it and regulate Qi channels, or are there any other purposes than these?

15. How does acupuncture actually correct the Qi flow? We need a more complete explanation through modern experimentation and scientific study.

16. Su Wen (素問) said our lives run in cycles of 7 years for women and 8 years for men. When the book was written, boys reached puberty around the age of 16, and girls around 14. Now that puberty comes 2 to 4 years earlier, have the cycles changed? Did they have objective reality, or were they more philosophical ideas?

**About Mutual Qi Nourishment**

1. Two people can practice together to balance their Qi through mutual Qi nourishment. The one with the stronger Qi gives his Qi while the weaker one gains it. Two people with weak Qi can help each other build it up. In this kind of mutual Qi nourishment, each must be able to coordinate with the other in every aspect, especially in breathing. Emotionally, they must be willing to share with each other. In this kind of practice, is it inevitable that they will fall in love? If not, how are they to touch and share Qi with each other? If the answer is "Yes," isn't it contrary to the principle of meditation that the mind should be calm and peaceful, without emotional disturbance?

2. When two people practice mutual Qi nourishment, do they actually share Qi, or do they stimulate each other's minds to enhance the brain's EMF and thereby increase their own Qi circulation, or both?

3. Love is a natural way of promoting mutual Qi nourishment and helping the other one recover from illness. Could this be a form of Qigong?

4. Is sexual activity the ultimate natural way of mutual Qi nourishment? Sex is a natural human desire. Through regular sexual activity, a person achieves mental calmness and peace, and releases the pressure generated by emotional disturbance. Could this be a form of Qigong practice?

5. When a man ejaculates, he loses Qi to the woman. How does this happen? Is this why women live longer? If she has reached a higher level of Qigong, could the man receive Qi instead of losing it?

6. How is it that Essence and Qi are lost during ejaculation? In certain Qigong practices, men avoid ejaculation. How is Qi transmitted under such circumstances?

7. If sex is beneficial for Qigong practice, why did all Buddhist monks and many of the Daoists hide in the mountains to avoid sexual contact? Were they afraid that sex and love would destroy the calm and peaceful mind they were cultivating?

8. Why did the Daoists develop so many techniques which used sexual activity for Qi nourishment? Could these techniques have been developed by those whose minds could not be calm? Or did they want, on the one hand to reach enlightenment, and the other hand to enjoy a natural, normal human life?

## About Health and Longevity

1. Could we use external electromagnetic stimulation to cure sickness in the same way that Qigong and acupuncture reinstate normal bioelectric circulation? Qigong cures many kinds of cancer. Could this be achieved with modern electric and magnetic technology?

2. Could the immune system be strengthened through electromagnetic stimulation to cure AIDS and cancer? The immune system is related closely to the body's bioenergy system. Could we increase the EMF of the brain and strengthen the bioenergetic circulation in the body?

3. Is it dangerous to use electricity and magnetism in acupuncture when we do not understand Qi science completely? So far, there is no conclusive report on the use of electricity and magnetism in acupuncture, even though they are widely used. Are they safe for general practice, or do we need more research?

4. Is practicing Qigong to obtain a longer life the correct goal? I believe that if someone really wants a much longer life, he needs to leave society to avoid emotional disturbance. However, when he does this, he loses the ordinary meaning of human life. I believe the correct purpose of Qigong practice is to achieve a healthy body and mind, while still experiencing life. You extend your lifespan somewhat because you are healthy, and you are still able to experience life.

5. What is the meaning of life? Could Qigong help humanity understand it? Does a long life mean more to you than a happy one? If you want both, what should you do? Qigong practice has helped me understand nature, and myself. It has stopped me wondering and being confused. Do you expect the same?

6. Could we use modern technology to reach the same goal as marrow washing training and obtain a longer life without sacrificing our emotions? I feel certain that once we understand exactly how marrow washing training works, we will be able to use modern technology to quickly reach the same goal.

## About Qi and Modern Living

1. Could we use ice to maintain the body's Qi balance during the summer? It was not possible to research this before refrigerators were invented. In summertime, when the heart is on fire (Yang), could placing ice in the palm of your hand cool the heart, or would it quench the heart fire too quickly and cause problems? What if we were to use alcohol instead of ice?

2. How does working night shifts affect one's Qi circulation? In ancient times, few people worked at night, so there are no documents available today which discuss this. Since the time of day has to be taken into account when giving acupuncture treatments, would being on night shift affect the treatment?

3. How is Qi circulation affected when you travel several time zones in a short time? Does jet lag indicate that the body's Qi is disturbed?

## About the Human Magnetic Field

1. Theoretically, there are two magnetic poles in the human body, matching that formed by the Earth's magnetic field. Do these two poles reverse when you move from the Northern to the Southern Hemisphere?

2. The Earth's magnetic field starts at the South Magnetic Pole and goes to the North Magnetic Pole. Since one's south magnetic pole seems to be on the head if one is in the Northern Hemisphere, does this mean his brain constantly receives energy nourishment? If the human magnetic poles are reversed in the Southern Hemisphere, does this mean that the brains of people there constantly lose nourishment?

3. Does this explain why the most highly developed technology has been created in the Northern Hemisphere?

4. If those in the Southern Hemisphere have their south magnetic poles in the Lower Dan Tian, do they have more energy, and does this help them live longer?

5. When people are sick, could they speed their recovery by flying to the equator, where the effect of the Earth's magnetic field is minimized? I believe many illnesses are caused or worsened by disturbances in the body's electromagnetic field. The earth energy can worsen the situation, since your body loses its natural balance. Could you remove this hindrance by moving to the Equator?

6. We are surrounded by energy fields, both natural and man-made. Could we insulate a room against them to help people convalesce? Would this also be a good place to meditate?

## Others

1. Are there specific spots on earth where natural energy is especially beneficial for Qigong? Many practitioners believe there are places where Heaven or Earth Qi nourishes your Qi and speeds up your training. Is this true? Would these areas be good for hospitals?

2. What happens when we are exposed to a strong electromagnetic field for a long time? How does it affect the body? Could it energize our vital force and improve our health?

3. Since ancient times, Qigong practitioners have claimed that there is a practice which makes the body light. Is this true? Is this beyond scientific explanation?

4. The Chinese have used jade for generations to regulate Qi in their bodies or absorb excess Qi. Has this ever been investigated scientifically?

5. Could we use electromagnetic means to increase the Qi on the scalp to prevent hair loss or increase its growth?

6. Meditators talk about absorbing energy from the earth through the feet. Is this different from magnetic energy?

7. Could a highly trained Qigong practitioner predict the future, or is this simply a matter of judgment, combined with experience and wisdom? Some Qigong masters are said to read your mind and even predict your future. I believe it is possible to read minds through brainwave correspondence, but predicting the future needs more than this. Intelligence and wisdom are needed, and a lot of experience. One's personality is the main factor in success, and it can be read in the face and even in the palms. Is this how the future is read, or is there another way?

8. How does the material your clothing is made of, affect your health? Natural materials such as cotton and wool dissipate some energy to the surrounding environment. Most man-made materials generate a Qi shield which does not allow your Qi to exchange with nature. This affects your body's electromagnetic field and perhaps even disturbs your Qi circulation. This needs to be investigated.

9. How does the weather affect our moods? Moods may be caused by the electric fields generated between low clouds and the ground. These strong, natural, electric fields affect your body's electromagnetic field and may cause sickness or emotional disturbance.

10. Is there a way to energize the muscles to a higher level via external electromagnetic stimulation, or must we rely on traditional practices? If it were possible, would it be fair in competitive sports such as boxing or football? Could it be safe for bodybuilders to use electrical stimulation of the muscles?

11. Would there be any danger in these experiments? We don't understand the human body very well, and we are such delicate and complicated creatures. Naturally, many experiments could be performed on other animals first,

but since the inner energy field is closely related to emotions, it is probable that most need to be conducted directly on humans.

12. Why do many Qigong practitioners hide themselves in caves for their cultivation? Is it because a cave shields one from external energy disturbances, such as electromagnetic fields or ions in the clouds?

13. Have there been several human civilizations on earth in the past, before the beginning of our recorded history? If there were, what happened? Did they destroy each other? How many cycles of civilization have there been? Is there some truth to the legend of Atlantis?

14. Will our human civilization survive or will we destroy ourselves, or be destroyed by natural disasters like those which came before us?

15. Will the development of our spiritual science ever match that of our material science? Although material science has advanced to a level capable of leading us to self-destruction, our spiritual development remains disappointingly stagnant.

16. While we frantically search for the origin of the material world, we have ignored the origin of our spiritual world. What is the root of our spiritual being?

17. We are increasingly playing the role of God in material science. Will we attempt to play the role of God in spiritual science as well?

18. Since the study of science such as mathematics and physics is a way of meditation, will humanity be able to open our third eye in the next few generations?

19. Did people from an earlier civilization go to Mars? Did Mars once have a similar climate to that on earth. If so, what happened? Did the settlers destroy each other, and the planet with them?

20. Will the 21st century be a spiritual century?

21. If modern medical science progresses to a point which allows humans to live for centuries, will we gain new understanding of the meaning of human life?

22. Would we obtain a harmonious life if we could live for several hundred years while still wasting this time searching for wealth and glory, whose importance gets instilled in us from an early age? Would we find new meaning in life?

23. Could we reach the stage of Wuwei (無為) in human society? Wuwei means doing nothing and regulating without regulating, ruling without ruling, a matrix without order. To achieve this, we would need to communicate telepathically. Would the whole of mankind need to open the third eye?

24. If we had been visited by intelligent aliens, this would mean their understanding of spiritual and material science would be far more advanced then our own. Have they opened their third eyes? Have they experienced a similar historical pattern as that of the human race?

25. If aliens had any intention of invading and taking over the earth, why would they have waited until now? Human technology is advancing rapidly. If they had intended taking over the earth, they could easily have done so in the past.

26. Were aliens in the past taken for Gods in the West or Immortals in the East? If our technology advanced to a level which allowed us to visit other undeveloped planets, would the local population consider us Gods?

27. If there were aliens amongst us, would they help us? Is it important for us to learn everything the hard way so we can gradually evolve spiritually by ourselves? If we were helped by intelligent aliens, would we appreciate it? Or would we be greedy and take their help for granted? We have not protected nature which provides for us. We simply take it for granted and destroy it.

28. How could we help each other to wake up and start building a spiritual connection with nature?

These are some questions I have. I have found some answers during forty years of study, but many of them need to be verified. You also have many unanswered questions in your mind. You should not ignore them but continue searching for the answers. This is the way and the meaning of our lives.

CHAPTER 10

# Conclusion
結論

If we attempt to comprehend any profound philosophy, we must first be calm. When the mind is calm and clear, judgment becomes logical and accurate. Through thousands of years of meditation and profound thought, science has developed. Unfortunately, most of this effort has been on developing material science, while spiritual development has been widely ignored. Since the eighteenth century, the gap between these two has increased rapidly. Most people seek glory, power, and wealth, becoming bogged down in the emotional bondage of material satisfaction, while the Yin spiritual side has been degraded.

To save humanity, we need to spend more effort contemplating spirituality instead of concentrating solely on material science. The various religious organizations must recognize their role and teach their followers the correct methods of meditation and spiritual development. This requires them to make revolutionary changes in policy. They must teach their followers that meditation is for self-awakening and enlightenment, not for worship. If they continue to educate their followers to worship and follow blindly, then we follow the same destructive paths as we have in the past, remaining in the domain of spiritual abuse.

Meditation has been widely practiced in the East. Often these meditators lived in obscurity in the mountains. Through meditation, they comprehended the Dao of mankind and of nature. I believe the documents written by these pioneers are amongst the most precious treasures mankind possesses. That is why I continue to study and translate them into English. Unfortunately, my progress has been very slow. I sincerely hope that an organization with a good financial foundation can sponsor and host the conversion of these ancient Eastern philosophical texts into English. If this study were introduced into every level of education I believe it would be very successful in gradually changing the view that Western society has as a whole on the world of spirituality.

I would like you to keep a few things in mind in the course of your study and research. These are:

**Avoid prejudice.** Any culture and tradition which has survived must have had some benefits to offer. Perhaps some of them do not fit in with our view of the world today, but they still deserve our respect. If you deny your past, you pull out your root. You should not be stubborn and claim that traditional culture is absolutely correct, or that a foreign culture must be better than your own. What you should do is keep the good of your own tradition and absorb the best of the foreign.

**Be objective in your judgment.** You should consider everything from the viewpoint of both sides to analyze it objectively. Your emotional responses should be taken into account, but should not dominate your judgment.

**Be scientific.** Although many things still cannot be explained by science, you should always judge scientifically. New sciences are constantly being developed. Phenomena which could not be tested before, should be examined with modern techniques.

**Be logical.** Whenever you read or study, always ask "Is it logical and does it make sense?" Contemplate and understand, instead of blindly believing.

**Do not ignore prior experience.** Prior experience which has been passed down is the root of research. You should always be sincere and respectful when you study the past. From it, you come to understand the present. By understanding the present, you create the future. The accumulation of experience is the best teacher. You should respect the past, be cautious about the present, and challenge the future.

China has more than 7000 thousand years of culture. There have been many incredible accomplishments, of which Qigong is only one. There has never been such open communication between the different cultures as there is today. It is our responsibility to encourage the general public to accept, study, and research other cultures. In this way, humanity can adopt the good aspects of each and live in a more peaceful and meaningful way.

Chinese Qigong is part of traditional Chinese medical science. It has sought to achieve calm, peace, and happiness for thousands of years. I believe this aspect of Chinese culture can help Westerners, especially in spiritual training. Further publications need to be encouraged, and scholastic and scientific study, research, and testing need to be conducted, especially by universities and medical organizations. We should not fear to face the truth and challenge old beliefs and ways of thinking.

I predict that the study of Chinese medical science and internal, meditative Qigong will produce great results in the next few decades. I invite you to join me and become a pioneer in this new field in the Western world.

# Translation and Glossary of Chinese Terms
# 中文術語之翻譯與解釋

**Ai** 哀 Sorrow.

**Ai** 愛 Love, kindness.

**An Lu** 安爐 To install a furnace, by establishing abundant Qi at the Real Lower Dan Tian (Zhen Xia Dan Tian, 真下丹田), using Embryonic Breathing (Tai Xi, 胎息).

**An Mo** 按摩 Press and rub. Together they mean massage.

**An Tian Le Ming** 安天樂命 Peace with heaven and delight in your destiny.

**Ba Chu** 八觸 The Eight Touches, which are sensations often felt during Qigong practice, such as heat, touch, or heaviness.

**Ba Duan Jin** 八段錦 Eight Pieces of Brocade. A Wai Dan Qigong (外丹氣功) practice said to have been created by Marshal Yue, Fei (岳飛) during the Southern Song Dynasty (1127-1280 A.D., 南宋).

**Ba Mai** 八脈 The Eight Extraordinary Vessels. These are considered to be Qi reservoirs, which regulate the Qi in the primary Qi channels.

**Bai Hao** 白毫 Tiny white beams of spiritual light, emitted from the head or third eye.

**Bai He** 白鶴 White Crane. A well known southern Chinese martial style which originated in the Shaolin Temple (少林寺).

**Bagua (Ba Gua or Ba Kua)** 八卦 Eight Divinations, also called Eight Trigrams. In Chinese philosophy, the eight basic variations in the *Yi Jing* (易經, *The Book of Change*) designated as groups of solid and broken lines.

**Baguazhang (Ba Kua Zhang)** 八卦掌 Eight Trigrams Palm. One of the internal martial styles, believed to have been created by Dong, Hai-Chuan (董海川) between 1866 and 1880 A.D.

**Bai Ri Zhu Ji** 百日築基 One Hundred Days to Build the Foundation. In Yi Jin Jing (易筋經) and Xi Sui Jing (洗髓經), the training of the first hundred days is the most important because it lays the foundation for further progress.

**Baihui (Gv-20)** 百會 Hundred Meetings. An important acupuncture cavity located on top of the head. It belongs to the Governing Vessel (Du Mai, 督脈).

**Baihui Hu Xi** 百會呼吸 Baihui Breathing, also called Spiritual Breathing (Shen Xi, 神息).

**Bao** 抱 Embrace, hold together, stick together, enfold, harbor, or cherish.

**Bao Xi (2852-2737 B.C.)** 包義 An ancient ruler of China.

**Bao Yi** 抱一 Embracing the state of oneness. To keep the spirit (or mind) and Qi at the central energy line, and unify spirit and Qi at the Real Lower Dan Tian (Zhen Xia Dan Tian, 真下丹田).

**Bao Yuan** 抱元 Embrace the origin. That means to keep your spirit at its residence, the Mud Pill Palace (Ni Wan Gong, 泥丸宮), and keep the Qi at the Real Lower Dan Tian (Zhen Xia Dan Tian, 真下丹田).

**Bi** 閉 To close, namely to close and hold up the Huiyin (Co-1, 會陰), or to hold the breath.

**Bi Hu** 閉戶 The closed door, also called Mi Hu (密戶) implying the Mingmen (Gv-4, 命門) cavity between L2 and L3.

**Bian Que** 扁鵲 A well known physician who wrote the book, *Nan Jing* (難經, *Classic on Disorders*) during the Chinese Qin and Han Dynasties (255 B.C.-220 A.D., 秦·漢).

**Bo Yang** 伯陽 A nickname of Lao Zi (老子).

**Bu** 補 Nourishment.

**Bu Tiao Er Tiao** 不調而調 Regulating without regulating. The stage of doing nothing (Wuwei, 無為), when regulating is no longer necessary, and all regulating processes cease.

**Cai Yao** 采藥 Picking up the herb. A Daoist term that means to receive the generated Qi.

**Cha Nu** 姹女 The shy lady (mother), implying Qi.

**Chan** 禪 Buddhist practices, which include cultivating, refining, and studying Buddhahood. It is also a Buddhist term for meditation, and means to regulate the Xin (心) until it is calm and steady. Chan is called Zen (忍) in Japan. It also refers to a Chinese school of Mahayana Buddhism that asserts enlightenment can be attained through meditation, self-contemplation, and intuition.

**Chan Yao** 產藥 Produce the herb (Qi).

**Chang** 長 Long.

**Chang Chuan (Changquan)** 長拳 Long fist or long sequence. Chang Chuan includes all northern Chinese long range martial styles. Taijiquan is called Chang Chuan because its sequence is long.

**Chang Zai** 常在 The name of the spleen's spirit, which is related to the soul.

**Changqiang (Gv-1)** 長強 Weilu (尾閭, Coccyx) in Daoist society or Long Strength in acupuncture.

**Chen** 沈 Sink.

**Chen Tu** 塵土 Dust. According to Buddhism, secular society is filled with emotions and desires, regarded as emotional mud or dust.

**Cheng Fo** 成佛 Achieving Buddhahood.

**Cheng, Gin-Gsao (1911 to 1976)** 曾金灶 Dr. Yang, Jwing-Ming's White Crane master.

**Chi (Qi)** 氣 The general definition of Qi is universal energy, including heat, light, electromagnetic energy, and any other type of energy. A narrower definition of Qi refers to the bioenergy (bioelectricity) circulating in human or animal bodies.

**Chi Kung (Qigong)** 氣功 The Gongfu (功夫), or study, of Qi.

**Chi Lao Huan Ji Yun Dong** 遲老返機運動 Qigong exercises to slow aging and return the function to a healthy state.

**Chin Na (Qin Na)** 擒拿 Seize Control. A type of Chinese Gongfu which emphasizes grabbing techniques to control the opponent's joints, while attacking certain acupuncture cavities. One of the four main fighting categories in Chinese martial arts. The four categories are kicking (Ti, 踢), striking (Da, 打), wrestling (Shuai, 摔), and controlling (Qin Na, 擒拿).

**Chong Lou** 重樓 Multi-towers, means layers of stories, which refers to the throat area.

**Chong Mai** 衝脈 Thrusting Vessel. One of the Eight Extraordinary Vessels.

**Chong Qi** 充氣 To accumulate Qi in the Real Lower Dan Tian.

**Chou Pi Nang** 臭皮囊 Smelly skin bag, a Buddhist term for the human body.

**Chu Gan** 觸感 Touch Feel, also called Moving Touch (Dong Chu, 動觸). A sensation which occurs in meditation.

**Chun Qiu** 春秋 Spring and Autumn. One of the Chinese warring periods (722 to 484 B.C.).

**Confucius (551-479** B.C.**)** 孔子 A Chinese scholar, during the Spring and Autumn Period, whose philosophy significantly influenced Chinese culture.

**Cuo** 撮 To condense, focus, or concentrate. It means to concentrate the mind and Qi.

**Da Ding** 大定 Great Steadiness. Profound steadiness of body and mind.

**Da Ding Lu** 大鼎爐 Large tripod and furnace. The final stage of conceiving a Spiritual Embryo (Shen Tai, 神胎 at the Huang Ting (黃庭) cavity is to unite the Shen with the Qi at the Huang Ting. The head is a tripod while the Huang Ting is a furnace.

**Da Fan** 大返 Great Return. To return the human temperament to the natural state.

**Da Huan Dan** 大還丹 Large Returning Elixir. The meditation which is used to lead Qi up, to nourish the brain for spiritual enlightenment.

**Da Mo** 達磨 The Indian Buddhist monk credited with creating the Yi Jin Jing (易筋經) and Xi Sui Jing (洗髓經) at the Shaolin monastery (少林寺) during the Liang Dynasty (502-557 A.D., 梁朝). His last name was Sardili (剎地利), and he was also known as Bodhidarma. He had been a minor prince in southern India.

**Da Qiao (Da Que Qiao)** 搭橋（搭鵲橋）To build the magpie bridge. Touching the roof of the mouth with the tip of the tongue to form a Qi bridge between the Governing and Conception Vessels.

**Da Zhou Tian** 大周天 Grand Cyclic Heaven or Grand Circulation, called Macrocosmic Meditation in Indian Yoga. After a Nei Dan practitioner completes Small Circulation (Xiao Zhou Tian, 小周天), he circulates Qi throughout the body or exchanges it with nature.

**Da Zuo** 打坐 Meditation is called Da Zuo in Daoism, which means engaging in sitting.

**Dai Mai** 帶脈 Girdle Vessel. One of the Eight Extraordinary Vessels.

**Dai Mai Xi** 帶脈息 Girdle Vessel Breathing. Also known as Skin Breathing (Fu Xi, 膚息) or Body Breathing (Ti Xi, 體息).

**Dan** 丹 Elixir.

**Dan Ding Dao Gong** 丹鼎道功 The Elixir Cauldron Way of Qigong. A form of Daoist Qigong training.

**Dan Jia** 丹家 Elixir Family, meaning Daoist Qigong society.

**Dan Lu** 丹爐 Elixir Furnace. Abdominal area (False Lower Dan Tian) which produces elixir.

**Dan Tian** 丹田 Elixir Field. Locations in the body which store and generate Qi in the body. The Upper, Middle, and Lower Dan Tians are located respectively in the brain, at the sternum (Jiuwei, Co-15, 鳩尾), and just below the navel.

**Dan Tian Hu Xi** 丹田呼吸 Dan Tian Breathing.

**Dan Yuan** 丹元 The name of the heart's spirit. It contains the Ling (靈) and maintains its activities.

**Dao** 道 The Way, or Natural Way.

*Dao De Jing* 道德經 *Classic on the Virtue of the Dao.* Written by Lao Zi (老子) during the Zhou Dynasty (1122-255 B.C., 周朝).

**Dao Jia (Dao Jiao)** 道家〔道教〕Daoism. Created by Lao Zi (老子) during the Zhou Dynasty (1122-255 B.C., 周朝). During the Han Dynasty (58 A.D., 漢朝), it was mixed with Buddhism to become the Daoist religion (Dao Jiao, 道教).

**Dao Jia Hu Xi** 道家呼吸 Daoist breathing, also called Reversed Abdominal Breathing (Fan Fu Hu Xi or Ni Fu Hu Xi, 反腹呼吸・逆腹呼吸).

**Dao Wai Cai Yao** 道外採藥 To pick the herb outside the Dao (道). A form of Daoist Qigong training.

**Dao Yin** 導引 Direct and lead. Another name for Qigong.

**Dazhui (Gv-14)** 大椎 Acupuncture name for a cavity on the Governing Vessel. It means Big Vertebra.

**De** 德 The manifestation of the Dao or the activities of nature.

**Di** 地 The Earth. Earth (Di, 地), Heaven (Tian, 天), and Man (Ren, 人) are the Three Natural Powers (San Cai, 三才).

**Di** 抵 To press up. The tongue presses up against the palate of the mouth.

**Di** 蒂 The stalk of a fruit or flower, connecting to the root of life.

**Di Li Shi** 地理師 Di Li (地理) means geomancy, and Shi (師) means teacher. Therefore Di Li Shi is a master who analyzes geographic locations according to the formula in the *Yi Jing* (易經, *The Book of Change*) and the energy distribution in the Earth. Also called Feng Shui Shi (風水師).

**Di Qi** 地氣 Earth Qi.

**Di Wu Xin Hu Xi** 第五心呼吸 Fifth Gate Breathing, also called Baihui Breathing (百會呼吸), or Upper Dan Tian Breathing (Shang Dan Tian Hu Xi, 上丹田呼吸).

**Dian Mai** 點脈 Mai means the blood vessel (Xue Mai, 血脈) or the Qi channel (Qi Mai, 氣脈). Dian Mai means to press the blood vessel or Qi channel.

**Dian Qi** 電氣 Dian means electricity, so Dian Qi means electrical energy. In China, a word is often placed before "Qi" to identify the different kinds of energy.

**Dian Xue** 點穴 Cavity Press. Qin Na (Chin Na, 擒拿) techniques that attack acupuncture cavities to immobilize or kill an opponent.

**Diao** 掉 Shake.

**Ding** 定 To stabilize or firm. The goal is to reach steadiness, the firmness of the body, mind, and spirit.

**Ding Lu** 鼎爐 Furnace Tripod, also called Elixir Furnace (Dan Lu, 丹爐). A Daoist term.

**Ding Shen** 定神 To stabilize the spirit. To keep the spirit at one place (usually the Shang Dan Tian at The Third Eye). An exercise for regulating Shen (神, spirit) in Qigong.

**Ding Xin** 定心 To stabilize the mind from emotional disturbance.

**Dong** 動 Moving.

**Dong Chu** 動觸 Moving Touch, or Touch Feel (Chu Gan, 觸感). A sensation in meditation.

**Dong Mian Xi** 冬眠息 Hibernation Breathing.

**Dou Niu** 斗牛 Big Dipper. Condensing the Shen at the Upper Dan Tian.

**Du Mai** 督脈 Governing Vessel. One of the Eight Extraordinary Vessels.

**Duan Pin** 端品 Straighten the behavior. Keep good habits.

**Emei Shan** 峨嵋山 Name of a mountain in Sichuan province (四川).

**Ezhong (M-HN-2)** 額中 The acupuncture name for the center of the forehead, above the mid-point of the eyebrows, also called Mingtang (明堂).

**Fa Lun** 法輪 Wheel of Law. Buddhist translation of Indian term Dharmachakra. The common name for Buddhism.

**Fan Fu Hu Xi** 反腹呼吸 Reversed Abdominal Breathing. A Qigong breathing method, also called Reverse Breathing (Fan Hu Xi, 反呼吸) or Daoist breathing (Dao Jia Hu Xi, 道家呼吸).

**Fan Hu Xi** 反呼吸 Reverse breathing. Also called Daoist Breathing.

**Fan Jing Bu Nao** 返精補腦 To return the Jing to nourish the brain, a special Daoist Qigong term.

**Fan Tong Hu Xi** 返童呼吸 Back to Childhood Breathing, also called Abdominal Breathing. A Nei Dan practice through which one regains control of the muscles in the lower abdomen.

**Fei Sheng** 飛升 Spiritual Ascending. Separation of the spiritual body from the physical body.

**Fen Sui Xu Kong** 粉碎虛空 To crush the nothingness. Daoist training for enlightenment which destroys the illusion connecting the physical world and the spiritual plane.

**Fen Xiang** 焚香 Burning incense.

**Feng Lu** 風路 Wind Path. The reverse of the Fire Path (Huo Lu, 火路) of Small Circulation.

**Feng Shui** 風水 Wind Water. Geomancy. Divination of natural energy relationships in a location, especially the interrelationships of wind and water, hence the name.

**Feng Shui Shi** 風水師 Wind Water Teacher. Master of divination. Also called Di Li Shi (地理師).

**Fengchi (GB-20)** 風池 Wind Pond. An acupuncture cavity on the Gall Bladder Primary Channel.

**Fengfu (Gv-16)** 風府 Wind's Dwelling. An acupuncture cavity on the Governing Vessel.

**Fo** 佛 The stage of enlightenment of truth, the stage of Buddhahood.

**Fo Jia (Fo Jiao)** 佛家（佛教）Buddhist family or religion. Jiao means religion.

**Fo Jia Hu Xi** 佛家呼吸 Buddhist Breathing or Normal Abdominal Breathing (Zhen Fu Hu Xi, 正腹呼吸).

**Fu** 符 Fu Water (Fu Shui, 符水), the magic water for curing diseases.

**Fu** 符 To accord, match, harmonize, coordinate, or cooperate.

**Fu** 浮 Float.

**Fu Qi** 伏氣 Tame the Qi. To govern Qi at will.

**Fu Shi Hu Xi** 腹式呼吸 Abdominal Way of Breathing. As you breathe, the muscles in the lower abdomen control the diaphragm. Also called 'Back to Childhood Breathing'.

**Fu Shui** 符水 Fu water, the magic water for curing diseases.

**Fu Xi** 膚息 Skin breathing. A Nei Dan Qigong (內丹氣功) breathing practice.

**Gao, Tao** 高濤 Dr. Yang, Jwing-Ming's first Taijiquan master.

**Gao Wan Yun Dong** 睪丸運動 Testicle exercises. Qigong exercises.

**Gong (Kung)** 功 Energy or hard work.

**Gongfu (Kung Fu)** 功夫 Energy Time. Any study, learning, or practice which requires patience, energy, and time to accomplish. Chinese martial arts require a great deal of time and energy, so they are commonly called Gongfu.

**Gu** 固 To solidify and to firm.

**Gu Dao** 穀道 Grain path, anus.

**Gu Jing** 固精 To solidify the Essence. A Qigong exercise for firming the Essence.

**Gu Shen** 谷神 Valley Spirit.

**Gu Shen** 固神 Regulate the Shen (神), firm and strengthen the spirit at its residence.

**Guan** 觀 To look, observe, pay attention. To feel and to sense.

**Guan Nian** 觀念 Observing the Thoughts.

**Guan Xin** 觀心 Observing the Xin. Pay attention to the activities of the emotional mind.

**Guan Yuan** 關元 Key Origin. Lower Dan Tian, where Pre-Birth Qi, or Original Qi, is converted from Original Essence (Yuan Jing, 元精).

**Guan Zhi** 觀止 Observation is stopped and no longer necessary. Once you have regulated your emotional mind, then no more regulating is necessary. The observation of Xin stops by itself.

**Guanyuan (Co-4)** 關元 Hinge at the Source. An acupuncture cavity on the Conception Vessel.

**Gui** 鬼 Ghost. When you die, if your spirit is strong, your soul's energy does not decompose and return to nature. This soul energy is a ghost.

**Gui Qi** 鬼氣 The Qi residue of a dead person or ghost.

**Gui Xi** 龜息 Turtle breathing. A turtle lives long because it breathes deep and slowly. This breathing leads Qi to the skin surface and to the marrow.

**Guo** 國 Country.

**Haidi** 海底 Sea Bottom. Martial arts name for the Huiyin (Co-1, 會陰), or perineum.

**Han (206 B.C.-221 A.D.)** 漢 A Chinese dynasty.

**Han, Ching-Tang** 韓慶堂 A well known Chinese martial artist, especially in Taiwan in the last forty years. Long Fist grandmaster of Dr. Yang, Jwing-Ming.

**He** 和 Harmony or peace.

**He Che** 河車 River Vehicles. The means of transporting Qi in Small Circulation Meditation.

**Hen** 恨 Hate.

**Hen** 哼 A Yin Qigong sound that is the opposite of the Yang Ha (哈) sound. This sound leads the Qi inward to the bone marrow. It can also be used for attack when only partial manifestation of power is desired. One of two sounds used in Taijiquan.

**Heng Ge Mo** 橫膈膜 Diaphragm.

**Hou Tian Qi** 後天氣 Post-Birth Qi or Post-Heaven Qi. This is converted from the Essence of food and air, and classified as Fire Qi, since it makes your body Yang.

**Hu** 虎 Tiger.

**Hua** 滑 Slippery.

**Hua Hao** 華皓 The name of the spirit of the lungs. Associated with the nose which takes in air (insubstantial material) and fills the body with life.

**Hua Tuo** 華佗 A famous doctor during the Jin Dynasty (晉) during the 3rd century A.D.

**Huan** 緩 Slow.

**Huan Jing Bu Nao** 還精補腦 To Return the Essence to Nourish the Brain. A Daoist Qigong process wherein Qi produced from Essence is led to nourish the brain.

**Huang Po** 黃婆 Old Yellow Lady. The match-maker who brings Yin and Yang together.

**Huang Ting** 黃庭 Yellow Yard. The area at the solar plexus, called Jade Ring (Yu Huan, 玉環) in Daoist society. It is the place where Fire and Water Qi blend to generate a spiritual embryo (Shen Tai, 神胎). Huang Ting can also refer to the Middle Dan Tian.

**Hui Guo** 悔過 Confess.

**Hui Neng** 慧能 Sixth Chan (禪) ancestor during the Tang Dynasty (713-907 A.D., 唐朝). He changed some meditation methods and philosophy, and was long considered a traitor.

**Huiyin (Co-1)** 會陰 Meet Yin. The perineum, an acupuncture cavity on the Conception Vessel.

**Hun** 魂 The Soul. Commonly used with the word Ling (靈), which means spirit. Daoists believe one's Hun (魂) and Po (魄) originate with his Original Qi (Yuan Qi, 元氣), and separate from the physical body at death.

**Huo Lu** 火路 Fire Path. The regular path of Small Circulation which follows the natural Qi circulation of the body.

**Huo Qi** 火氣 Fire Qi or Post-Heaven Qi. From the Middle Dan Tian. Makes the body Yang.

**Huo Qi** 活氣 Living Qi or Vital Qi. When something is alive, it has Vital Qi.

**Ji Xing** 積行 Accumulate good deeds. Doing good things for others.

**Jia Guan** 假觀 Observation of falseness or illusion.

**Jia Xia Dan Tian** 假下丹田 False Lower Dan Tian. Called Qihai (Co-6, 氣海, Qi ocean) in Chinese medicine. Daoists believe that the Lower Dan Tian in front of the abdomen is not the Real Dan Tian or center of gravity.

**Jia Zuo** 跏坐 A special Buddhist meditation term, which means to sit with crossed legs.

**Jian** 堅 Hard or strong.

**Jiaji** 夾脊 Squeezing Spine. Daoist name for the cavity between the shoulder blades. Called Lingtai (靈臺) in acupuncture.

**Jiang Gong** 絳宮 Crimson Palace. The space under the heart, or Middle Dan Tian. A term often used as an alternative for heart (Xin, 心). The Middle Dan Tian provides you with Post-birth Qi converted from food and air.

**Jie Jia Fu Zuo** 結跏趺坐 Buddhist term for sitting with crossed legs.

**Jie Tai** 結胎 Conceive the embryo.

**Jie Tuo** 解脫 Liberate yourself from spiritual bondage.

**Jin Dan** 金丹 Golden Elixir. Precious Qi.

**Jin Dan Da Dao** 金丹大道 Golden Elixir Large Way. Major Daoist Qigong training. The elixir is produced in the body and used to extend life.

**Jin Dian** 金殿 Golden Palace, also called Jin Shi (金室). The lungs or brain.

**Jin Gong** 金公 Golden Male. Original Essence (Yuan Jing, 元精).

**Jin Guan** 金關 Golden Gate. Upper Dan Tian.

**Jin Niao** 金鳥 Golden Bird. Original Spirit (Yuan Shen, 元神).

**Jin Pin** 金品 Golden Material. Spiritual Embryo.

**Jin Que** 金闕 Golden Palace. The space under the heart. The Middle Dan Tian.

**Jin Shi** 金室 Golden Residence. Also called Jin Dian (金殿). Upper Dan Tian or the lungs.

**Jin Zhong Zhao** 金鐘罩 Golden Bell Cover. A high level of Iron Shirt training.

**Jin, Shao-Feng** 金紹峰 Dr. Yang, Jwing-Ming's White Crane grandmaster.

**Jing** 經 Channels or meridians. Twelve organ-related rivers which circulate Qi throughout the body.

**Jing** 靜 Calm and silent.

**Jing** 精 Essence. The most refined part of anything. What is left after something has been refined and purified. In Chinese medicine, Jing can mean semen, but it generally refers to the basic substance of the body enlivened by the Qi and Shen.

**Jing Lian** 精煉 To refine or purify a liquid to a high quality.

**Jing Liang** 精良 Pure and Good. Excellent quality.

**Jing Ming** 精明 Keen and clever.

**Jing Qi** 景氣 Qi scenery or Qi view, a feeling generated in meditation by the Qi.

**Jing Qi** 精氣 Essence Qi or semen Qi, converted from Original Essence (Yuan Jing, 元精).

**Jing Shen** 精神 Essence Spirit. Spirit of Vitality, raised by Qi but restrained by Yi (意).

**Jing Xi** 精細 Pure and Fine. Delicate and painstaking.

**Jing Zi** 精子 Son of Essence. A man's most refined essence. The sperm.

**Jing Zuo** 靜坐 To sit quietly in meditation.

**Jiu Gong** 九宮 Nine palaces. A Daoist name for the brain.

**Jiu Nian Mian Bi** 九年面壁 Nine years of facing the wall. The last stage of Xi Sui Jing (洗髓經) training for enlightenment or Buddhahood.

**Jiuwei (Co-15)** 鳩尾 Wide Pigeon's Tail. An acupuncture cavity at the lower sternum on the Conception Vessel. Called Xinkan (心坎, Heart Pit) by martial society.

**Jizhong (Gv-6)** 脊中 Middle of the Spine, an acupuncture cavity on the Governing Vessel.

**Ju Jing Hui Shen** 聚精會神 Gathering Jing to meet Shen. Concentration.

**Jun Qing** 君倩 A Daoist doctor during the Jin Dynasty (265-420 A.D., 晉朝). Credited with creating the Five Animal Sports (Wu Qin Xi, 五禽戲) Qigong practice.

**Kai Qiao** 開竅 Opening the tricky gate. Opening the gate of the Upper Dan Tian.

**Kan** 坎 Water. One of the Eight Trigrams.

**Kan Gong** 坎宮 Kan Palace. Qihai (氣海, Qi ocean) or Lower Dan Tian (Xia Dan Tian, 下丹田).

**Kan-Li** 坎離 Kan represents water and Li represents fire. Kan and Li means to use water and fire to adjust the body's Yin and Yang.

**Kong Guan** 空觀 Observation of emptiness.

**Kong Qi** 空氣 The air is called Kong Qi, which means the Qi in space.

**Kong Zi (551-479** B.C.) 孔子 Confucius. A famous scholar and philosopher during the Spring and Autumn Period (722-484 B.C., 春秋).

**Kongdong** 崆峒 There are three mountains called Kongdong, located in Henan (河南), Jiangxi, (江西) and Gansu (甘肅) provinces.

**Kou Chi** 扣齒 Biting the teeth.

**Kung Fu (Gongfu)** 功夫 Energy Time. Any study, learning, or practice which requires patience, energy and time to accomplish. Chinese martial arts require a great deal of time and energy, so they are commonly called Kung Fu.

**Kunlun** 崑崙山 One of the highest mountains in China, located in the west.

**La Ma** 喇嘛 Tibetan priests are called Lamas.

**Lao Dan** 老聃 Lao Zi (老子).

**Lao Jun** 老君 Lao Zi. Lao Jun is the name given by his followers.

**Lao Zi (604-531** B.C.) 老子 The creator of Daoism, also called Li Er (李耳), Lao Dan (老聃), or by his nickname, Bo Yang (伯陽).

**Laogong (P-8)** 勞宮 Labor's Palace. A cavity on the Pericardium Primary Channel in the center of the palm.

**Le** 樂 Joy or happiness.

**Lei** 雷 Thunder.

**Leng** 冷 Cold.

**Li** 離 Fire. One of the Eight Trigrams (Bagua, 八卦).

**Li** 立 To establish.

**Li Er** 李耳 Lao Zi.

**Li Gong** 離宮 Li Palace. The heart. Li means fire in the Eight Trigrams.

**Li Zhi** 立志 To establish or build strong willpower.

**Li, Mao-Ching** 李茂清 Dr. Yang, Jwing-Ming's Long Fist master.

**Li, Shi-Zhen (1518-1593** A.D.**)** 李時珍 A famous doctor and Qigong master who wrote a book about the eight Qi vessels, titled *Qi Jing Ba Mai Kao* (奇經八脈考, *The Study of Strange Meridians and Eight Vessels*) in the 16th century.

**Lian** 練 To refine, train, or discipline.

**Lian Ji** 煉己 Train the self. Self-discipline.

**Lian Jing Hua Qi** 練精化氣 To refine the Essence and convert it into Qi. A Qigong training process.

**Lian Qi** 練氣 To train, strengthen, and refine. Daoist training to strengthen and increase Qi.

**Lian Qi Hua Shen** 練氣化神 To refine the Qi to nourish the spirit. Qigong training to lead Qi to nourish the brain and Shen (神, spirit).

**Lian Qi Sheng Hua** 練氣昇華 To train the Qi and sublimate it. Xi Sui Jing (洗髓經) training to lead Qi to the Huang Ting (黃庭) or the brain.

**Lian Shen** 練身 To train the body.

**Lian Shen** 練神 To train the spirit. To refine, strengthen, and focus the Shen.

**Lian Shen Fan Xu** 練神返虛 To train the spirit to return to nothingness, to attain freedom from emotional bondage. An advanced stage of enlightenment and Buddhahood training to lead the spirit to separate from the body.

**Lian Shen Liao Xing** 練神了性 To refine the spirit and end human nature. The final stage of enlightenment training where you keep your emotions neutral, undisturbed by human nature.

**Lian Yao** 煉藥 Refine or purify the herb (Qi).

**Liang (502-557** A.D.**)** 梁 A Chinese dynasty.

**Liang** 涼 Cool.

**Lianquan (Co-23)** 廉泉 Modesty's Spring. An acupuncture cavity on the Conception Vessel.

**Liao** 了 The end or completion of the cultivation.

**Liao Wu** 了悟 The end of comprehension. Enlightenment.

**Ling** 靈 1. The spirit of being, which acts upon others. Ling only exists in highly spiritual animals such as humans and apes. It represents an emotional comprehension and understanding. When you are alive, it is your intelligence and wisdom.

When you die, it is the spirit of the ghost. Ling also means divine or supernatural. Together with Shen (Ling Shen, 靈神) it means supernatural spirit. Qi is the source which nourishes it, called Ling Qi (靈氣), meaning supernatural energy, power, or force.

2. Supernatural Shen is called Ling. Ling describes someone who is sharp, clever, nimble, and able to quickly empathize with others. Ling can also be a supernatural psychic capability which allows you to communicate with nature or other spiritual beings. Often, it means Divine Inspiration which allows you to comprehend and understand changes or variations in nature.

**Ling Guang** 靈光 Supernatural divine light.

**Ling Gui** 靈鬼 Spiritual ghost.

**Ling Hun** 靈魂 Spiritual soul.

**Ling Shan** 靈山 Spiritual Mountain. A Buddhist term equivalent to the Spiritual Valley (Shen Gu, 神谷) of the Daoists.

**Ling Shen** 靈神 Supernatural spirit or Divine.

**Ling Tai** 靈胎 Spiritual embryo.

**Lingtai** 靈臺 Spiritual Platform or Station, meaning Spiritual Valley (Shen Gu, 神谷).

**Lingtai (Gv-10)** 靈臺 Spiritual Platform. An acupuncture cavity on the Governing Vessel. Called Jiaji (夾脊, Squeeze the Spine) by Daoists and Mingmen (命門, Life Door) by martial arts society.

**Liu** 流 Flow.

**Liu He Ba Fa** 六合八法 Six Combinations Eight Methods. One of the Chinese internal martial arts. Its techniques combine Taijiquan (太極拳), Xingyiquan (形意拳), and Baguazhang (八卦掌). This style was reportedly created by Chen, Bo (陳博) during the Song Dynasty (960-1280 A.D., 宋朝).

**Liu Zu Shuo Chuan Fa** 六祖說傳法 Sixth Ancestor Disrupting the Passed Down Method. The sixth Chan (禪) ancestor of Chan (禪), Hui Neng (慧能), who lived during the Tang Dynasty (713-907 A.D., 唐朝), changed some of the meditation methods and philosophy and was long considered a traitor. Because of this, the Chan divided into Northern and Southern styles. This is well known in Buddhist society.

**Long** 龍 Dragon.

**Long Hu Jiao Gou** 龍虎交媾 Intercourse of dragon and tiger. Implies the interaction of Yin and Yang.

**Long Yan** 龍煙 The name of the liver's spirit, which is associated with the eyes. When the liver is healthy, the eyes are bright and sharp.

**Long Yao** 龍曜 The name of the gall bladder's spirit, which is associated with the liver.

**Longmen (M-CA-24)** 龍門 Dragon's Gate. An acupuncture cavity in a miscellaneous category. Also called Xiayin (下陰, Low Yin) which implies the groin area.

**Lower Dan Tian** 下丹田 Lower Elixir Field.

**Lu Che** 鹿車 Deer Vehicle. The way of leading Qi from Jiaji (夾脊) to Yuzhen (玉枕). The leading of Qi should be fast like a deer.

**Lulu Guan** 轆轤關 Windlass Gate. A cavity located at the center of the back where the shoulders turn. Also called Jiaji (夾脊, squeezing spine) by Daoists and Mingmen (命門, Life Door) by martial artists. Also called Lingtai (Gv-10)(靈臺, spiritual platform) in acupuncture. (Note: Mingmen cavity in acupuncture is located on the lower back.)

**Luo** 絡 The small Qi channels which branch out from the primary ones, and which connect to the skin and bone marrow.

**Ma** 馬 Horse.

**Mai** 脈 Vessel or Qi Channel. The Eight Vessels involved with transporting, storing, and regulating Qi.

**Mencius (372-289 B.C., Meng Zi)** 孟子 A famous follower of Confucius during the Chinese Warring States Period (403-222 B.C., Zhan Guo, 戰國).

**Mi Hu** 密戶 Concealed Door. The Mingmen (Gv-4, 命門) cavity located between L2 and L3 vertebrae. Also called Bi Hu (閉戶).

**Mi Zong** 密宗 (秘宗) Secret style. Tibetan Qigong is called Mi Zong because it is kept secret from outside people.

**Mian** 綿 Soft.

**Mian Bi** 面壁 Face the wall.

**Ming** 命 The physical body is called Ming, which means life.

**Ming Tian Gu** 鳴天鼓 To Beat the Heavenly Drum. The head is regarded as heaven. Using the tips of the fingers to tap it, is called Ming Tian Gu, one of the exercises in the Eight Pieces of Brocade (Ba Duan Jin, 八段錦).

**Ming Xin Jian Xing** 明心見性 Understand your Xin to see your human nature.

**Mingmen** 命門 Mingmen (Life Door) often means navel or Qihai (Co-6, 氣海 ) in Daoist society.

**Mingmen (Gv-4)** 命門 Life Door. An acupuncture cavity on the Governing Vessel on the lower back (between L2 and L3). Sometimes, it means the two kidneys in Qigong society. In Chinese martial arts, Mingmen is the area between the shoulder blades. It also implies the Lower Dan Tian.

**Mingtang** 明堂 The space between the two eyebrows, one inch inward is called Mingtang.

**Mu** 母 Mother.

**Mu Mu** 木母 Wood Mother or liver (Shen).

**Mu Zi Xiang He** 母子相合 Mutual Harmonization of Mother and Son. Qi is referred to as mother and the spirit as the son. When the spirit is led down to unite with the Qi at the Real Lower Dan Tian, it is called Mu Zi Xiang He, the state of Embryonic Breathing.

**Mu Zi Xiang Yi** 母子相依 Mutual Dependence of Son and Mother.

**Naohu (Gv-17)** 腦戶 Brain's Household. An acupuncture cavity on the Governing Vessel. Also called Jade Pillow (Yuzhen, 玉枕 ) by Daoist society.

**Nei Dan** 內丹 Internal Elixir. A form of Qigong in which Qi (elixir) is built up in the body and spread out to the limbs.

**Nei Gong** 內功 Internal Gongfu. All training in which the mind leads the circulation of Qi, either for manifestation or enlightenment.

**Nei Qi** 內氣 Lower Level Qi, also called Inner Qi (Xia Ceng Qi, 下層氣 ).

**Nei Shen** 內腎 Internal Kidneys. In Chinese medicine and Qigong, the real Kidneys. Wai Shen (外腎, External Kidneys) refers to the testicles.

**Nei Shi Gongfu** 內視功夫 To look inside to determine your state of health and the condition of your Qi.

**Ni Fu Hu Xi** 逆腹呼吸 Reversed Abdominal Breathing. Also called Fan Fu Hu Xi (反腹呼吸 ) or Daoist Breathing (Dao Jia Hu Xi, 道家呼吸 ).

**Ni Wan Gong** 泥丸宮 Mud Pill Palace. Qigong term for the brain or Upper Dan Tian. Mud pills refer to the pineal and pituitary glands.

**Ni Xing** 逆行 Reversed Path. The direction of Qi circulation is the opposite of normal Qi circulation (Fire Path). Reversed path is also called Feng Lu (風路, Wind Path).

**Nian** 念 The thoughts which linger in your mind and is hard to get rid of.

**Ning** 凝 To concentrate, condense, refine, focus, and strengthen.

**Ning Shen** 凝神 To condense or focus the spirit. Once you can keep your spirit in one place, you condense it into a tiny spot to make it stronger.

**Niu Che** 牛車 Bull Vehicle. When leading the Qi from Yuzhen (玉枕) to Niwan (泥丸, Baihui), the Qi movement should be strong as a bull.

**Niu Lang** 牛郎 Cowherd. A legendary love story in heaven. The cowherd falls in love with the weaving lady (Zhi Nu, 織女). But their union is forbidden, and they are only allowed to meet once a year.

**Niwan** 泥丸 A Daoist name for the crown, brain, or Upper Dan Tian.

**Nu** 怒 Anger.

**Nuan** 暖 Warm.

**Peng Lai Xian Dao** 蓬萊仙島 Peng Lai Immortal Island. An island in the East Sea where the immortals resided, according to Chinese legend.

**Peng, Zu** 彭祖 A legendary Qigong practitioner during the period of Emperor Yao (2356-2255 B.C., 堯), who was said to have lived for 800 years.

**Pin** 牝 Female Animals, or Mothers.

**Pin Chang Hu Xi** 平常呼吸 Normal regular breathing.

**Ping** 平 Peace and harmony.

**Po** 魄 Vigorous life force. The Po is considered to be the inferior animal soul. It is the sentient animal life which is an innate part of the body. At death, it returns to the earth with the rest of the body. When someone is in high spirits and gets vigorously involved in some activity it is said he has Po Li (魄力), which means he has vigorous strength or power.

**Qi (Chi)** 氣 The general definition of Qi is universal energy, including heat, light, and electromagnetic energy. A narrower definition refers to the energy circulating in human or animal bodies. A current popular model is that Qi in the body is bioelectricity.

**Qi An Mo** 氣按摩 Qi massage. One of the high levels of massage techniques in which a massage doctor uses his own Qi to remove Qi stagnation in the patient's body. Also called Wai Qi Liao Fa (外氣療法) which means healing with external Qi.

**Qi Huo** 起火 To start the fire. Build up Qi at the Lower Dan Tian (Xia Dan Tian, 下丹田).

**Qi Hua Lun** 氣化論 Theory of Variations of Qi. An ancient book on changes in natural energy.

**Qi Jing** 奇經 The extraordinary vessels or strange meridians They function like reservoirs and regulate the distribution and circulation of Qi in your body.

**Qi Jing Ba Mai** 奇經八脈 Strange Channels Eight Vessels. The Eight Extraordinary Vessels. Called strange because they are not well understood, and some do not exist in pairs.

**Qi Qing Liu Yu** 七情六慾 The seven passions and six desires. The seven passions are happiness (Xi, 喜), anger (Nu, 怒), sorrow (Ai, 哀), joy (Le, 樂), love (Ai, 愛), hate (Hen, 恨), and desire (Yu, 慾). The six desires are the six sensory pleasures derived from the eyes, ears, nose, tongue, body, and mind.

**Qi Shi** 氣勢 Shi means the way something looks or feels. Qi Shi is the feeling of Qi as it expresses itself. For example, the spiritual state or morale of an army is called its energy state.

**Qi-Xue** 氣血 Qi Blood. According to Chinese medicine, Qi and blood cannot be separated, and the two words are commonly used together.

**Qian Shan** 遷善 Shift into goodness. Change from bad to good.

**Qiangjian (Gv-18)** 強間 Between Strength. An acupuncture cavity on the Governing Vessel. This and the third eye are located at the exit of the Spiritual Valley.

**Qiao** 竅 The changes or variations of nature.

**Qiao Men** 竅門 A secret way of learning and practicing.

**Qigong (Chi Kung)** 氣功 Gong (功) means Gongfu (功夫). Qigong is the study and training of Qi.

**Qihai (Co-6)** 氣海 Qi Ocean. An acupuncture cavity on the Conception Vessel, about two inches below the navel.

**Qin and Han Dynasties** (255 B.C.-223 A.D.) 秦、漢 Two dynasties in Chinese history.

**Qin Na (Chin Na)** 擒拿 Seize Control. Gongfu which emphasizes grabbing techniques to control the opponent's joints, while attacking certain acupuncture cavities. One of the four main fighting categories in Chinese martial arts. The four categories are kicking (Ti, 踢), striking (Da, 打), wrestling (Shuai, 摔), and controlling (Qin Na, 擒拿). Qin Na specializes in controlling the enemy through misplacing the joint (Cuo Gu, 錯骨), dividing the muscle (Fen Jin, 分筋), sealing the breath (Bi Qi, 閉氣), and cavity press (Dian Xue, 點穴).

**Qing** 輕 Light.

**Qing Dynasty (1644-1912** A.D.**)** 清朝 The last Chinese dynasty.

**Qing Xiu Pai** 清修派 Peaceful Cultivation Style. A branch of Daoist Qigong.

**Qingcheng** 青城 A mountain in Sichuan province (四川省).

**Qu Jiang** 曲江 Curved Rivers. Intestines, Real Lower Dan Tian.

**Que Qiao** 鵲橋 Magpie bridge or tongue which bridges the Conception and Governing Vessels.

**Re** 熱 Hot.

**Re Qi** 熱氣 Re means warmth or heat. Re Qi represents heat Qi.

**Ren** 仁 Humanity, kindness, or benevolence. When Dao and De are applied in human society, it is benevolence (Ren, 仁) and righteousness (Yi, 義).

**Ren** 人 Man or mankind. One of the Three Powers (San Cai, 三才), which are Heaven (Tian, 天), Earth (Di, 地), and Man (Ren, 人).

**Ren (Zen)** 忍 To endure. The Japanese name for Chan.

**Ren Mai** 任脈 Conception Vessel. One of the Eight Extraordinary Vessels.

**Ren Qi** 人氣 Human Qi.

**Ren Shi** 人事 Human Relations. Human events, activities, and relationships.

**Renzhong (Gv-26)** 人中 Philtrum. An acupuncture cavity on the Governing Vessel. Also called Shuigou (水溝), meaning water ditch.

**Ru Dao** 入道 Enter the Dao. Means getting involved in Daoist study and practice.

**Ru Ding** 入定 Enter the state of mental and physical steadiness.

**Ru Guan** 入觀 Enter the observation. The mind is calm and clear, which allows you to enter a profound state of observation and analysis.

**Ru Jia** 儒家 Confucian family. Those followers of Confucian precepts.

**Ru Jing** 入景 Enter the scenery. When you meditate profoundly, you experience all kinds of phenomena. This is called Ru Jing.

**Ru Mo** 入魔 Enter the devil. Wrong feeling or perception can lead you into fascination, illusion, and imagination.

**Ruan** 軟 Soft.

**Ruo Cun** 若存 As if it were existing.

**San Bao** 三寶 Three Treasures. Jing (Essence, 精), Qi (energy, 氣), and Shen (spirit, 神). Also called San Yuan (三元, three origins).

**San Ben** 三本 The Three Foundations.

**San Cai** 三才 The Three Powers. Heaven (Tian, 天), Earth (Di, 地), and Man (Ren, 人).

**San Che** 三車 Three Vehicles. Three ways of leading Qi in the course of Small Circulation practice. Sheep vehicle, deer vehicle, and bull vehicle.

**San Gong** 散功 Energy Dispersion. Premature degeneration of the body where Qi cannot effectively energize it, generally caused by excessive training.

**San Guan** 三關 Three Gates in Small Circulation. They are Weilu, Jiaji, and Yuzhen.

**San Guan** 三觀 Three observations in Buddhist meditation. 1. Observing Emptiness (Kong Guan, 空觀)—to observe the emptiness of all natural laws and events, 2. Observing Falseness (Jia Guan, 假觀)—to observe the falseness of all natural laws, 3. Observing Double Reflections (Zhong Guan, 中觀)—to observe between the two.

**San Hua Ju Ding** 三花聚頂 Three flowers reach the top. One of the final goals of Qigong, whereby the Three Treasures are led to the top of the body to nourish the spirit at the Upper Dan Tian.

**San Jiao** 三教 Three Schools. Buddhism, Daoism, and Confucianism.

**San Jie** 三界 Three Worlds. The secular matrix. 1. The world of desires, 2. The world of colors (material world), 3. The world of no color (extreme calmness through meditation).

**San Mei Yin** 三昧印 San Mo Di (三摩地, Samadhi), a special Indian Buddhist term which means steadiness of the mind and body (Ding, 定). The Buddhist name for Small Circulation. Also called Yin-Yang Xun Huan Yi Xiao Zhou Tian, 陰陽循環一小周天) which means Yin-Yang Circulation Small Heavenly Cycle in Daoist society.

**San Mo Di** 三摩地 San Mei Yin

**San Nian Bu Ru** 三年哺乳 Three years of nursing.

**San Qi Gui Yuan** 三氣歸元 The three Qi's (essence, Qi, and spirit) all return to their origins.

**San Yuan** 三元 Three origins. Also called San Bao (三寶, Three Treasures).

**Sanyinjiao (Sp-6)** 三陰交 Three Yin Junctions. An acupuncture cavity on the spleen channel. The junction of the three Yin channels, namely spleen, liver, and kidneys.

**Se** 澀 Harsh.

**Seng Bing** 僧兵 Monk Soldiers. Shaolin martial monks.

**Shang Ceng Qi** 上層氣 Upper Level Qi. Also called Wai Qi (外氣, External Qi).

**Shang Dan Tian** 上丹田 Upper Dan Tian in the brain at the Third Eye, the residence of Shen.

**Shang Dan Tian Hu Xi** 上丹田呼吸 Upper Dan Tian Breathing. Spiritual Breathing (Shen Xi, 神息).

**Shang E** 上顎 Palate of the mouth.

**Shang Que Qiao** 上鵲橋 Upper magpie bridge, the tongue, which bridges the Conception and Governing Vessels.

**Shanzhong (Co-17)** 膻中 The central area between the nipples. Some Qigong practitioners consider Shanzhong to be the Middle Dan Tian. Its acupuncture name is Penetrating Odor.

**Shaolin** 少林 Young Woods. A Buddhist temple in Henan, famous for its martial arts.

**She Jing** 攝精 Absorb the essence.

**Shen** 深 Deep.

**Shen** 神 When a spirit becomes divine, it is called Shen.

**Shen** 神 Spirit. The conscious functioning of mind and thought. It resides at the Upper Dan Tian (Shang Dan Tian, 上丹田).

**Shen Bu Shou She** 神不守舍 The Spirit is not kept at its Residence.

**Shen Gu** 神谷 Spirit valley. Formed by the two hemispheres of the brain, with the Upper Dan Tian at the exit.

**Shen Gui** 神龜 Spiritual Turtle.

**Shen Hun** 神魂 The spirit of a dying person, between Shen and Hun.

**Shen Jiao** 神交 Spiritual communication.

**Shen Ming** 神明 Spiritually divine or enlightened beings.

**Shen Qi Xiang He** 神氣相合 Mutual Harmony or Unification of Shen and Qi. The final regulating of Shen.

**Shen Tai** 神胎 Spiritual embryo. Also called Ling Tai (靈胎).

**Shen Xi** 神息 Spirit breathing. The stage of Qigong training where the spirit is coordinated with the breathing.

**Shen Xi Xiang Yi** 神息相依 Mutual Dependence of Spirit and Breathing.

**Shen Xian** 神仙 Xian originates with Shen, sometimes called Shen Xian, or immortal spirit.

**Shen Xin Ping Heng** 身心平衡 Body and heart are balanced. There is balance body and the mind.

**Shen Ying** 神嬰 Spiritual baby or spiritual embryo.

**Shen Zhi** 神志 The mind generates the will, which keeps the Shen firm. The Chinese commonly write Shen and Zhi (will) together as Shen Zhi, because they are so closely related.

**Shen Zhi Bu Qing** 神志不清 The spirit and the will (generated from Yi) are not clear. The mind is confused and unsteady.

**Sheng Men** 生門 Life Door. Implies navel.

**Sheng Ming Zhi Ben** 生命之本 The root of our lives.

**Sheng Qi** 生氣 To produce Qi.

**Sheng Tai** 聖胎 Holy embryo. Another name for the spiritual embryo (Shen Tai, 神胎).

**Shenshu (B-23)** 腎俞 Kidney's Admittance or Kidney Hollow. Two acupuncture cavities on the bladder channels. They are the immediate entrance and exit of kidney Qi to the outside through the back.

**Shenzhu (Gv-12)** 身柱 Body Pillar. An acupuncture cavity on the Governing Vessel.

**Shi Er Di Zhi** 十二地支 The Twelve Terrestrial Branches, the traditional Chinese divisions of the day: Zi (子, 11 P.M. to 1 A.M., Rat), Chou (丑, 1 to 3 A.M., Ox), Yin (寅, 3 to 5 A.M., Tiger), Mao (卯, 5 to 7 A.M., Hare), Chen (辰, 7 to 9 A.M., Dragon), Yi (巳, 9 to 11 A.M., Snake), Wu (午, 11 A.M. to 1 P.M., Horse), Wei (未, 1 to 3 P.M., Sheep), Shen (申, 3 to 5 P.M., Monkey), Qiu (酉, 5 to 7 P.M., Cock), Shu (戌, 7 to 9 P.M., Dog) and Hai (亥, 9 to 11 P.M., Boar).

**Shi Er Jing** 十二經 The Twelve Primary Qi Channels in Chinese medicine.

**Shi Er Jing Luo** 十二經絡 The Twelve Primary Qi Channels and Their Branches.

**Shi Er Shi** 十二時 Twelve Timings. Shi Er Di Zhi, The Twelve Terrestrial Branches.

**Shi Jie** 世界 The world.

**Shi Tian Gan** 十天干 The Ten Celestial Stems. The Chinese use The Ten Celestial Stems together with the Twelve Terrestrial Branches (Shi Er Di Zhi, 十二地支) to form a cycle of sixty. From this, they distinguish the different natural cycles of the year. The Ten Celestial Stems are: Jia (甲), Yi (乙), Bing (丙), Ding (丁), Wu (戊), Ji (己), Geng (庚), Xin (辛), Ren (壬), and Gui (癸).

**Shi Yue Huai Tai** 十月懷胎 Ten months of pregnancy. The stage in Yi Jin Jing training during which the spiritual embryo is nourished.

**Shiqizhuixia (M-BW-25)** 十七椎下 An acupuncture cavity located below the 17th vertebra.

**Shou** 守 To keep and protect.

**Shou Jue Yin Xin Bao Luo Jing** 手厥陰心包絡經 Arm Absolute Yin Pericardium Primary Qi Channel. One of the twelve primary Qi channels.

**Shou Shao Yang San Jiao Jing** 手少陽三焦經 Arm Lesser Yang Triple Burner Primary Qi Channel. One of the twelve primary Qi channels.

**Shou Shao Yin Xin Jing** 手少陰心經 Arm Lesser Yin Heart Primary Qi Channel. One of the twelve primary Qi channels.

**Shou Shen** 守神 To focus the mind on the spirit. Qigong meditation training.

**Shou Tai Yang Xiao Chang Jing** 手太陽小腸經 Arm Greater Yang Small Intestine Primary Qi Channel. One of the twelve primary Qi channels.

**Shou Tai Yin Fei Jing** 手太陰肺經 Arm Greater Yin Lung Primary Qi Channel. One of the twelve primary Qi channels.

**Shou Yang Ming Da Chang Jing** 手陽明大腸經 Arm Yang Brightness Large Intestine Primary Qi Channel. One of the twelve primary Qi channels.

**Shou Yin** 手印 Hand stamp. Hand forms that assist meditation. Stamp here means to press.

**Shu Tou** 梳頭 Combing the Hair. A Qigong practice using the same movement.

**Shuang Xiu** 雙修 Double cultivation. A Qigong training method in which Qi is exchanged with a partner to balance the Qi of both. It also means dual cultivation of the body and the spirit.

**Shuang Zhao** 雙照 The observation of double reflections, or relative comparison. A Buddhist terminology which implies comparison with the opposite position.

**Shui Huo Zhi Ji** 水火之際 The Junction of Water and Fire. Weilu ( 尾閭, tailbone) is where Qi enters the water or fire path. It is called Changqiang (Gv-1, 長強, long strength) in acupuncture.

**Shui Lu** 水路 Water Path. One Qi path in which Qi is led up through the Thrusting Vessel to the brain for nourishment. It can calm down the excitement of your body. It is also the path of spiritual enlightenment cultivation.

**Shui Qi** 水氣 Water Qi. Qi created from Original Essence, which can calm your body.

**Shuigou** 水溝 Water Ditch. Another name for Renzhong (Gv-26, 人中) acupuncture cavity.

**Shun Xing** 順行 Following the Natural Path. Fire Path (Huo Lu, 火路) in Small Circulation.

**Si Da** 四大 Four Greatnesses or Four Larges. These are the earth (Di, 地), water (Shui, 水), fire (Huo, 火), and wind (Feng, 風, air).

**Si Da Jie Kong** 四大皆空 Four Larges are Empty. A stage of Buddhist training where all four elements (earth, water, fire, and air) are absent from the mind, so that one is completely indifferent to worldly temptations.

**Si Qi** 死氣 Dead Qi. The Qi remaining in a dead body. Also called ghost Qi (Gui Qi, 鬼氣).

**Si Zi Jue** 四字訣 Four Secret Words, are Cuo (撮, condensing or concentrating), Di (抵, pressing up), Bi (閉, closing) and Xi (吸, drawing in).

**Song and Yuan Dynasties (960-1367** A.D.) 宋、元 Two dynasties in Chinese history.

**Suan Ming Shi** 算命師 Calculate Life Teacher. A fortune teller who calculates your future and destiny.

**Sui Qi** 髓氣 Marrow Qi.

**Ta** 塔 Pagoda.

**Tai Chi Chuan (Taijiquan)** 太極拳 Great Ultimate Fist. An internal Chinese martial art.

**Tai Xi** 胎息 Embryonic Breathing. A Qigong breathing technique which stores Qi in the Lower Real Dan Tian.

**Tai Xi Jing Zuo** 胎息靜坐 Embryonic Breathing Meditation.

**Tai Xu** 太虛 Grand Emptiness. The great nature of the universe (Dao, 道).

**Taiji** 太極 Grand Ultimate. Taiji is the invisible force which makes Wuji (無極, no extremity) derive into Yin and Yang poles, and into which the two once again resolve into one. Also often called Xuan Pin (玄牝).

**Taijiquan (Tai Chi Chuan)** 太極拳 A Chinese internal martial style based on the theory of Taiji.

**Taipei Xian** 台北縣 A county in the north of Taiwan.

**Taiwan** 台灣 An island to the southeast of mainland China. Also called Formosa.

**Taiwan University** 台灣大學 A well known university in Taipei.

**Taizuquan** 太祖拳 A southern style of Chinese external martial arts.

**Tamkang** 淡江 A university in Taiwan.

**Tang Dynasty** (**713-907** A.D.) 唐朝 One of the Chinese dynasties.

**Tang Yan** 燙眼 Iron the Eyes. A Qigong practice which keeps the eyes in a healthy condition.

**Ti Xi** 體息 Body Breathing. Also called Skin Breathing (Fu Xi, 膚息). This Qigong breathing technique enables you to lead Qi to the skin surface, to strengthen Guardian Qi.

**Tian** 天 Heaven or Sky. One of the Three Powers (San Cai, 三才). In ancient China, people believed Heaven to be the most powerful force in the universe.

**Tian Chi Shui** 天池水 Heavenly Water. Saliva.

**Tian Di** 天地 The physical body is often called Heaven and Earth in Qigong.

**Tian Gu** 天谷 Heavenly Valley. The space between the two hemispheres of the brain. It has many other names, such as Spiritual Valley (Shen Gu, 神谷), Yellow Yard (Huang Ting, 黃庭), Mud Pill Palace (Ni Wan Gong, 泥丸) or Kunlun (崑崙).

**Tian He Shui Ni Liu** 天河水逆流 Reversed Flow of the Heavenly River Water. To lead Qi up from Huiyin to the crown is called reversed flow of the heavenly river water.

**Tian Ling Gai** 天靈蓋 Heavenly Spiritual Cover. The crown, or Baihui (Gv-20, 百會) in acupuncture.

**Tian Mu** 天目 Heavenly Eye. Called the Third Eye by Western society. The Chinese believe that prior to our evolution into humans, our race possessed an additional sense organ in our forehead. This third eye provided a means of spiritual communication between one another, and with the natural world. As we evolved and developed means to protect ourselves from the environment, and as societies became more complex and human vices developed, this third eye gradually closed and disappeared.

**Tian Qi** 天氣 Heaven Qi. Commonly refers to the weather, which is governed by Heaven Qi.

**Tian Ren He Yi** 天人合一 Heaven and Man Unified as One. A high level of Qigong meditation in which one can communicate with the Qi of Heaven.

**Tian Shi** 天時 Heavenly timing. The repeated natural cycles generated by the heavens, such as seasons, months, days, and hours.

**Tian Ting** 天庭 Heavenly yard. The Third Eye. Called Yintang (M-HN-3, 印堂) in acupuncture.

**Tian Yan** 天眼 Heaven Eye. The Third Eye or Yintang cavity in acupuncture.

**Tianshan** 天山 Sky Mountain. The name of a mountain in Xinjiang province (新疆省).

**Tiantu (Co-22)** 天突 Heaven's Prominence. An acupuncture cavity on the Conception Vessel. This cavity connects with the Dazhui cavity (Gv-14, 大椎) on the back, and they are regarded as a pair of corresponding cavities.

**Tiao** 調 A gradual regulating process, resulting in that which is regulated achieving harmony with others.

**Tiao Qi** 調氣 To regulate the Qi.

**Tiao Shen** 調神 To regulate the spirit.

**Tiao Shen** 調身 To regulate the body.

**Tiao Xi** 調息 To regulate the breathing.

**Tiao Xin** 調心 To regulate the emotional mind.

**Tie Bu Shan** 鐵布衫 Iron shirt. Gongfu training which toughens the body externally and internally.

**Tie Sha Zhang** 鐵砂掌 Iron Sand Palm. A special martial arts conditioning for the palms.

**Tong San Guan** 通三關 Pass through Three Gates. The Three gates are Weilu, Jiaji, and Yuzhen.

**Tu-Na** 吐納 Qigong is commonly called Tu-Na, which means to utter and admit. This implies uttering and admitting the air through the nose in respiration.

**Tui Na** 推拿 To push and grab. Chinese massage for healing and treating injuries.

**Tuo Yue** 橐龠 Bellows. A tube used to fan the fire in a furnace.

**Wai Dan** 外丹 External Elixir. External Qigong exercises to build up Qi in the limbs and lead it into the center of the body for nourishment.

**Wai Jia** 外家 External Family. Those schools which practice external styles of Chinese martial arts.

**Wai Qi** 外氣 External Qi. Also called Upper Level Qi (Shang Ceng Qi, 上層氣).

**Wai Qi Liao Fa** 外氣療法 External Qi Healing. A high level of Qi massage, in which you use your own Qi to remove Qi stagnation in the patient.

**Wai Shen** 外腎 Chinese define the kidneys as internal kidneys and external kidneys. Internal kidneys (Nei Shen, 內腎) are the kidneys defined by Western medicine. External kidneys are the testicles or ovaries.

**Wan Zhuan** 宛轉 Soft, gradual, and gentle.

**Wei Qi** 衛氣 Protective Qi or Guardian Qi. The Qi at the surface of the body forms a shield to protect the body from negative external influences such as cold.

**Weilu** 尾閭 Coccyx. Called Changqiang (Gv-1, 長強, Long Strength) in medical society.

**Wilson Chen** 陳威伸 Dr. Yang, Jwing-Ming's martial arts friend.

**Wo Gu** 握固 To hold and firm.

**Wu** 午 Noon. One of the twelve Terrestrial Branches (11 A.M. to 1 P.M.)

**Wu Nian** 無念 The mind of no mind, or the thought of no thought.

**Wu Qi Chao Yuan** 五氣朝元 Five Qi's Return to their Origins. When Qi has been regulated to its normal original level in the five Yin organs, it is called Wu Qi Chao Yuan. The five internal organs are the heart, lungs, liver, spleen, and kidneys.

**Wu Qin Shi** 五禽戲 Five Animal Sports. A set of medical Qigong practice created by Jun Qing (君倩) during the Jin Dynasty (265-420 A.D., 晉朝). It imitates the movements of the tiger, deer, bear, ape, and bird. Others say it was created by Dr. Hua Tuo (華佗).

**Wu Tiao** 五調 Five regulating methods in Qigong practice, namely regulating the body, the breathing, the mind, the Qi, and the spirit.

**Wu Tiao Er Tiao** 無調而調 The regulating of no regulating. All actions are so natural that no more regulating is necessary.

**Wu Xin** 無心 When there is no emotional mind generated, it is called Wu Xin.

**Wu Xin Hu Xi** 五心呼吸 A Nei Dan Qigong practice in which one uses the mind in coordination with breathing, to lead Qi to the center of the palms, feet, and head.

**Wu Xing** 五行 Five Phases or Five Elements, namely metal (Jin, 金), wood (Mu, 木), water (Shui, 水), fire (Huo, 火), and earth (Tu, 土).

**Wu Xing** 悟性 To comprehend the temperament. One requirement for spiritual cultivation.

**Wu Zhen** 悟真 To comprehend the truth. Implies reaching spiritual enlightenment.

**Wudang Mountain** 武當山 Located in Hubei province (湖北省).

**Wuji** 無極 No Extremity. The state of undifferentiated emptiness before beginning.

**Wushu** 武術 Martial Techniques. A common name for Chinese martial arts. Many other terms are used, including Wuyi (武藝, martial arts), Wugong (武功, martial Gongfu), Guoshu (國術, national techniques) and Gongfu (功夫, energy-time). Because Wushu has been modified in mainland China over recent decades into gymnastic martial performance, many traditional Chinese martial artists have given up this name, to avoid confusing modern Wushu with traditional Wushu. Recently, mainland China has attempted to bring modern Wushu back to its traditional roots and practice.

**Wuwei** 無為 Doing Nothing. Regulating without regulating.

**Wuxing** 五行 Five Elements. Metal (Jin, 金, Lungs, Fall), Wood (Mu, 木, Liver, Spring), Water (Shui, 水, Kidneys, Winter), Fire (Huo, 火, Heart, Summer), and Earth (Tu, 土, Spleen, Four Seasons).

**Xi** 息 Embryonic Breathing.

**Xi** 喜 Joy, delight, and happiness.

**Xi** 吸 To draw in or to suck in. Leading Qi up the spine together with inhalation.

**Xi** 細 Slender.

**Xi Huo** 熄火 Cease the fire.

**Xi Lian** 洗臉 Washing the face. A practice in which both hands brush downward on the face.

**Xi Sui Gong** 洗髓功 Marrow and brain washing Qigong practice.

*Xi Sui Jing* 洗髓經 *Marrow and Brain Washing Classic.* Qigong training to lead Qi to the marrow to cleanse it, or to the brain to nourish the spirit for enlightenment. It is regarded as the key to longevity and spiritual enlightenment.

**Xi Xin** 息心 To cease the activity of Xin is called Xi Xin.

**Xi Yuan** 息緣 To cease the affinity which connects with secular affairs is called Xi Yuan.

**Xia Dan Tian** 下丹田 Lower Dan Tian.

**Xia Que Qiao** 下鵲橋 Lower magpie bridge. Huiyin, which joins Conception and Governing Vessels.

**Xia Zhen Dan Tian** 下真丹田 Real Lower Dan Tian, or the second brain. Called the Enteric Nervous System in current Western medical science.

**Xian** 仙 An Immortal. One who has attained enlightenment or Buddhahood and whose spirit can separate from and return to his physical body at will.

**Xian Ren** 仙人 Those who have reached spiritual immortality or enlightenment.

**Xian Tai** 仙胎 Immortal Embryo.

**Xian Tian Qi** 先天氣 Pre-Birth Qi or Pre-Heaven Qi. Also called Dan Tian Qi (丹田氣). The Qi which is converted from Original Essence and stored in the Lower Dan Tian. Considered to be Water Qi, it calms the body.

**Xian Tian Zhi Zhen** 先天之真 Pre-Heaven Truth. The truthful mind before birth.

**Xiao** 孝 Filial Piety.

**Xiao Ding Lu** 小鼎爐 Small Tripod and Furnace. Huang Ting (黃庭) is a tripod, while the Real Lower Dan Tian is a furnace.

**Xiao Tong** 小通 Small smoothness. The smooth circulation of Qi.

**Xiao Zhou Tian** 小周天 Small Cyclic Heaven or Small Circulation Meditation. Called Microcosmic Orbit in Yoga, or Turning the Wheel of Natural Law (Zhuan Fa Lun, 轉法輪) by Buddhist society. A Nei Dan Qigong (內丹氣功) training in which Qi is generated at the Dan Tian (丹田) and then moved through the Conception and Governing Vessels.

**Xiao Zhou Tian Jing Zuo** 小周天靜坐 Small Circulation Meditation.

**Xiayin** 下陰 Low Yin. The groin. Also called Longmen (M-CA-24, 龍門, Dragon's Gate) in Chinese medicine.

**Xie** 洩 Releasing.

**Xin** 心 Heart. The mind generated from emotional disturbance, desire.

**Xin** 信 Trust.

**Xin Shen Bu Ning** 心神不寧 The (emotional) mind and spirit are not at peace. The mind is scattered.

**Xin Xi Xiang Yi** 心息相依 Heart (mind) and breathing are mutually dependent.

**Xin Yuan Yi Ma** 心猿意馬 Heart Monkey Yi Horse. Xin (heart) represents the emotional mind, which acts like a monkey, unsteady and disturbing. Yi is the wisdom mind generated from calm, clear thinking and judgment. The Yi is like a horse, calm and powerful.

**Xin Zhai** 心齋 Purified Xin, which implies a calm, sincere mind.

**Xing** 性 Human nature or temperament.

**Xing Gong** 行功 To carry out the Gong. To train.

**Xing Ming Shuang Xiu** 性命雙修 Double Cultivation of Human Nature and Life.

Originally a Buddhist, though now predominantly a Daoist, approach to Qigong, it emphasizes the cultivation of both spirituality and the physical body.

**Xing Qi** 行氣 Transporting or circulating the Qi.

**Xinkan** 心坎 Heart Pit. Martial arts name for Jiuwei (Co-15, 鳩尾, Wide Pigeon's Tail).

**Xingyiquan (Xingyi)** 形意拳 Shape-Mind Fist. An internal style of Gongfu in which the mind determines the shape or movement of the body. Its creation is attributed to Marshal Yue, Fei (岳飛) during the Chinese Southern Song Dynasty (1127-1280 A.D., 南宋).

**Xinzhu Xian** 新竹縣 Birthplace of Dr. Yang, Jwing-Ming in Taiwan.

**Xiong Bu Hu Xi** 胸部呼吸 Chest breathing.

**Xiu Qi** 修氣 Cultivate the Qi. Buddhist Qigong training to protect, maintain, and refine.

**Xiu Shen** 修身 Cultivating the physical body.

**Xu** 虛 Emptiness, nothingness.

**Xu Mi** 須彌 The Daoist term for the human spiritual being in the fullness of human virtue.

**Xu Qi** 蓄氣 Store the Qi to an abundant level.

**Xu Wu** 虛無 Nothing.

**Xuan** 玄 marvelous, incredible, or mysterious. It also means original (Yuan, 元).

**Xuan Guan** 玄關 Tricky Gates. Key places in Qigong training.

**Xuan Ming** 玄冥 The spirit of the kidneys. It produces sperm so a baby can be born.

**Xuan Pin** 玄牝 The marvelous and mysterious Dao, mother of creation of millions of objects.

**Xun Dao Zhe** 尋道者 Dao searcher. One who studies the truth of the Dao.

**Yamen (Gv-15)** 啞門 Door of Muteness. An acupuncture cavity on the Governing Vessel.

**Yan** 言 Speaking or negotiating.

**Yan Guan Bi** 眼觀鼻 To use the eyes to look at the tip of the nose. To pay attention to the breathing.

**Yan Xi** 晏息 Meditation or profound breathing.

**Yang** 養 To nourish, increase, raise up, or to cultivate.

**Yang** 癢 Itching.

**Yang** 陽 One of the two poles (Liang Yi, 兩儀). The other is Yin. In Chinese philosophy, the active, positive, masculine polarity is classified as Yang. In Chinese medicine, Yang means excessive, overactive, or overheated. The Yang (or outer) organs are the Gall Bladder, Small Intestine, Large Intestine, Stomach, Bladder, and Triple Burner.

**Yang Che** 羊車 Sheep Vehicle. The way to lead Qi from Weilu to Jiaji. The Qi movement should be slow.

**Yang-Huo** 陽火 Yang Fire. The way of increasing the body's fire so it becomes more Yang.

**Yang Jian** 陽間 Yang World. The material world in which we live.

**Yang Qi** 養氣 Nourishing and protecting the Qi.

**Yang Shen** 養神 Yang means to raise, nourish, and maintain. Shen means spirit. Yang Shen is the main Buddhist approach to regulating the Shen.

**Yang Shen** 陽神 When Shen manifests Qi into action, it is powerful. Though Shen itself is considered Yin, it is called Yang Shen.

**Yang Style Taijiquan** 楊氏太極拳 A style of Taijiquan created by Yang, Lu-Shan (楊露禪, 1799-1872 A.D.).

**Yang Ying** 養嬰 Nursing the baby.

**Yang, Jwing-Ming** 楊俊敏 Author of this book.

**Yangqiao Mai** 陽蹻脈 Yang Heel Vessel. One of the eight Qi vessels.

**Yangwei Mai** 陽維脈 Yang Linking Vessel. One of the Eight Extraordinary Vessels.

**Yao (2356 B.C.)** 堯 Ancient Chinese emperor said to have lived to be 800 years old.

**Yi** 一 Oneness, singularity.

**Yi** 義 Justice, righteousness.

**Yi** 狩 Ripple.

**Yi** 意 Mind. (Pronounced "ee") Specifically, the mind generated by clear thinking and judgment, which can make you calm, peaceful, and wise.

*Yi Jin Jing* 易筋經 *The Muscle/Tendon Changing Classic*, credited to Da Mo (達磨) around 550 A.D. It describes Wai Dan Qigong training for strengthening the physical body.

*Yi Jing* 易經 *The Book of Changes.* A book of divination written during the Zhou Dynasty (1122-255 B.C., 周).

**Yi Qi Xiang He** 意氣相合 Harmonization of the Yi and Qi.

**Yi Shen Yu Qi** 以神馭氣 Use spirit to govern and manage the Qi.

**Yi Shou Dan Tian** 意守丹田 Keep your Yi at your Lower Dan Tian (Xia Dan Tian, 下丹田). In Qigong training, you keep your mind at the Lower Dan Tian to accumulate Qi. When you circulate it, you always lead it back to your Lower Dan Tian at the end of practice.

**Yi Yi Yin Qi** 以意引氣 Use the Yi to lead the Qi.

**Yin** 陰 In Chinese philosophy, this is the passive, negative, feminine polarity. In Chinese medicine, Yin means deficient. The Yin organs are the Heart, Lungs, Liver, Kidneys, Spleen, and Pericardium.

**Yin He** 陰核 Yin center. The weak Yin which exists within the great Yang. This Yin stabilizes the Yang's manifestation.

**Yin Jian** 陰間 Yin world. The spirit world after death is considered Yin.

**Yin Qi** 引氣 To lead the Qi.

**Yin Shen** 陰神 Yin Spirit. The Yin center of the Upper Dan Tian.

**Yin-Fu** 陰符 Yin magic water. The way to enhance the body's water, so its Yang can be made more Yin.

**Yin-Yang Xun Huan Yi Xiao Zhou Tian** 陰陽循環一小周天 A Yin-Yang Circulation Small Heaven Cycle. Daoist name for Small Circulation. Called San Mei Yin (三昧印) or San Mo Di (三摩地) in Buddhist society.

**Ying Er** 嬰兒 Baby (son), which implies the Spiritual Embryo.

**Ying Gong** 硬功 Hard Gongfu. Any martial training which emphasizes strength and power.

**Ying Qi** 營氣 Managing Qi. The Qi which manages the functions of the body and its organs.

**Ying Zhou** 瀛洲 A legendary mountain in the East Sea where the Chinese immortals dwell.

**Yinjiao (Co-7)** 陰交 Yin junction. The junction of two vessels, Conception Vessel and Thrusting Vessel. Yinjiao is on the Conception Vessel. It is also considered a paired cavity with Mingmen (Gv-4, 命門, Life's Door), located between L2 and L3 vertebrae.

**Yinjiao (Gv-28)** 齦交 Gum's Junction. An acupuncture cavity at the mouth, on the Governing Vessel.

**Yinqiao Mai** 陰蹻脈 Yin Heel Vessel. One of the Eight Extraordinary Vessels.

**Yintang (M-HN-3)** 印堂 Seal Hall. A miscellaneous acupuncture cavity, located at the Third Eye area.

**Yinwei Mai** 陰維脈 Yin Linking Vessel. One of the Eight Extraordinary Vessels.

**Yongquan (K-1)** 湧泉 Gushing Spring. An acupuncture cavity on the Kidney Primary Qi Channel.

**Yongquan Hu Xi** 湧泉呼吸 Yongquan breathing. The mind leads Qi to the Yongquan (K-1, 湧泉) cavities on the bottom of the feet.

**You** 悠 Continuous.

**Yu** 慾 Desire or lust.

**Yu Huan Xue** 玉環穴 Jade ring cavity. The space inside the solar plexus (Huang Ting).

**Yu Men** 玉門 Jade Gate. The Third Eye.

**Yu Tang** 玉堂 Jade Hall. Implies the palate of the mouth.

**Yu Tu** 玉兔 Jade Rabbit. Implies Original Essence (Yuan Jing, 元精).

**Yuan Jing** 元精 Original Essence. The fundamental, original essential substance inherited from your parents. It is converted into Original Qi (Yuan Qi, 元氣).

**Yuan Qi** 元氣 Original Qi. Created from the Original Essence (Yuan Jing, 元精) inherited from your parents.

**Yuan Shen** 元神 Original Spirit. The spirit you already had when you were born.

**Yue** 曰 To speak.

**Yue, Fei** 岳飛 A Chinese hero of the Southern Song Dynasty (1127-1280 A.D., 南宋). Said to have created Ba Duan Jin (八段錦), Xingyiquan (形意拳), and Yue's Ying Zhua (岳家鷹爪).

**Yun** 勻 Uniform.

**Yuzhen** 玉枕 Jade Pillow. The Daoist name for the acupuncture cavity Naohu (Gv-17, 腦戶, Brain's Household). This cavity is the third gate of Small Circulation.

**Zai Jie Pai** 栽接派 Plant and Graft Style. A style of Daoist Qigong training.

**Zen (Ren)** 忍（禪）To endure. The Japanese name for Chan (禪).

**Zhan Guo** 戰國 Warring States Period in Chinese history (403-222 B.C.).

**Zhang, Dao-Ling** 張道陵 A Daoist who combined scholarly Daoism with Buddhist philosophies to create Religious Daoism (Dao Jiao, 道教) during the Chinese Eastern Han Dynasty (25-220 A.D., 東漢).

**Zhang, Xiang-San** 張祥三 A well known martial artist in Taiwan during the 1960s.

**Zhen Nian** 念 The real righteous mind or thought.

**Zhen Ren** 真人 Real Person or Truthful Person. A Daoist.

**Zhen Ru** 真如 Real Buddhahood.

**Zhen Xi** 真息 The real breathing or true breathing. Breathing that has been regulated to a deep and profound level. It implies Embryonic Breathing.

**Zhen Xia Dan Tian** 真下丹田 Real Lower Dan Tian, the main Qi reservoir or bio-electric battery in the body.

**Zhen Yi** 真一 Real One, Real Singularity, or Real Oneness. One, or Singularity refer to one's main energy polarity comprising the spiritual center and the Qi center.

**Zheng Fu Hu Xi** 正腹呼吸 Abdominal Breathing, commonly called Buddhist Breathing (Fo Jia Hu Xi, 佛家呼吸).

**Zheng Nian** 正念 Righteous mind or thought.

**Zheng Qi** 正氣 Righteous Qi. When one is righteous, he is said to have righteous Qi which evil Qi cannot overcome.

**Zhi** 止 Stop.

**Zhi Guan** 止觀 To stop the observation, which implies stopping the observation of the activities of the Xin.

**Zhi Nu** 織女 Weaving Lady and Cowherd. A legendary love story in Heaven. The weaving lady falls in love with a cowherd (Niu Lang, 牛郎), but their union is forbidden by heaven, and they are only allowed to meet each other once each year.

**Zhong** 重 Heavy.

**Zhong** 忠 Loyalty.

**Zhong Dan Tian** 中丹田 The Middle Dan Tian located at the Shanzhong (膻中) area at the center between the nipples.

**Zhong Gong** 中宮 Central Palace, or Huang Ting (黃庭) area located between the Real Lower Dan Tian and the Middle Dan Tian. It means the solar plexus.

**Zhong Guan** 中觀 Observation of neutral (neither empty nor illusory). That means to observe events from a neutral point of view.

**Zhong Xi** 踵息 Sole breathing.

**Zhongji (Co-3)** 中極 Middle Summit. An acupuncture cavity on the Conception Vessel.

**Zhongwan (Co-12)** 中脘 Middle Cavity. Solar plexus. An acupuncture cavity on the Conception Vessel.

**Zhou** 周 To be complete, perfect, or round.

**Zhu** 注 Tendency. It also means major flow or pouring.

**Zhu Ji** 築基 Build a foundation.

**Zhuan Fa Lun** 轉法輪 Turning the Wheel of Natural Law. A Buddhist term for Small Circulation.

**Zhuang Zhou** 莊周 Zhuang Zi. A Daoist scholar during the Warring States Period (403-222 B.C.) He wrote a book called *Zhuang Zi* (莊子).

*Zhuang Zi* 莊子 The book written by the Daoist scholar Zhuang Zhou during the Chinese Warring States Period.

**Zi** 子 Son.

**Zi** 子 Midnight. One of the twelve Terrestrial Branches. 11 P.M. to 1 A.M.

**Zi Jue** 自覺 Self-awareness.

**Zi Shi** 自識 Self-recognition.

**Zi Tuo** 自脫 Freedom from emotional or spiritual bondage.

**Zi Wu** 自悟 Self-awakening.

**Zi Wu Liu Zhu** 子午流注 Zi (子) refers to the period around midnight (11 P.M. to 1 A.M.), and Wu (午) refers to midday (11 A.M. to 1 P.M.). Liu Zhu (流注) means the tendency to flow. The term refers to a schedule of Qi circulation showing which channel has the predominant Qi flow at any particular time, and where the predominant Qi flow is, in the Conception and Governing Vessels.

**Zi Xing** 自醒 Self-awakening.

**Zou Huo** 走火 Entering the fire path. False and unrealistic feelings can lead you to a state of emotional disturbance, and away from the correct practice of Qi cultivation.

**Zou Huo Ru Mo** 走火入魔 Walk into the fire and enter the devil. If you lead your

Qi into the wrong path, it is called walking into the fire. If your mind has been led into confusion, it is called entering the devil.

**Zu Jue Yin Gan Jing** 足厥陰肝經 Leg Absolute Yin Liver Primary Qi Channel. One of the twelve primary Qi channels.

**Zu Shao Yang Dan Jing** 足少陽膽經 Leg Lesser Yang Gall Bladder Primary Qi Channel. One of the twelve primary Qi channels.

**Zu Shao Yin Shen Jing** 足少陰腎經 Leg Lesser Yin Kidney Primary Qi Channel. One of the twelve primary Qi channels.

**Zu Tai Yang Pang Guang Jing** 足太陽膀胱經 Leg Greater Yang Bladder Primary Qi Channel. One of the twelve primary Qi channels.

**Zu Tai Yin Pi Jing** 足太陰脾經 Leg Greater Yin Spleen Primary Qi Channel. One of the twelve primary Qi channels.

**Zu Yang Ming Wei Jing** 足陽明胃經 Leg Yang Brightness Stomach Primary Qi Channel. One of the twelve primary Qi channels.

**Zuo Chan** 坐禪 Meditation is called Zuo Chan by Buddhists, which means to sit for Chan.

# Index

# BOOKS FROM YMAA

*more products available from...*

**YMAA Publication Center, Inc.** 楊氏東方文化出版中心

1-800-669-8892 • ymaa@aol.com • www.ymaa.com

## BOOKS FROM YMAA (continued)

## VIDEOS FROM YMAA

## DVDS FROM YMAA

*more products available from...*

**YMAA Publication Center, Inc.** 楊氏東方文化出版中心

1-800-669-8892 • ymaa@aol.com • www.ymaa.com